NOV 1 4 2001	DATE DUE		

Mechanisms in
Hematology

Lyonel G. Israels
Distinguished Professor, University of Manitoba
Senior Scientist, Manitoba Institute
of Cell Biology

Esther D. Israels
Associate Professor, Department of Pediatrics & Child Health
University of Manitoba

Printed in Canada

Third Edition - January 2002
ISBN 1-894481-19-4

Published by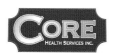

Core Health Services Inc.
1800 Steeles Avenue West, 2nd Floor
Concord, Ontario, Canada L4K 2P3
www.core-che.com
E-mail: mechanisms@core-che.com
Toll-Free Tel.: 1-888-862-8722

The development and production has been made possible by
an unrestricted educational grant from

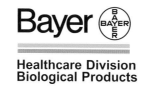

CONTRIBUTORS

Asher Begleiter, PhD (Section 23)
Professor, Department of Pharmacology
University of Manitoba
Associate Director, Manitoba Institute of Cell Biology
Winnipeg, Manitoba

Bonnie Cham, MD (Section 6)
Assistant Professor, Department of Pediatrics and Child Health
University of Manitoba
Winnipeg, Manitoba

Sara Israels, MD (Section 30)
Professor and Head, Section of Hematology & Oncology
Department of Pediatrics and Child Health
University of Manitoba
Winnipeg, Manitoba

Frixos Paraskevas, MD (Section 17-21)
Former Professor of Medicine, University of Manitoba and
Head of the Laboratory of Clinical Immunology
Health Sciences Centre
Winnipeg, Manitoba

Marlis Schroeder, MD (Section 11)
Professor, Department of Pediatrics and Child Health
University of Manitoba
Director of the Pediatric Bone Marrow Transplant Program
Health Sciences Centre
Winnipeg, Manitoba

ACKNOWLEDGEMENTS

We are indebted to Lynne Savage for her secretarial expertise, to Cynthia Chuckree our medical artist, and to Tim Spencer at Biomedical Communications, Health Sciences Centre, Winnipeg.

Photomicroscopy was provided by Danielle Milette. Blend Media Group brought the images "to life" on the CD-ROM. The reviews and comments of Jim Davie, Spencer Gibson, Don Houston, Archie McNicol, Mike Mowat, and Gaynor Williams are greatly appreciated. Visual material was supplied by Neil Crowson, Colin Merry, and Carmen Morales.

Our publisher David Searle and his staff at Core Health Services, as in the past, have been a source of support and encouragement.

None of this would have been possible without an unrestricted educational grant from Bayer Inc. (Canada). Our special thanks to Rena Battistella, Biological Products, Bayer Inc., whose confidence in, and support of, the project have been indispensible.

PREFACE – Third Edition

The third edition of Mechanisms in Hematology has been amplified to afford a more comprehensive description of basic molecular biological processes that impact upon the discipline of hematology. Once again, we have made broad use of illustrations to complement the text. The accompanying CD ROM has been expanded to provide a clarity beyond the written word.

The book and CD are intended as an introduction or re-introduction to the basic biology of clinical hematology. For some readers each Section may be complete in itself – for others it will provide an update or entreé to further reading.

January 2002

LGI
EDI

PREFACE – First Edition

Modern medicine is a science of mechanisms. Our understanding of disease is predicated on our knowledge of the normal physiological process and the perturbations that cause dysfunction. In assembling a logical understanding of function and dysfunction many of us do so in a series of visual images; we return to our text, reviews, or original articles and frequently sketch a diagrammatic or tabular representation of the process.

We have assembled the basic mechanisms of normal and abnormal hematology within a relatively compact space. The diagrams and tables are primary. The descriptions are short, intended to lead the reader through the mechanisms as displayed in the diagrams, and to assemble diffuse information as a brief compendium. It is intended as a rapid introduction or re-introduction to the subject. The references at the end of each section are primarily reviews selected to further expand and consolidate the knowledge base.

The first three sections are dedicated to basic mechanisms that apply across a number of systems and are recurring themes in hematological cell function and dysfunction. The incorporation of new or complex mechanisms into the language of the student or clinical practitioner is not always easy. It is more difficult to distil the essence than to assemble a lengthy treatise. The reader will find that the sections, although brief by textbook standards, are a highly concentrated look at the basic biology of the subject.

This book has been designed for senior students, residents, fellows, and physicians with the purpose of introducing, clarifying, and perhaps simplifying the subject – with the final goal of luring the reader into further exploration of the area.

April 1996

TABLE OF CONTENTS

Sections

CELL SIGNALING

"One, if by land, or two, if by sea."
Paul Revere's Ride, Longfellow

Cell activation and response depend on external signals and stimuli reaching the cell from its proximate environment or from a more distant source. Signals may arrive via the blood stream from specialized endocrine cells (hormonal stimuli), from neighbouring cells (paracrine stimuli), or from the cell itself (autocrine stimuli). The signal may be a small hydrophobic molecule (steroid and thyroid hormones) that transits the lipid membrane, binds directly to and activates its intracellular receptor which, in turn, regulates the transcription of specific genes; some signals are gases (NO and CO) that pass unhindered through the membrane to activate intracellular enzymes; other signals are transmitted by direct cell-cell contact. However, many signals are large hydrophilic molecules that do not enter the cell but bind to their specific cell-surface receptor and, on docking, activate the receptor and transduce a message to its cytoplasmic tail. Cell surface receptors are of four primary types: (1) ion-channel-linked receptors governing ion permeability, particularly important to synaptic neurotransmission and muscle contractility – they will not be considered here, (2) G protein-coupled receptors, (3) enzyme-linked receptors, (4) integrins – discussed in Section 3. The signaling molecules are ligands for specific receptors that initiate cell responses manifest by activation, secretion, motion, cell cycle progression or other intracellular events. The transmitted signal is propagated within the cell by a series of mediators that include proteins and phospholipids, as well as small molcules such as cyclic AMP and calcium ions (Figure1-1).

SIGNAL TRANSDUCTION BY CELL SURFACE RECEPTORS

The signaling ligand docks on its specific receptor which may be a serpentine seven-pass receptor linked to a trimeric G-protein or a single-pass transmembrane receptor. The latter are of two types: (1) those with intrinsic protein tyrosine kinase (PTK) activity – these are referred to as receptor tyrosine kinases (RTKs), and (2) those that lack intrinsic kinase activity but activate an associated PTK; this group includes the cytokine receptors. Ligand binding initiates signals that pass from the receptor to the nucleus via a cascade of phosphorylations mediated through a selected series of cytoplasmic proteins and phospholipids.

Trimeric G Proteins and Their Receptors

The G protein-coupled receptor family, with over a thousand members, is activated by diverse stimuli. Upon ligand binding, these cell-surface receptors interact directly with

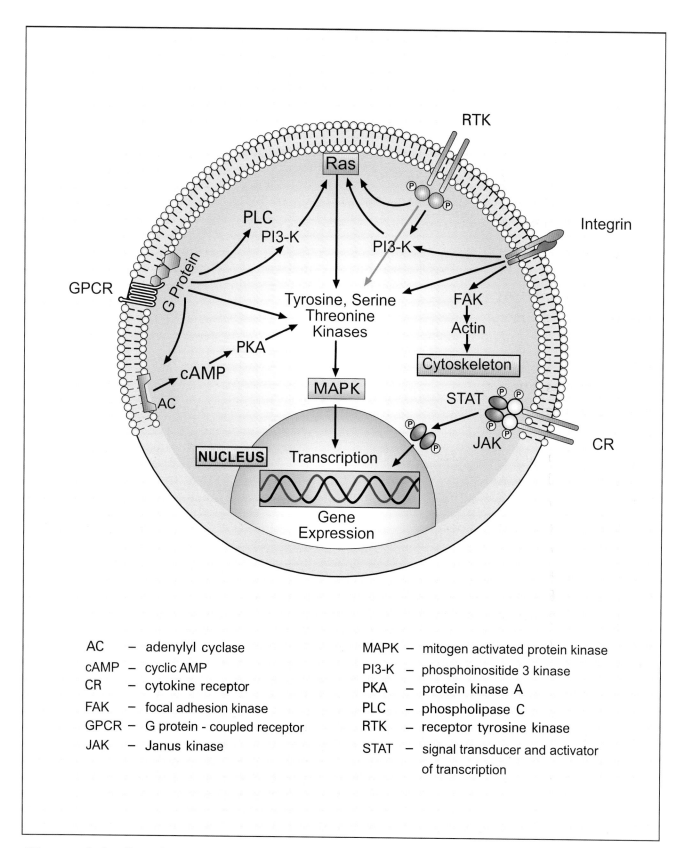

Figure 1-1 Cell Surface Receptor Signaling

guanosine triphosphate (GTP)-binding proteins (G proteins) that serve as intermediates in the signal-transduction chain (Figure 1-2).

The G Protein-Coupled Receptor (GPCR). G protein-linked receptors are all structurally similar: a single polypeptide chain with an extracellular N-terminus joined to the intracellular C-terminus by a serpentine transmembrane region that weaves back and forth through the cell membrane seven times. The ligand-binding domains include the N-terminal segment and those segments of the transmembrane chain that protrude through the exterior surface of the membrane. The message is transmitted into the cell where the C-terminus and the intracellular portions of the transmembrane loops of the receptor interact with and activate the G protein located on the inner surface of the membrane.

The Trimeric G Proteins. These proteins either stimulate or inhibit effector enzymes, thus altering the activity of the signaling mediators. Located on the inner plasma membrane in juxtaposition to the receptor, the heterotrimeric GTP-binding proteins consist of non-covalently linked α, β, and γ subunits. The α unit is bound firmly to guanosine diphosphate (GDP) but linked less tightly to the β and γ units; these form a more closely associated $\beta\gamma$ dimer.

In the basal unstimulated state (the "OFF" position), the α subunit is linked to GDP. On stimulation of the receptor, GDP is displaced by cytosolic GTP; the process is induced and accelerated by the activated receptor – functioning as a **guanine nucleotide exchange factor**. The GTP-α complex dissociates from the $\beta\gamma$ subunits. Both the GTP-α complex and the abandoned $\beta\gamma$ dimer are capable of stimulating substrates; the system is now turned "ON". GTP-α may interact with multiple downstream effectors exposed on the inner surface of the plasma membrane, thereby initiating cell activation. The duration and intensity of the signal is dependent on, and limited by, the bound GTP. The **intrinsic GTPase** activity of the α subunit hydrolyzes the bound GTP to GDP turning the signal off. This GTPase activity is enhanced by the binding of **RGS (regulator of G protein signaling)** proteins to the α subunit. The RGS proteins are **GTPase-activating proteins (GAPs)** which function as negative regulators of the signal. Binding of these proteins to the GTP-α subunit accelerates hydrolysis of the bound GTP to GDP. GDP-α then recombines with the $\beta\gamma$ complex; with reconstitution of GDP-$\alpha\beta\gamma$, the system resumes its basal state.

The activated G protein may: (1) activate protein kinases that phosphorylate tyrosine, serine or threonine sites on cytoplasmic proteins rendering them active transmitters of message, (2) interact with membrane-associated adenylyl cyclase to synthesize cyclic AMP (cAMP), (3) activate the phosphoinositide pathways, (4) activate the Ras/MAP kinase pathways.

The Enzyme-Linked Cell-Surface Receptors (Figure 1-1)

These receptors have an external ligand-binding domain, a single pass transmembrane segment and a cytoplasmic domain. Most of these receptors belong to the **receptor tyrosine**

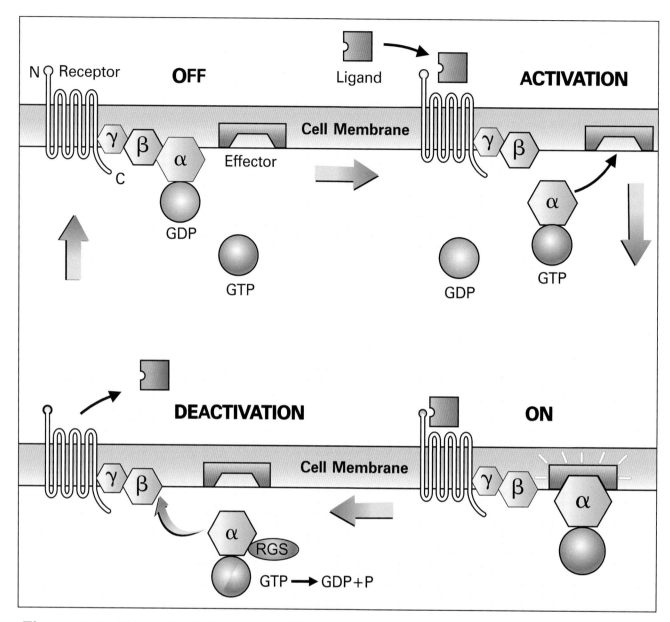

Figure 1-2   Trimeric G-Protein and Receptor Complex

kinase (RTK) family in which the cytoplasmic tail has intrinsic kinase activity. (Kinases are the enzymes that add phosphate groups to selected amino acids in a protein). The docking of ligand induces receptor dimerization; the juxtaposition of two cytoplasmic catalytic domains allows transphosphorylation of the catalytic sites followed by autophosphorylation of additional tyrosine residues and further activation of the receptor. This sets in motion a cascade of protein phosphorylations via a series of serine, threonine and tyrosine kinases – resulting in cell activation. Many of the ligands are growth factors, eg, epidermal growth factor (EGF) and platelet derived growth factor (PDGF). The downstream phosphorylation of enzymes and structural proteins regulates the cell cycle, differentiation, shape and adhesion.

Receptors that lack intrinsic kinase activity are coupled to a nonreceptor protein tyrosine kinase. These include the **cytokine receptors** for erythropoietin on red cell precursors, interleukins on lymphoid cells, and G-CSF and GM-CSF on hematopoietic cells. Cytokines binding to these receptors produce dimerization and a conformational change that induces phosphorylation and activation of an associated protein tyrosine kinase, a member of the Janus family of PTKs – **JAK 1, 2 or 3**. (The Roman deity Janus, guardian of the gate of heaven, is represented with two faces – one face directed outwards, the other inwards to the temple). The aptly named JAK PTKs are intermediates in the transfer of signal: they first phosphorylate receptor subunits then activate a transcription pathway through phosphorylation of **STAT** (signal transducers and activators of transcription). Phosphorylated STATs dimerize and migrate to the nucleus as inducers and regulators of transcription of specific genes. The cytokine signal also articulates with the Ras and PI3-K pathways.

Integrins

The integrins are cell surface receptors that interact with complementary adhesion molecules to "integrate" the external environment with the interior of the cell. They transmit signals from the extracellular environment to activate intracellular responses. They are discussed in Section 3.

INTRACELLULAR MEDIATORS

Signal transmission and amplification involves a network of proteins that transform external stimuli into the appropriate cellular response. Propagation may proceed by protein phosphorylation of tyrosine, serine and threonine sites through a network of protein kinases. Termination of the signal depends upon dephosphorylation by specific phosphatases or proteolysis.

The Small G Protein Family (Figure 1-3)

This includes the Ras superfamily, a group of smaller 21 kD monomeric GTP-binding proteins anchored to the cytoplasmic surface of the cell membrane. Three Ras proteins, H-Ras, Ki-Ras, and N-Ras, as well as a number of closely related proteins (Rho, Rac), are expressed in most mammalian cells. Signals from a variety of activated cell-surface receptors induce Ras activation. Ras binding to cytosolic GTP is catalyzed by **GTP/GDP exchange factors** (eg, the cytoplasmic **Sos** protein). An activated RTK recruits an **adapter protein Grb2** through its linker SH2 domains. SH2 (src protein homology sites) can serve as recognition and coupling domains for tyrosine phosphorylated signaling proteins. Because Grb2, through its SH3 domains, is constitutively associated with Sos, the RTK-Grb2 interaction brings Sos to the cell membrane in proximity to Ras, setting in motion a process similar to that for the trimeric G

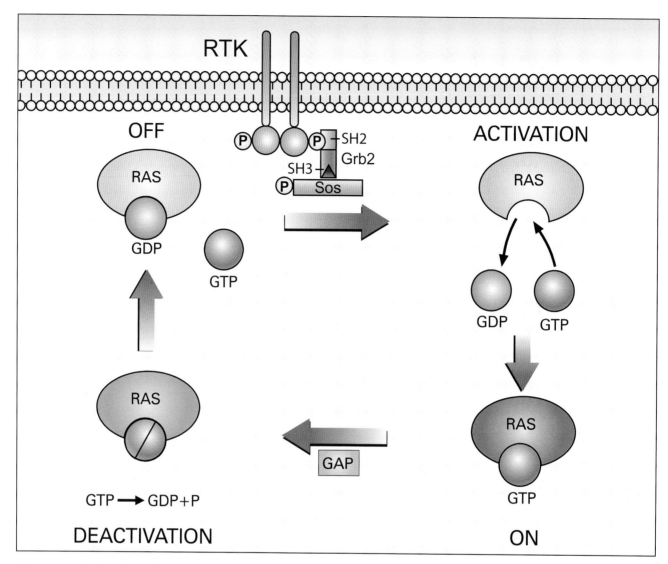

Figure 1-3   Ras GTP-Binding Protein

proteins. Sos increases the dissociation rate of GDP by several orders of magnitude; GDP leaves Ras and is replaced by free cytosolic GTP. Ras-GTP is the active complex capable of inducing a cascade of intracellular phosphorylation events that result in cell activation, proliferation or differentiation. Ras-GTP is returned to its inactive state by GTPase activity which splits off phosphate to reform Ras-GDP. Because Ras hydrolyzes GTP slowly, turning off this system requires the participation of GTPase-activating proteins (GAPs) to accelerate the conversion of GTP to GDP. The Ras proteins function as molecular switches: cycling between the active GTP-based "on" state and the inactive GDP "off" state.

    The propagation of signal from Ras travels through both Ras associated protein kinases and lipid kinases. One final common pathway is via the MAP kinases (mitogen activated protein kinases). The sequence of activation is: MAPKKK to MAPKK and finally to MAPK.

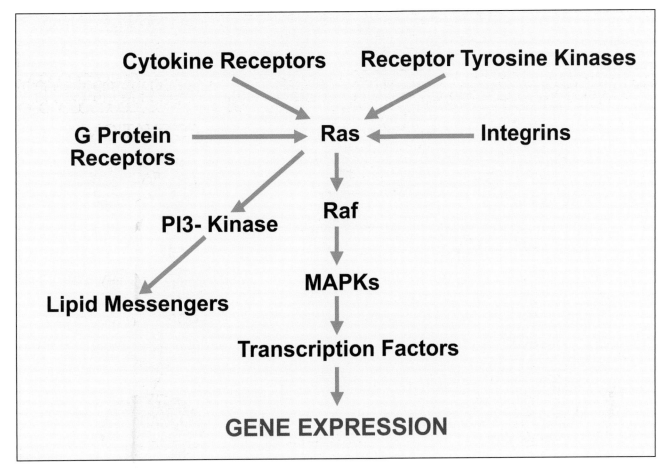

Figure 1-4 The Centrality of Ras

Activation of these three kinases requires phosphorylation of both tyrosine and threonine sites. MAPK then phosphorylates transcription factors (eg, Myc, Jun, Fos) that induce gene expression. The centrality of Ras signaling is shown in Figure 1-4.

Stimulation of cell growth by Ras occurs during the G_1 phase of the cell cycle. The *ras* gene can be altered by a number of oncogenic mutations. Many of these tumour-associated Ras mutants are resistant to the GTPase amplification by GAP – Ras therefore remains in its active GTP conformation (i.e. a turned on signal), resulting in deregulated cell stimulation, proliferation and transformation.

Protein Signaling Modules

Receptor-induced recruitment of proteins relays the activation message along specific signaling pathways. Activated receptors or their targets interact with adapter proteins that contain specific domains or modules – these non-catalytic modules serve as intermediate linkers in the transmission chain. By recruiting specific proteins, adapters organize the signaling pathway into macromolecular complexes that determine the specificity of signal transduction;

they recruit enzymes and bring them into close proximity with their substrates. One example is the SH2 (src homology 2) module that is present in at least 100 adapter proteins; SH2 binds to phosphorylated tyrosine sites. The specificity of the linkage is dictated by SH2 recognition of a particular amino acid sequence adjacent to the phosphorylated tyrosine. Similar SH3 domains also function as linkers between specific proteins. Signaling pathways involve large numbers of proteins that contain these or other linker modules. The modules connect one protein to another, determining the specificity of the interactions necessary for a precise signaling route.

Second Messengers

A rapid propagation of signal is achieved by the diffusion of small molecules released into the cytoplasm; these include cAMP, cGMP, IP3, and DAG. The release of these "second messengers" follows the activation of specific enzymes, eg, adenylyl cyclase, phospholipase C and nitric oxide synthase.

Adenylyl Cyclase (AC). This membrane bound enzyme, when activated by a G protein, produces a molecular rearrangement of ATP, with the loss of two phosphate groups, to form cyclic AMP (cAMP); cAMP in turn activates protein kinase A (PKA). cAMP serves as a second messenger for a number of hormonal signals in multiple target tissues; in the platelet it is an inhibitor of aggregation. The signal is turned off when cAMP is degraded to 5 AMP by phosphodiesterase (Figure 1-1).

Phosphatidylinositol. Phosphatidylinositol, a minor component of cell membranes, can be phosphorylated at multiple free hydroxyls on the inositol ring. Phosphoinositides, the phosphorylated derivatives of phosphatidylinositol, are precursors of second messengers that regulate a variety of intracellular processes: proliferation, survival, cytoskeletal organization and vesicle trafficking (Figure 1-5). Phosphatidylinositol 4,5-bisphosphate (PIP2) is the major substrate for two enzymes, phospholipase C (PLC) and phosphoinositide 3 kinase (PI3-K).

PLC, activated by stimulated G protein-coupled receptors (GPCRs), cleaves membrane PIP2, generating two second messengers: inositol triphosphate (IP3) and diacylglycerol (DAG). IP3 mobilizes calcium from the endoplasmic reticulum which then associates with the protein calmodulin. The Ca^{2+}/calmodulin complex binds to and alters the conformation of a variety of intracellular proteins and activates a series of protein kinases. Removal of the 5-phosphate from the inositol ring by an inositol phosphatase terminates the IP3 signal. DAG activates protein kinase C (PKC) which in turn initiates a phosphorylation cascade resulting in propagation of an intracellular signal. DAG activity is shut off by a kinase that adds a phosphate to DAG, converting it to phosphatidic acid.

Phosphoinositide 3 kinases (PI3-K)

PI3 kinases are activated by ligand-bound growth factor receptors (GPCRs, RTKs and

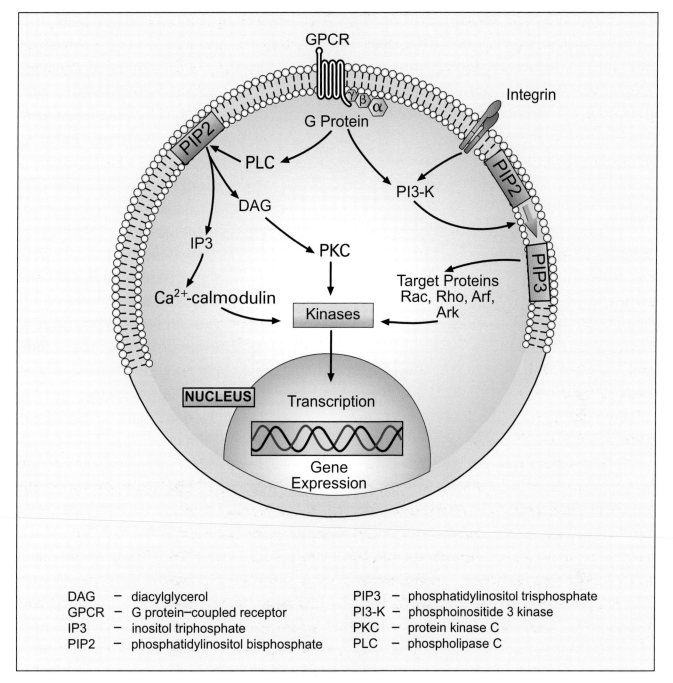

DAG   – diacylglycerol   PIP3 – phosphatidylinositol trisphosphate
GPCR – G protein–coupled receptor   PI3-K – phosphoinositide 3 kinase
IP3   – inositol triphosphate   PKC   – protein kinase C
PIP2 – phosphatidylinositol bisphosphate PLC   – phospholipase C

Figure 1-5 Phosphoinositol Signaling Pathways

integrins). Activated PI3-Ks phosphorylate inositol lipids at the 3-position of the inositol ring
to generate the 3-phosphoinositides. The major substrate for PI3-K is phosphatidylinositol 4,5
phosphate – PIP2; the product is phosphatidylinositol 3,4,5 phosphate – PIP3. Levels of these
3-phosphoinositides are very low in quiescent cells but rapidly increase upon activation of
PI3-K. These lipids function in signal transduction by interacting with a variety of proteins
containing 3-phosphoinositide-binding motifs and recruiting the target proteins to cell

membranes. The protein domains that recognize the 3-phosphoinositides include the pleckstrin homology (PH) domains and FYVE domains. PH domains are found in a wide range of guanidine nucleotide exchange factors for small G proteins (Rac, Rho and Arf). Proteins containing the FYVE domain have been implicated in a variety of vesicular trafficking events. Maintenance of 3-phosphoinositides at a low level is the primary function of the inositol phosphatase **PTEN** – dephosphorylation of these phospholipids switches off the signal. PTEN is the product of the *PTEN* tumor suppressor gene.

Nitric Oxide Synthase (NOS)

Three isoenzymes of this haemoprotein have been identified: nNOS constitutively expressed in neuronal cells; iNOS typically expressed in inflammatory macrophages, and eNOS constitutively expressed in endothelial cells. Nitric oxide (NO), synthesized by NOS from L-arginine, is a diffusible intracellular messenger with multiple physiological functions, including a critical role in regulating blood pressure. NO diffuses out of the endothelial cell and enters the vessel smooth muscle cells where it stimulates soluble guanylyl cyclase to form cGMP. The increased levels of cGMP result in smooth muscle cytoskeletal changes and vascular dilatation (Sections 13, 31).

TRANSCRIPTION FACTORS

Transcription factors are signaling proteins that regulate gene expression. Some reside in an inactive form in the cytoplasm and on activation (phosphorylation), enter the nucleus; others reside within the nucleus. On activation, they bind to regulatory elements of DNA and turn on DNA transcription. They may bind to the promoter region in juxtaposition to the gene or to a more distant enhancer region. They form the link between the receipt of message and its translation into the cellular response.

Transcription factors of primary interest in hematopoietic cells include:

STAT (signal transducer and activator of transcription) relays information from a number of cytokines. Cytokine binding to a cell-surface receptor results in activation (phosphorylation) of JAK, which in turn recruits and phosphorylates tyrosine residues on STAT. Activated STAT dimerizes and moves to the nucleus where it regulates gene expression. (This is the JAK-STAT pathway: Figure 1-1).

GATA-1 regulates the expression of genes required for erythropoiesis. GATA-1 recognizes conserved DNA (G-A-T-A) nucleotide motifs in regulatory regions of a number of erythroid-expressed genes, including genes for heme synthetic enzymes, globin, and membrane proteins (Section 9).

NF-κB (nuclear factor κB) is a cytoplasmic protein widely distributed in a variety of cell types. It is a transcription factor for the leukocyte adhesion molecules ICAM-1, VCAM-1 and E-selectin, as well as for a number of cytokines and growth factors including G-CSF and GM-CSF. In unstimulated cells, NF-κB dimers are bound non-covalently to the inhibitor IκB – an association which prevents nuclear translocation. Upon receipt of a stimulatory signal, the complex dissociates; IκB is phosphorylated and degraded, and NF-κB enters the nucleus.

E2F is a transcription factor held within a pocket of the retinoblastoma (Rb) protein. Upon phosphorylation of Rb, E2F is released; unbound E2F activates expression of specific genes. Proteins encoded by these genes trigger the cell to move past the G_1 restriction point and proceed into S phase (Section 2).

TURNING OFF THE SIGNAL

The dynamic state of cell structure and function depends upon regulation of both protein synthesis and protein degradation. Temporal and spatial activation of signaling pathways are regulated by mechanisms that modify or terminate the signal.

Protein phosphatases may be divided into two groups based on substrate specificity Tyrosine phosphatases specifically hydrolyze protein phosphotyrosines; they are important in the regulation of signal transduction pathways. The second group of phosphatases specifically hydrolyze serine/threonine phosphoesters that are essential to the regulation of cell cycle progression, DNA replication and transcription.

Intracellular Proteolysis. The proteasome and ubiquitin are the principal components of an energy (ATP)-dependent proteolytic system that controls the intracellular concentration of many regulatory proteins. Proteins are targeted for degradation by covalent conjugation to ubiquitin, a 76 amino acid protein. Ubiquitin belongs to a family of shuttle proteins. The attachment of ubiquitin to its target protein requires the sequential action of three proteins: an activating enzyme (E1), a conjugating enzyme (E2), and a protein ligase (E3) (Figure 1-6). E1 forms a thioester bond with the carboxyl terminus of ubiquitin in an ATP-dependent reaction. Activated ubiquitin is transferred to the cysteine in the active site of E2. E3 binding to both E2-ubiquitin and the target protein results in formation of an isopeptide bond between ubiquitin and a specific lysine residue on the protein. Successive ubiquitin molecules are linked through isopeptide bonds to form a polyubiquinated chain. The polyubiquination provides the biological signal for protein degradation by the proteasome.

The proteasome is a 26S cylindrical structure containing a catalytic core capped by one or two regulatory complexes. The proteolytic complex consists of multiple catalytic sites that degrade targeted proteins by ATP-dependent hydrolysis, releasing small peptides and free ubiquitin. Proteolytic degradation targets proteins engaged in processes that maintain cell function, differentiation and mitosis. There is selective degradation of a variety of proteins,

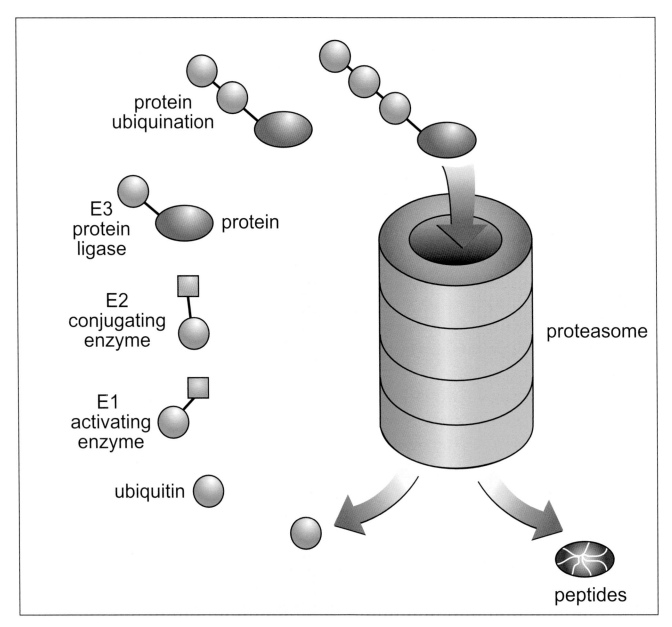

Figure 1-6   Proteolysis by Ubiquination

including components of the cell cycle (cyclins and inhibitors of CDKs), transcription factors (NF-κB and its inhibitor IκB, and p53).

CLINICAL CORRELATES

Proto-oncogenes/Oncogenes. Deregulation of cell signaling or the cell cycle is associated with oncogenesis. Proto-oncogenes encode a variety of proteins: the EGF receptor, the GTP-binding protein Ras, src protein kinase, the growth factor PDGF, and nuclear transcription factors myc, jun and fos. Over 100 proto-oncogenes have been identified;

mutations usually result in a dominant phenotype. Oncogenes are derived from their normal cell precursor, the proto-oncogene, by a number of mechanisms: (1) point mutations or deletions resulting in increased activity (eg, ras), (2) gene amplification with increased cell proliferation (eg, cyclin D1), (3) translocation and fusion to produce a new protein with increased proliferative activity (eg, bcr/abl in chronic myelocytic leukemia – Section 22), (4) translocation of a proliferative gene placed under the control of an enhancer gene (eg, the translocation of myc from chromosome 18 to the vicinity of the immunoglobulin (Ig) heavy chain enhancer on chromosome 14 in Burkitt's lymphoma – Section 18).

The G proteins. Mutations that alter G protein activation result in a variety of diseases including: (1) the pituitary adenomas associated with acromegaly due to impaired GTP hydrolysis with prolonged transmission of signal, and (2) pseudohypoparathyroidism characterized by resistance to the parathyroid hormone due to deficient signaling caused by genetic loss of the α subunit of a G protein subtype (G_s).

Vibrio cholera toxin attaches to the $G\alpha$ subunit and markedly slows GTP hydrolysis – the G protein is locked into its active GTP-bound form. The prolonged signaling results in increased cAMP synthesis with excessive loss of salt and water from intestinal mucosal cells.

The Ras Proteins. Acquired point mutations of *ras* are associated with increased oncogenesis. They are present in some 20% of patients with myelodysplastic syndrome and are associated with more rapid progression of the disease and shortened survival. Mutations are present in 20% to 30% of acute myeloblastic leukemias. Point mutations are found in over 20% of cases of myeloma, chronic myelomonocytic leukemia and large cell lymphomas. There is also a high incidence of mutations in solid tumors – up to 40% in colorectal tumors and almost 100% in pancreatic carcinoma.

The tumor suppressor gene PTEN. Somatic deletions or mutations of this gene that governs dephosphorylation of 3-phosphoinositides are present in a large number of tumors, including glioblastomas, endometrial and prostate cancers. The mutation frequency of PTEN approximates that of p53. Germline mutations are present in Cowden disease, an autosomal dominant disorder associated with developmental defects and an increased incidence of cancer.

————— •••●●●••• —————

SUGGESTED READING

Berridge MJ. Calcium signaling and cell proliferation. Bioessays 17:491-500, 1995.

Bourne HR. How receptors talk to trimeric G proteins. Curr Opin Cell Biol 9:134-142, 1997.

Czech MP. PIP2 and PIP3: Complex roles at the cell surface. Cell 100:603-606, 2000.

Di Cristofano A. Pandolfi PP. The multiple roles of PTEN in tumor suppression. Cell 100: 387-390, 2000.

DeVries L, Zheng B, Fischer T, Elenko E, Farquhar G. The regulator of G protein signaling family. Annu Rev Pharmacol Toxicol 40:235-271, 2000.

Farfel Z, Bourne HR, Iiri T. The expanding spectrum of G protein diseases. N Eng J Med 340:1012-1020, 1999.

Garrington TP, Johnson GL. Organization and regulation of mitogen-activated protein kinase signaling pathways. Curr Opin Cell Biol 11:211-218, 1999.

Hilt W, Wolf DH. Proteasomes: destruction as a programme. Trends Biochem Sci 21: 96-102, 1996.

Hunter T. Oncoprotein networks. Cell 88:333-346, 1997.

Hunter T. Signaling – 2000 and beyond. Cell 100:113-127, 2000.

Hurley JH. Structure, mechanism, and regulation of mammalian adenylyl cyclase. J Biol Chem 274:7599-7602, 1999.

Ihle JN. Cytokine receptor signaling. Nature 377: 591-594, 1995.

Mercurio F, Manning AM. Multiple signals converging on NF-kB. Curr Opin Cell Biol 11:226-232, 1999.

Oren M. Regulation of the p53 tumor suppressor protein. J Biol Chem 274:36031-36034, 1999.

Pawson T, Scott JD. Signaling through scaffold, anchoring, and adapter proteins. Science 278:2075-2080, 1997.

Shields JM, Pruitt K, McFall A, Shaub A, Der CJ. Understanding Ras: 'it ain't over 'til it's over'. Trends Cell Biol 10:147-154, 2000.

Yamamoto T, Taya S, Kaibuchi K. Ras-induced transformation and signaling pathway. J Biochem 126:799-803, 1999.

Zwerschke W, Jansen-Dürr P. Cell transformation by the E7 oncoprotein of human papillomavirus type 16: interactions with nuclear and cytoplasmic target proteins. Adv Cancer Res 78:3-29, 2000.

THE CELL CYCLE

"Cycle – A series of events which recur
everlastingly in the same order."
Brewer's Dictionary of Phrase and Fable – 1870

The cell cycle is a highly ordered process that results in the duplication and transmission of genetic information from one cell generation to the next. During the process, DNA must be replicated accurately and identical chromosomal copies distributed to two daughter cells. The cell cycle is divided into discrete phases: G_1 (gap 1) is the interval or gap between mitosis (M phase) and DNA synthesis (S phase). During G_1 the cell is subject to stimulation by extracellular mitogens and growth factors; in response to these stimuli, the cell passes through G_1 and proceeds with DNA synthesis in S phase; G_2 (gap 2) is the interval between the completion of DNA synthesis (S) and mitosis; M phase is marked by the generation of bipolar mitotic spindles, segregation of sister chromatids and cell division. Regulation of the cell cycle ensures that the events in each phase are completed before there is advancement to the next. Checkpoints for monitoring the integrity of DNA are strategically placed in late G_1 and at the G_2/M interface to prevent progression and propagation of mutated or damaged cells. G_0 refers to cells that are quiescent (temporarily or permanently out of cycle). The normal cell is dependent on external stimuli (mitogens or growth factors) to move it out of G_0 and through the early part of G_1. The cell responds to these external stimuli, communicated through a cascade of intracellular phosphorylations, by upregulating expression of the **cyclins** which associate with the **cyclin-dependent kinases (CDKs)**. The time periods shown in Figure 2-1 are generic and only indicate the relative duration of each phase.

REGULATION

The cell cycle is propelled by a series of protein kinases: the cyclin-dependent kinases (CDKs) form complexes with specific cyclins and, subsequently, are activated through phosphorylation by an activating kinase. Cyclin is the regulatory unit, CDK its catalytic partner. Cyclins, with their bound and activated CDKs, function during distinct stages of the cell cycle. As the name suggests, the level of each cyclin independently increases or decreases with the phases of the cycle. Cyclin/CDK complexes phosphorylate specific protein substrates to move the cell through the cycle with activation of DNA synthesis (in late G_1 and S), and formation of the structural components associated with mitosis (in late G_2 and M). The periodicity of the cyclins, mediated by their synthesis and subsequent proteolytic degradation, ensure the well-delineated transitions between cell cycle stages. Because errors encoded in the

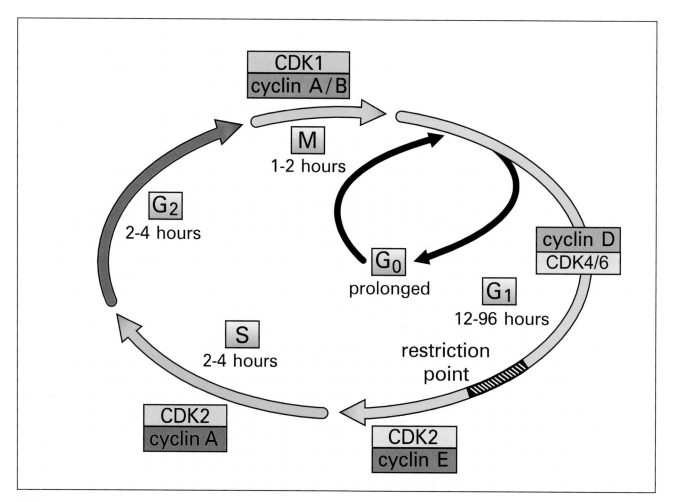

Figure 2-1   The Cell Cycle - Times are Relative

genome may result in defective clones, monitoring of the cell cycle for abnormal programming is imperative. The best understood and probably the most important regulatory site is a checkpoint referred to as the "restriction point" (R) in the latter third of G_1. An error occurring later in the cell cycle, in S or at G_2/M, is recognized by other checkpoints. Depending upon the degree of damage, either the defect will be repaired or mitosis will be aborted.

In response to growth or mitotic signals, the cell moves out of G_0 and through G_1. In the absence of mitotic signaling, the cell may undergo differentiation, apoptosis, or enter the quiescent state (G_0); the mechanisms responsible for taking the cell out of cycle into G_0 or inducing differentiation are unclear. The cycle begins in G_1 with increased expression of the D cyclins (D1, D2, D3). The D cyclins associate with CDK4 and CDK6; formation of the cyclin/CDK complexes results in phosphorylation and activation of the CDKs. The activated CDKs then phosphorylate the retinoblastoma protein (Rb). The Rb protein has a critical role in regulating G_1 progression through the restriction point – in the event of genomic damage, the cycle may be delayed or abandoned (Figure 2-2).

Rb PROTEINS

The Rb family members are "pocket proteins" that sequester the E2F transcription proteins; E2Fs are complexed with DNA – unphosphorylated or hypophosphorylated Rb tightly binds E2F and inhibits transcription. Upon Rb phosphorylation by CDK4/6, Rb dissociates from E2F, allowing E2F to transcribe a number of responder genes (including cyclin E) required for passage through the restriction point (R). Rb is the gatekeeper of the cycle. Hypophosphorylated Rb guards the restriction point preventing cell cycle progression; hyperphosphorylation of Rb is associated with release of E2F and cell passage through R. Rb is maintained in the hyperphosphorylated state throughout the remainder of the cycle – it may play a role in guiding the cell through S, G_2 and M. Rb is not dephosphorylated until mitosis is complete.

As the cell progresses through late G_1, there is increased expression of cyclin E. The cyclin E/CDK2 complex is required for the transition from G_1 into S. Increased expression of cyclin A occurs at the G_1/S transition and persists through S phase. With the binding of cyclin A to CDK2, DNA synthesis proceeds. In the latter part of S, cyclin A associates with CDK1. A checkpoint in G_2 responds to DNA damage or incomplete DNA synthesis: progression into mitosis is delayed to allow DNA repair or the cycle is aborted. Increased levels of cyclins A and B complexed with CDK1 propel the cell though mitosis. (Note: historically, CDK1 is referred to as cdc2).

ROLE OF p53

The integrity of the cell's genome is monitored by the transcription factor p53. In the presence of genomic damage, p53 interrupts cycling to allow time for DNA repair. This is accomplished by p53 inhibition of Rb phosphorylation. In normal dividing cells, levels of p53 are low or undetectable and replication proceeds unimpeded. p53 is negatively regulated by MDM2 (murine double-minute 2) protein; MDM2, reciprocally, is regulated by p53. MDM2 functions at two sites: at the level of the gene it downregulates p53 transcription; it also binds to p53 protein, inhibiting p53 activity, and mediating its export from the nucleus, ubiquination and proteasomal degradation. In the presence of DNA damage, p53 binds to its sequence-specific DNA site – gene induction results in increased p53 protein synthesis. The subsequent phosphorylation of p53 activates the protein; phosphorylated p53 is more resistant to binding and inactivation by MDM2 – consequently, the p53 half-life ($t_{1/2}$) is doubled. As a result, p53 protein activity may increase a hundredfold (Figure 2-2).

p53 control of the cell cycle operates through transcriptional upregulation of the CDK inhibitor (CKI), p21, an active inhibitor of CDKs 4, 6 and 2. The inhibition of kinase activity

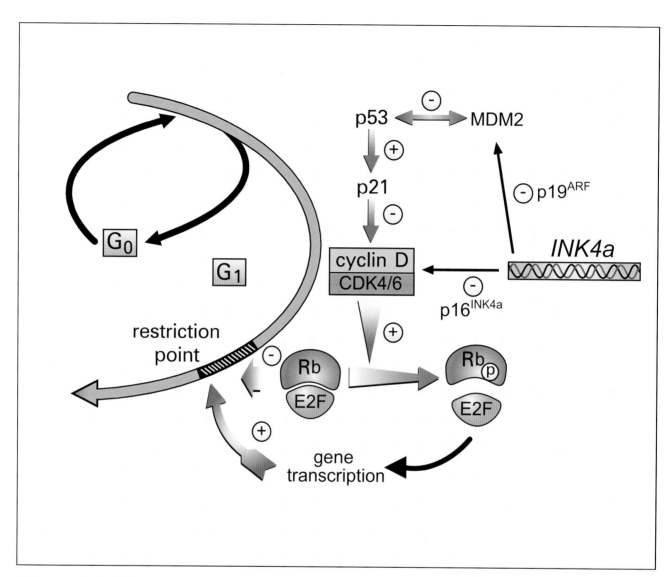

Figure 2-2 The p53 - Rb Axis in the Regulation of the Cell Cycle

prevents phosphorylation of Rb and, as a result, the cell remains in G_1 to allow time for DNA repair. When DNA damage exceeds the capacity of the cell for repair, p53 guides the corrupt cell into apoptosis by inducing the expression of the pro-apoptotic protein Bax (Section 4).

Two families of CDK inhibitors (CKIs) are involved in cell cycle regulation. The Cip/Kip family includes the inhibitors p21 and p27; they function at several sites in the cell cycle, targeting CDKs 4, 6 and 2. The second family includes the constitutively expressed INK4a (inhibitor of cyclin dependent kinase 4) gene. The INK4a gene encodes two distinct transcripts, p16[INK4a] and p19[ARF]. The CKI p16[INK4a] specifically inhibits CDK4/6; p19[ARF] binds to MDM2 and blocks p53 degradation. In response to upregulation of p53, there is an increase in p21 followed by inhibition of CDK4 and CDK6. The action of these CKIs (p21 and the INK4a proteins) inhibits Rb phosphorylation and the cell remains in G_1.

CLINICAL CORRELATES

Cancer cells tend to remain in cycle, insensitive to internal or external controls. Normally, G_1 cells are receptive to external growth signals and are subject to internal regulation; once the cell has passed through the G_1 restriction point, there is unhindered progression through S and M phases. Abnormal cells are able to evade the G_1 restriction point – the cell, no longer subject to normal internal control, continues to proliferate in the absence of external stimuli. Deletion or mutational silencing of p53, Rb or INK4a results in unregulated cell growth with an increased risk of tumor formation. Deregulation of growth also occurs with overexpression of the cyclins – particularly cyclin D which promotes Rb phosphorylation and E2F release.

p53

Because the tumor suppressor gene *p53* is recessive, malignant transformation requires the functional loss of both copies of the gene – either two somatic mutational events or, in the presence of one mutated germ-line gene, a single somatic mutation of its allele. There is a high incidence of tumor in kindred bearing the germ-line mutation, eg, the Li-Fraumeni syndrome characterized by primary tumors that develop in multiple organs at an early age.

p53 mutations – most commonly missense mutations that disrupt p53-DNA binding – are present in over 50% of carcinomas of the lung or bowel. Tumors that express a mutated p53 often have a poorer prognosis and are more resistant to chemotherapy. Amplification of MDM2, an inhibitor of p53, is present in a number of lymphomas and soft tissue sarcomas.

The normal protein kinase ATM (**m**utated in **a**taxia **t**elangiectasia), an activator of p53 phosphorylation, is induced by DNA double strand breaks. When ATM is mutated (as in ataxia telangiectasia), phosphorylation of p53 is reduced. Ataxia telangiectasia is associated with an increased tumor incidence.

Rb

Rb is a recessive gene; malignant cell transformation requires loss of function of both copies of the gene. A germ-line mutation in hereditary retinoblastoma is characterized by early onset (before 18 months of age); the tumors are usually bilateral. Loss of Rb function later in life (non-hereditary) is associated with osteogenic sarcoma and small cell lung cancer.

INK4a

The loss of INK4a has been documented in familial malignant melanoma. Deletion of $p16^{INK4a}$ is present in up to 50% of cases of T-cell acute lymphoblastic leukemia (ALL) and in over 20% of B-cell ALL, B-cell and T-cell lymphomas. Its loss is associated with gliomas and many solid tumors, including carcinoma of the lung, pancreas, bladder, biliary tract, ovary and esophagus.

Cyclin D1

Cyclin D1 has been identified as the Bcl1 oncogene associated with mantle cell lymphoma. The t(11:14) translocation transfers the gene for D1 into juxtaposition with the enhancer region of the immunoglobulin heavy (H) chain gene on chromosome 14 (Section 18). The result is enhanced cyclin D1 gene activation with subsequent cell cycle deregulation. Cyclin D1 amplification also is present in a range of solid tumors (lung, breast, bladder).

Virus Associated Tumors

Infection by human papilloma virus (HPV) subtypes 16 and 18 (which, respectively, produce the gene products E6 and E7) is associated with a high risk of cervical carcinoma. The E6 gene product (protein) inactivates and degrades p53. The E7 protein binds to Rb causing ubiquitin conjugation and subsequent proteasomal degradation. This release from cell cycle control is a significant factor in carcinoma of the cervix.

Human herpes virus 8 (HHV8) has been implicated as the causative agent of Kaposi's sarcoma. HHV8-encoded cyclins promote deregulation of the cell cycle. The viral cyclin, which resembles cyclin D, forms active kinase complexes with CDK6 that are resistant to inhibition by the CDK inhibitors p16^{INK4a}, p21 and p27. Expression of the viral cyclins allows progression through the restriction point R and unrestricted proliferation.

••••◉••••

SUGGESTED READING

Chin L, Pomerantz J, DePinho RA. The INK4a/ARF tumor suppressor: one gene – two products – two pathways. Trends Biochem Sci 23:291-296, 1998.

Jansen-Dürr P. How viral oncogenes make the cell cycle. Trends Genet 12:270-275, 1996.

Johnson DG, Walker CL. Cyclins and cell cycle checkpoints. Ann Rev Pharmacol Toxicol 39:295-312, 1999.

Levine AJ. p53, the cellular gatekeeper for growth and division. Cell 88:323-331, 1997.

Lohrum MAE, Vousden KH. Regulation and activation of p53 and its family members. Cell Death Diff 6:1162-1168, 1999.

Lundberg AS, Weinberg RA. Control of the cell cycle and apoptosis. Eur J Cancer 35:1886-1894, 1999.

Nakamura Y. ATM: the p53 booster. Nat Med 4:1231-1232, 1998.

Nigg EA. Cyclin-dependent protein kinases: key regulators of the eukaryotic cell cycle. Bioessays 17:471-480, 1995.

Oren M. Regulation of the p53 tumor suppressor protein. J Biol Chem 274:36031-36034, 1999.

Prives C, Hall PA. The p53 pathway. J Pathol 187:112-126, 1999.

Sherr CJ. Cancer cell cycles. Science 274:1672-1677, 1996.

Sherr CJ, Roberts JM. CDK inhibitors: positive and negative regulators of G1-phase progression. Genes Dev 13: 1501-1512, 1999.

Sidransky D, Hollstein M. Clinical implications of the p53 gene. Annu Rev Med 47:285-301, 1996.

Swanton C, Card GL, Mann D, McDonald N, Jones, N. Overcoming inhibitions: subversion of CKI function by viral cyclins. Trends Biochem Sci 24:116-120, 1999.

ADHESION MOLECULES

"But screw your courage to the sticking place, and we'll not fail."
Macbeth, Act I Scene VII

Cell-cell interactions, adhesion of cells to extracellular matrix, and binding of diffusable ligands to cell receptors are essential to the integrity and function of the vascular system. Adhesion of circulating leukocytes to endothelial cells, leukocyte migration, and platelet aggregation are required for inflammatory and immune responses, hemostasis and wound repair. Intracellular signaling, a consequence of these adhesive events, transduces internal messages which culminate in the appropriate cellular response. Deregulation of these mechanisms disrupts normal physiological processes and results in clinical disease.

Maintenance of an intact endothelial surface and the recruitment of blood cells to specific histological sites are dependent upon a series of events mediated by the interaction of cellular adhesion molecules with their specific ligands. Adhesion receptors can be divided into four generic classes: the integrins, the selectins, the immunoglobulin (Ig) superfamily, and the cadherins.

INTEGRINS

The integrins are cell surface receptors that interact with complementary adhesion molecules to provide and "integrate" connections between the outside environment and the inside of the cell. They recognize and bind specific plasma proteins, extracellular matrix (ECM) proteins, and cell surface macromolecular ligands – transmitting signals from the external environment to activate intracellular responses. These interactions mediate platelet activation and adhesion, neutrophil localization and migration, lymphocyte homing, and T-cell activation.

The integrins are heterodimers of non-covalently linked α and β subunits belonging to a supergene family in which 18 α and 8 β subunits have been identified. The resultant heterodimers have been arranged into families on the basis of the β subunit – the largest and best understood are the β_1, β_2, and β_3 families.

β_1 Integrins

The β_1 dimers, which consist of a β_1 subunit plus one of nine α subunits, are involved with cell-extracellular matrix adhesion and cell-cell adhesion. They are expressed on hematopoietic precursors, monocytes, T and B lymphocytes, and platelets. Their ligands are ECM proteins: collagen, fibronectin, vitronectin and laminin.

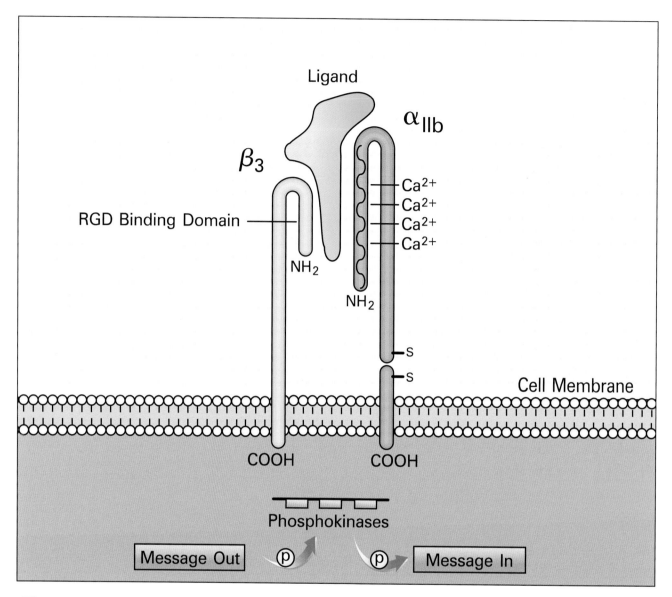

Figure 3-1　Integrin $\alpha_{IIb}\beta_3$ (GPIIb/IIIa)

β_2 Integrins

The β_2 family members have one β_2 subunit (also referred to as CD18) combined with one of four α subunits. These are the leukocyte-specific receptors that mediate neutrophil adhesion, tissue migration and phagocytosis, as well as T-cell response. Their ligands include the intercellular adhesion molecules (ICAM-1 and ICAM-2), the C3b component of complement, and fibrinogen. The two β_2 integrins, CD11a/CD18 ($\alpha_L\beta_2$) and CD11b/CD18 ($\alpha_M\beta_2$), are involved predominantly in leukocyte adhesion to endothelium.

β_3 Integrins

The β_3 family of integrins has one β_3 subunit combined with one of two α subunits. The integrin $\alpha_{IIb}\beta_3$, expressed exclusively on megakaryocytes and platelets, binds to fibrinogen, von Willebrand factor (vWF), fibronectin, collagen, and thrombospondin.

Structure

The α subunits vary in size from 120 to 180 kD and the β subunits from 90 to 100 kD; they combine to form a long slender extracellular stalk with a folded globular terminus. Each α and β subunit has a single transmembrane segment and a short cytoplasmic terminus. The C-terminal cytoplasmic tails are associated anatomically with the cytoskeleton of the cell and are associated functionally with a number of cytoplasmic phosphokinases.

The two expanded extracellular N-terminal regions of the integrin form a docking unit capable of binding macromolecular ligands. The platelet $\alpha_{IIb}\beta_3$ (GPIIb/IIIa) integrin, diagrammed in Figure 3-1, is presented as a general model. The extracellular portions of the α_{IIb} and β_3 subunits form the ligand binding pocket: α_{IIb} contains Ca^{2+} binding sites; β_3 recognizes a specific tripeptide, arginine-glycine-aspartic acid (the RGD sequence), on fibrinogen, vWF, thrombospondin, fibronectin, vitronectin and type I collagen. Interaction with an RGD sequence and dependence on divalent cation-binding is common to a number of integrins. Other integrins recognize different specific peptide sequences present on other ligands. The binding site of an integrin may be specific for a single ligand or it may be capable of binding more than one ligand. Conversely, one ligand may be recognized by several integrins.

Function

Integrins are both recipients and generators of cell signals; signal transduction may operate in either an "outside in" or an "inside out" mode. Ligand binding to the extracellular component primes the integrin – the intracellular region then associates with tyrosine kinases to induce a cascade of intracellular signals that result in cell activation (outside-in signaling). Conversely, cell activation by a variety of other stimuli activates a series of kinases that communicate intracellularly with the cytoplasmic tail of the integrin; this triggers a conformational change in the extracellular binding-site making it receptive to ligand binding (inside-out signaling).

Binding of ligand induces integrin clustering and lateral association with proximate membrane growth factor receptors (eg, PDGF, EGF, VEGF). The cytoplasmic tail of the integrin (lacking intrinsic tyrosine kinase activity) associates with kinase signaling pathways that may activate: (1) small G-proteins (Ras and Rho), (2) FAK (focal adhesion kinase) which interacts with actin and the cytoskeleton, (3) PI3-kinase, (4) the cyclins – regulators of the cell cycle. Depending on the cell type and the nature of the stimulus, integrin-ligand interaction

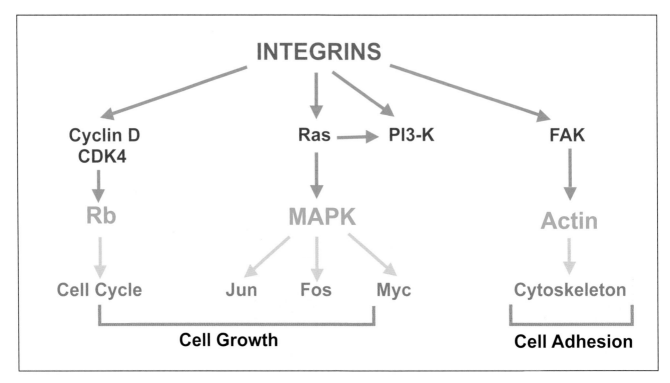

Figure 3-2 Integrin Signaling

may increase gene expression, cell proliferation, cell adhesion, and cytoskeletal changes (Figure 3-2).

Platelets - In unstimulated platelets, the integrin GPIIb/IIIa is unavailable to its ligands. When the platelet is activated by thrombin or other agonists, intracellular signaling stimulates the cytoplasmic tail of the integrin, transducing a conformational change in the extracellular binding-site that now becomes available to the circulating ligands vWF and fibrinogen (inside-out signaling). The integrin recognizes and binds the RGD sequences of these ligands, mediating platelet adhesion and aggregation. Conversely, vWF or fibrinogen in subendothelial tissues, at sites of vascular injury, can bind to GPIIb/IIIa of non-activated platelets to trigger intracellular signaling that results in cytoskeletal shape change, cytoplasmic phosphokinase activity, and release of granule contents (outside-in signaling) (Section 30).

Neutrophils – The β_2 integrins (primarily CD11b/CD18) of unstimulated neutrophils are maintained in an inactive state. In areas of inflammation, soluble inflammatory stimuli (chemokines and cytokines) bind to the neutrophil and induce intracellular signaling that primes the cytoplasmic tail of the integrin, increasing the affinity for its endothelial ligands ICAM-1 and ICAM-2. Tight adhesion of CD11b/CD18 to the endothelial surface precedes leukocyte transendothelial migration.

Lymphocytes - The β_2 integrins (primarily CD11a/CD18) expressed on lymphocytes have a major role in their tissue migration into inflammatory sites. Lymphocyte homing to peripheral lymph nodes takes place in postcapillary high endothelial venules (HEVs) and is mediated by L-selectin; transmigration into secondary lymphoid structures requires the participation of L-selectin and the integrin $\alpha_4\beta_7$.

SELECTINS

Selectins are a family of cellular glycoprotein adhesion molecules present in endothelial cells, leukocytes, and platelets. The three known members share a common structure. The extracellular component consists of an N-terminal lectin domain followed by an epidermal growth factor-like region and a series of complement receptor-like repeats; there is a single transmembrane domain and a short intracellular cytoplasmic C-terminal end. The N-terminal domain binds to a number of counter-adhesive oligosaccharides commonly present on cell surface glycoproteins and glycolipids. (Note: lectins are proteins that recognize carbohydrates). All three selectins are involved in the leukocyte rolling along the endothelium that initiates the physical leukocyte-endothelial interaction preceding the recruitment of lymphocytes and neutrophils into areas of inflammation. L-selectin is expressed on leukocytes and binds to carbohydrate ligands on endothelium; P-and E-selectins are expressed on endothelial cells and bind carbohydrate ligands on leukocytes (Figure 3-3).

L-selectin is expressed constitutively on the surface microvilli of neutrophils, lymphocytes and monocytes. Interaction with its carbohydrate ligand on activated endothelial cells initiates leukocyte rolling along the vessel wall. Expression of L-selectin is constitutive and therefore independent of leukocyte activation; however, its endothelial ligands are displayed only when endothelial cells are activated by inflammatory stimuli. The selectin bonds are formed and broken rapidly, resulting in a rolling progression of the cell along the endothelium. The reduced velocity of rolling leukocytes enhances their encounter with the endothelial surface. L-selectin also functions as a signaling receptor, transmitting an intracellular message that primes the leukocyte integrins, thus triggering firm adhesion of neutrophils and lymphocytes to the endothelium within areas of inflammation. L-selectin also mediates the homing of lymphocytes into lymph nodes by interacting with its ligands (GlyCAM1, CD34 and MadCAM-1) expressed on the HEVs of lymph nodes.

P-selectin is present in the α-granules of platelets and in the Weibel-Palade bodies of endothelial cells. On activation of the endothelial cell, the preformed P-selectin is redistributed to the cell surface where it mediates binding of circulating leukocytes. At sites of vascular injury, P-selectin released from α-granules of activated platelets is mobilized rapidly to the cell surface where it enhances adhesion of platelets to circulating leukocytes; it also may increase the expression of tissue factor on monocyte membranes, thus triggering or amplifying hemostasis. The major leukocyte ligand for P-selectin, PSGL-1 (P-selectin glycoprotein ligand-1), is

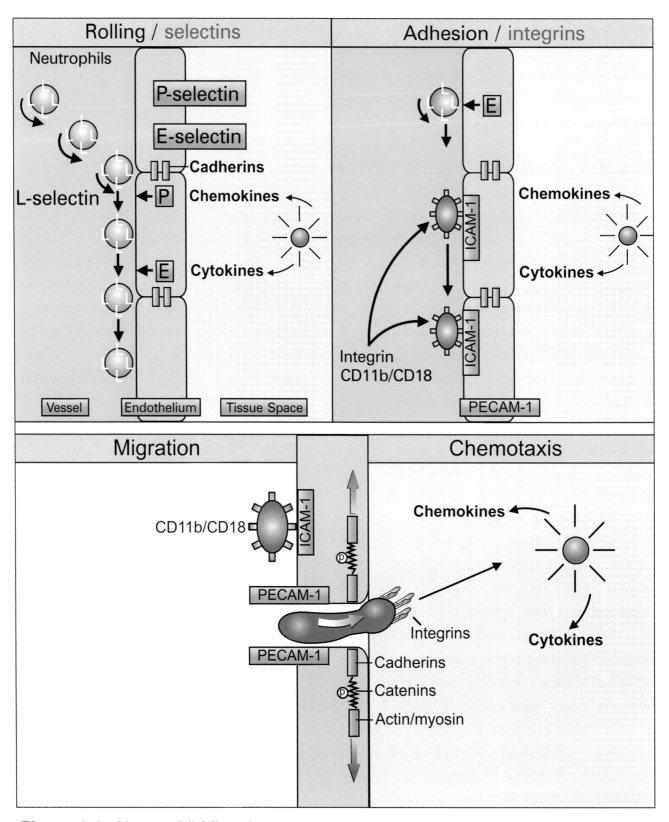

Figure 3-3   Neutrophil Migration

required for P-selectin binding to neutrophils and lymphocytes.

E-selectin is restricted to endothelial cells (ECs). It is expressed following cytokine stimulation of ECs in areas of inflammation. There is a delay of some hours before E-selectin appears on the cell surface – the time required for gene transcription, translation and protein synthesis. It may react with the PSGL-1 ligand on leukocytes.

IMMUNOGLOBULIN (Ig) SUPERFAMILY

The members of the immunoglobulin superfamily are transmembrane glycoproteins that share a common extracellular structure: they contain a varying number (2 to 9) of immunoglobulin-like domains that mediate heterophilic or homophilic cell-cell adhesion. This family includes the ICAMS, VCAM-1 and PECAM-1. The intercellular adhesion molecules (ICAMs) are cell surface proteins that serve as counterreceptors for integrins. Five ICAMs have been described: ICAM-1 on leukocytes, endothelial cells and other tissues; ICAM-2 confined to leukocytes and endothelial cells; ICAM-3 is leukocyte specific; ICAM-4 is red cell specific, originally described as the LW (Landsteiner-Weiner) blood group antigen; ICAM-5 is expressed in brain.

ICAM-1 is constitutively expressed at a very low level on endothelium – its synthesis is upregulated several fold by inflammatory agents such as interferon-α and interleukin-1. It interacts with the β_2 integrins CD11a/CD18 and CD11b/CD18 expressed on lymphocytes and neutrophils.

ICAM-2 is constitutively expressed on quiescent endothelial cells; its synthesis is non-inducible. It binds to the β_2 integrins CD11a/CD18 and CD11b/CD18.

VCAM-1 (vascular cell adhesion molecule-1) is upregulated on endothelial cells by inflammatory stimuli (IFN-α, IL-4). It binds to the integrin $\alpha_4 \beta_1$ expressed on lymphocytes, monocytes, eosinophils and basophils.

PECAM-1 (platelet endothelial cell adhesion molecule) is expressed on the surface of endothelial cells, platelets, neutrophils, monocytes and lymphocytes. On endothelial cells, it is present in highest concentration adjacent to intercellular junctions. It mediates neutrophil and monocyte transmigration (diapedesis) from the circulation into the subendothelial space through these endothelial junctions by interaction with its leukocyte homologue, PECAM-1.

The interactions of selectins, integrins and intercellular adhesion molecules mediate lymphocyte homing to immunological reactive sites, and guide neutrophils and monocytes to inflammatory foci. In areas of inflammation, the on-off tethering of leukocytes with margination and rolling along the endothelium is initiated by the selectins; firm adherence occurs through the interaction of endothelial ICAMs with leukocyte integrins, and extravascular migration is facilitated by PECAM-1 which moves the cells out of the circulation into the subendothelial space and towards the inflammatory focus.

CADHERINS

Cadherins are a class of adhesion molecules that promote Ca^{2+}-dependent cell to cell binding in the endothelium, skin and other tissues. The cells adhere to their neighbouring cells that express the identical cadherin molecule (homophilic binding). Clusters of cadherin molecules at sites of cell contact form "adherens junctions" which determine and maintain tissue organization (Section 31).

Cadherins are single pass transmembrane proteins. The extracellular region, consisting of five homologous repeats, determines the adhesive-binding specificity. The short cytoplasmic tail associates with cytoplasmic structural proteins, α and β catenins, which in turn mediate linkage to the actin cytoskeleton. At inflammatory sites, cytokine-induced activation of the endothelial cell results in phosphorylation of the catenins with disruption of the adherens junctions – the cadherins on adjacent endothelial cells separate to allow passage of leukocytes into the inflammatory site (Figure 3-3).

CLINICAL CORRELATES

Glanzmann Thrombasthenia is an autosomal recessive disease due to dysfunctional or absent GPIIb/IIIa ($\alpha_{IIb}\beta_3$) integrins on platelets and megakaryocytes. Mutation in either α_{IIb} or β_3 results in failure of the heterodimer assembly in the platelet membrane. This integrin is key to platelet binding of fibrinogen and von Willebrand factor. In the absence of functional GPIIb/IIIa, reduced platelet adhesion and aggregation is associated with a major bleeding diathesis (Section 30).

Therapeutic inhibitors of GPIIb/IIIa. A series of antithrombotic agents that block GPIIb/IIIa-mediated platelet aggregation are in clinical use or in clinical trial. These include: (1) monoclonal antibodies, or their Fab piece, specific for GPIIb/IIIa, (2) RGD-containing peptides capable of blocking the integrin RGD-binding site. Clinically, these agents may be of value following coronary angiography, coronary stenting or bypass surgery.

Disintegrins are potent anticoagulant toxins found in some viper venoms. These soluble proteins have an RGD sequence with a high affinity for the platelet GPIIb/IIIa integrin. Tight competitive binding by the disintegrin renders GPIIb/IIIa unavailable to the normal ligands – thus interfering with platelet function. The therapeutic value of these disintegrins as antithrombotic agents is of interest.

Leukocyte Adhesion Deficiency Syndrome (LAD). LAD-I is due to a variety of genetic mutations in the β_2 subunit (CD18) of the CD11/CD18 integrins – normal expression of these integrins is essential for neutrophil migration into extravascular sites. The defect is manifest by neutrophilia and life-threatening infections beginning shortly after birth; neutrophilia results from the inability of the cells to migrate out of the vasculature. Variant LAD-I syndromes have similar clinical features although the expression of β_2 integrins is only moderately reduced.

LAD-II is a rare congenital disorder due to a defect that involves the oligosaccharide ligands for all three selectins. The abnormality may be due to defects in fucose metabolism that result in deficiency of the fucosylated carbohydrate ligands necessary for selectin adhesion; α-fucose is an essential structural component of the normal ligands. Because the leukocytes cannot attach and roll along the endothelial surface, their recruitment into tissues is impaired. Episodes of infection are less severe and less frequent than in LAD-I (Section 7).

Integrins on Tumor Cells

Integrins may be missing or non-functional on cells undergoing malignant transformation. The loss of cell-cell surface adhesion and signaling results in deregulation of growth and facilitates tissue invasion and metastases.

———————— •••●●●•• ————————

SUGGESTED READING

Aplin AE, Howe A, Alahari SK, Juliano RL. Signal transduction and signal modulation by cell adhesion receptors: the role of integrins, cadherins, immunoglobulin-cell adhesion molecules, and selectins. Pharm Rev 40:197-263, 1998.

Boudreau NJ, Jones PL. Extracellular matrix and integrin signaling: The shape of things to come. Biochem J 339:481-488, 1999.

Chen S, Springer TA. An automatic braking system that stabilizes leukocyte rolling by an increase in selectin bond number with shear. J Cell Biol 144:185-200, 1999.

Dedhar S. Integrins and signal transduction. Curr Opin Haemat 6:37-43, 1999.

Etzioni A, Doerschuk CM, Harlan JM. Of man and mouse: Leukocyte and endothelial adhesion molecule deficiencies. Blood 94:3281-3288, 1999.

Hynes RO. Cell adhesion: Old and new questions. Trends in Cell Biol 9:M33-M37, 1999.

Petruzzelli L, Takami M, Humes HD. Structure and function of cell adhesion molecules. Am J Med 106:467- 476, 1999.

Vestweber D, Blanks JE. Mechanisms that regulate the function of the selectins and their ligands. Physiol Rev 79:181-213, 1999.

Vleminckx K, Kemler R. Cadherins and tissue formation: Integrating adhesion and signaling. BioEssays 21:211-220, 1999.

Yang J, Furie BC, Furie B. The biology of P-selectin glycoprotein ligand-1: Its role as a selectin counterreceptor in leukocyte-endothelial and leukocyte-platelet interaction. Thromb Haemost 81:1-7, 1999.

APOPTOSIS

"This is the way the world ends
Not with a bang but a whimper."
The Hollow Men – T.S. Eliot

Cells die by two primary processes: (1) necrosis, in which the release of intracellular proteases and lysozymes induce an inflammatory response, or (2) apoptosis, where the cell remnants quietly disappear as they are phagocytosed by surrounding cells.

Cell death by necrosis usually follows major pathological acute injury such as hypoxia, hyperthermia, viral invasion, exposure to various exogenous toxins, or attack by complement. Necrosis is characterized by early mitochondrial swelling and failure, dysfunction of the plasma membrane with loss of homeostasis, cell swelling and rupture. The loss of cell membrane integrity with release of cell contents, including proteases and lysozymes, induces an inflammatory response with cytokine release by the surrounding macrophages as they mop up the damaged cells and begin the process of repair.

The major physiological mechanism of cell removal is apoptosis – a Greek descriptive term for falling leaves or petals. Apoptosis describes the process by which cells are "silently" removed under normal conditions when they reach the end of their life span, are damaged, or are superfluous. It is a general tissue phenomenon necessary for development and homeostasis: elimination of redundant cells during embryogenesis, cell atrophy on endocrine withdrawal or loss of essential growth factors or cytokines, tissue remodelling and repair, and removal of cells that have sustained genotoxic damage. Externally-induced apoptosis occurs in thymocytes exposed to corticosteroids and in immune-mediated tumor-cell kill. Cells characterized by a normally short life span, such as neutrophils, undergo apoptosis as an intrinsic pre-programmed suicidal event. Examples of apoptotic cell removal include: (1) erythroid precursors upon withdrawal of erythropoietin, (2) removal of neutrophils outside the inflammatory response, (3) clonal selection of lymphocytes in the thymus, and (4) cell kill by anti-neoplastic chemotherapeutic agents. Normal apoptotic cell removal and cell replacement in tissue remodelling is estimated at some 1×10^{11} cells per day – equivalent to the turnover of an adult's total body weight every 18 to 24 months.

Morphologically, cells undergoing apoptosis exhibit ruffling, blebbing and condensation of the plasma and nuclear membranes and, subsequently, aggregation of nuclear chromatin. Mitochondria and ribosomes retain their gross structure and at least partial function. There is disruption of the cytoskeletal architecture, the cell shrinks and then fragments into a cluster of membrane-enclosed "apoptotic bodies" that are rapidly ingested by adjacent macrophages or other neighbouring phagocytic cells. As these apoptotic bodies induce no significant cytokine

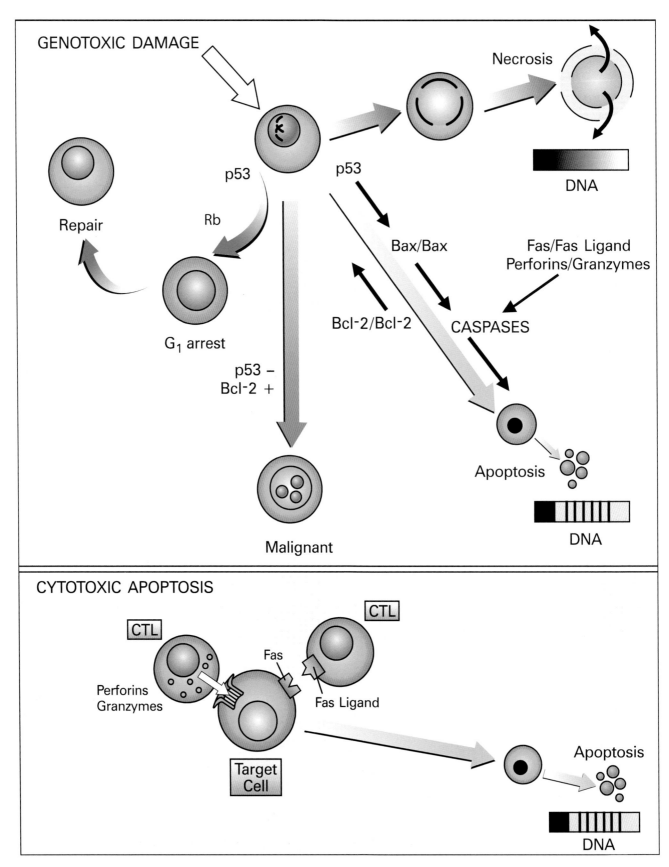

Figure 4-1 Pathways to Apoptosis

release by the phagocytic cell, the process progresses without concomitant induction of an inflammatory response (Figure 4-1).

Apoptosis is an active energy-dependent process requiring RNA and protein synthesis. It can be inhibited in a number of *in vitro* cell systems by either actinomycin D blockade of RNA synthesis or cyclohexamide interference with protein synthesis – an indication that these cells both activate and participate metabolically in their own death.

The hallmark of the end stage of apoptosis is endonuclease cleavage of DNA in the internucleosomal linker regions, yielding 180 base-pair fragments. This type of DNA fragmentation minimizes the possibility of intact gene or viral transfer to the phagocyte. (However, horizontal transfer of Epstein-Barr virus from apoptotic bodies to phagocyte has been observed in vitro). Separation of these fragments by agarose gel electrophoresis reveals the characteristic DNA ladder pattern of apoptosis; this is in contrast to the smudge pattern seen in cell necrosis that confirms the presence of fully degraded DNA.

The apoptotic process may be set in motion by: (1) genes responding to DNA damage, (2) death signals received at the cell membrane (Fas ligand), or (3) proteolytic enzymes entering directly into the cell (granzymes). The final events, evidenced by the changes in cell structure and disassembly, are the work of specific proteases (caspases).

GENE REGULATION OF APOPTOSIS

Regulation of apoptosis is highly conserved, with many of the same gene control processes operative in species from nematodes to humans. Although the cell death signal may be regulated by gene expression, the process can be set in motion by diverse stimuli such as genotoxic damage (eg, chemotherapy, radiation), or deprivation of cytokines (eg, erythropoietin). DNA single or double strand breaks or nucleotide deprivation activate a cascade beginning with the DNA-binding transcription factor p53; the downstream targets of p53 induce either growth arrest or entry of the cell into the apoptotic pathway.

The Role of p53

Cell injury resulting in genotoxic events activates *p53*, a transcription regulator gene. The p53 protein product is a regulator of DNA transcription; it binds directly to DNA, recognizes DNA damage (single or double strand breaks), and mediates at least two important cellular events: it can induce cell cycle arrest in G_1 or it can promote apoptosis. If cellular damage is reparable, p53-induced cell cycle arrest allows time for DNA repair. With more extensive damage, to prevent the cell with an impaired DNA sequence from proliferating as a defective or malignant clone, p53 moves the cell into the apoptotic pathway. p53 levels increase within minutes of DNA damage and the apoptotic process begins in a few hours.

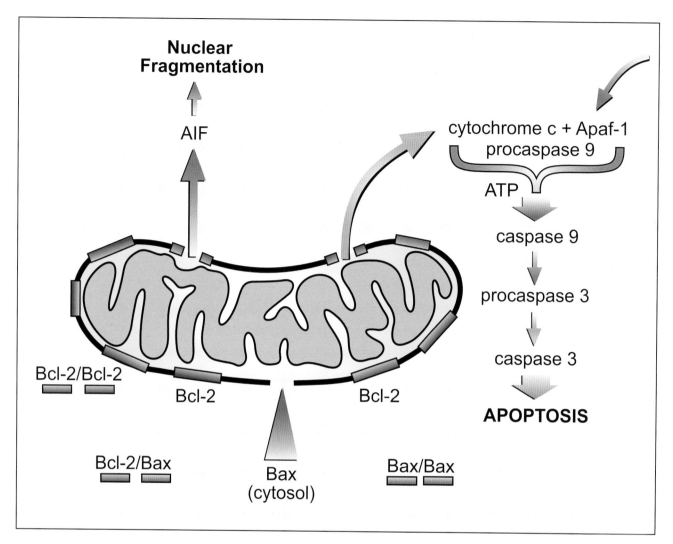

Figure 4-2 The Role of Mitochondria in Apoptosis

p53 protein, normally, is present in the cytosol in low concentration. It is negatively regulated by another transcription factor **MDM2** (murine double minute 2). MDM2 downregulates *p53* transcription; it also binds to the p53 protein, decreases its activity, and escorts it from the nucleus to the cytoplasm functioning as a ubiquitin protein ligase to accelerate p53 proteasomal degradation. In the event of DNA damage, *p53* gene induction is accompanied by increased synthesis and phosphorylation of p53. Phosphorylation renders the protein more active and reduces its binding and inactivation by MDM2, thereby doubling its half-life. As a result, p53 activity may increase a hundred-fold (Section 2).

p53 promotes cell cycle arrest in late G_1 at a restriction point guarded by the retinoblastoma (**Rb**) protein. Phosphorylation of Rb permits the cell to pass through this cell-cycle transition point and into S phase. p53 exerts control of the cell cycle through upregulation of **p21**, an inhibitor of the cyclin-dependent kinases (CDKs) responsible for moving the cell through G_1. The cyclinD/CDK4 complex normally promotes phosphorylation of Rb. Hypophosphorylated Rb sequesters **E2F,** a transcription factor required for passage through the G_1 restriction point. Upon Rb phosphorylation, E2F is released from Rb suppression and induces transcription of a number of proteins necessary for DNA replication, prompting the cell to move into S phase (Figure 2-2).

Cell injury results in increased expression of p53 followed by p53-regulated induction of p21 and, consequently, by the inhibition of cyclinD/CDK4 phosphorylation of Rb. Maintenance of Rb in its active hypophosphorylated state holds the cell in G_1, allowing time for repair. Two other important regulators of p53 and Rb are products of the INK4a gene: **p19**[ARF] blocks the MDM2 inhibition of p53; **p16**[INK4a], an inhibitor of CDK 4/6, blocks Rb phosphorylation and induces G_1 arrest. In the event that DNA damage is more severe and non-reparable, p53 performs its alternate role of moving the cell into apoptosis through the Bcl-2/Bax system.

Bcl-2 / Bax

The major downstream regulation of the apoptotic death signal resides with the *bcl-2/ bax* gene family. It plays an essential role in regulating the release of pro-apoptotic cytochrome c from the mitochondrial intermembranous space into the cytoplasm. Sixteen members of this family have been recognized: the Bcl-2 and Bcl-X_L members are apoptosis-inhibitory proteins, the Bax, Bad and Bid members are promoters of apoptosis. Areas of commonality of structure allow these proteins to homo- and hetero-dimerize. A high expression of the Bax group promotes apoptosis, a high expression of the Bcl-2 group inhibits apoptosis. Some members of the Bax group (eg, Bad) function by dimerizing with Bcl-2 and Bcl-X_L to reduce their anti-apoptotic potential and to alter the ratio in favour of apoptosis. p53 probably functions by regulating the ratios of the Bax/Bax, Bax/Bcl-2 and Bcl-2/Bcl-2 groups in favour of the Bax family.

Mitochondria (Figure 4-2)

Mitochondria are double-walled organelles that house the electron-transport and the energy-converting systems of the cell. In addition, there are a number of pro-apoptotic proteins within the intermembranous space. The Bcl-2 group of proteins associate with the outer mitochondrial membrane and are oriented towards the cytosol – they govern the transition pores in the membrane. The Bax monomers reside in the cytosol, but can move between the cytosol and the mitochondria. Upon receipt of the apoptotic signal, Bax proteins form dimers or oligomers that bind to the mitochondrial membrane "permeability transition pore" inducing loss of selective ion permeability. As a result of the outer membrane changes, there is release into the cytosol of the contents of the intermembranous space, including **cytochrome c** and apoptosis-inducing factor (**AIF**): AIF moves directly to the nucleus where it induces chromatin condensation and nuclear fragmentation; cytosolic cytochrome c sets in motion the terminal events of apoptosis. Cytochrome c binds to the cytoplasmic protein **Apaf-1** (apoptotic protease activating factor-1). Cytochrome c associates with Apaf-1 and procaspase-9 in the presence of

ATP in a complex referred to as the apoptosome. Formation of the apoptosome results in the activation of procaspase-9. Caspase-9 then activates downstream caspases, including procaspase-3. Caspase-3 is responsible for the cytological changes characteristic of apoptosis (Figure 4-2).

The Caspases

The caspases are cysteine proteases that are activated specifically in apoptotic cells; the constitutively expressed procaspases (enzymatically inert zymogens) are present in the cytosol. More than a dozen human caspases have been identified. Caspases activate other procaspases in a sequential cascade (reminiscent of the complement or the coagulation sequence); they also are activated by self-cleavage: autocatalytic processing of zymogens is facilitated by aggregation of caspases into large oligomeric structures. Caspases are classified as either 'initiators' (caspase 2,8, 9,10), or 'effectors' (caspase 3,6,7) of proteolysis – the effector caspases are activated downstream of the initiator caspases.

Proteolysis by caspases is restricted and limited: cleavage of peptide bonds occurs only following specific aspartic acid residues (thus c-asp-ases), producing disassembly of the protein – not general proteolysis. Caspase activity results in: cleavage of cytoskeletal proteins, disruption of the nuclear membrane, disruption of cell-cell contact, and the freeing of the DNA nuclease **CAD** (caspase-activated deoxyribonuclease) which is responsible for DNA fragmentation. CAD is present in cells as an inactive complex with the inhibitory protein **ICAD**. Caspase-3-mediated cleavage of ICAD results in the release and activation of CAD. This nuclease cleaves DNA between nucleosomes to generate the 180 base-pair fragments demonstrated by the DNA agarose gel ladder pattern that is the signature of apoptosis.

This restricted proteolysis does not result in cellular lysis but rather in the morphological changes, including the membrane-bound sealed apoptotic bodies, characteristic of apoptotic cells. The caspases, in addition, may permeablize the mitochondrial membrane with further release of cytochrome c and intramitochondrial procaspases. A family of caspase inhibitors, **IAPs** (inhibitors of apoptosis), selectively inhibit effector caspases, blocking the apoptotic process. In turn, the mitochondrial protein Smac/DIABLO binds to and neutralizes IAP anti-apoptotic activity; Smac/DIABLO is released into the cytosol, probably by the same route as cytochrome c. IAPs are overexpressed in many malignant cells. The IAP family also inhibits apoptosis through non-caspase mechanisms: by modulation of transcription factors, and by involvement in cell-cycle control.

CYTOTOXIC REGULATION OF APOPTOSIS

The Granzyme System (Figure 4-1)

This secretory apoptotic pathway is operative in removing pathogen-infected cells and tumor cells. **Perforins** and **granzymes** are proteins contained within the cytoplasmic secretory granules of cytotoxic lymphocytes (CTLs) and natural killer (NK) cells, Upon CTL receptor-mediated binding to a target cell, perforins are secreted and inserted into the membrane of the target cell where they assemble into a circular membrane-spanning pore similar to the membrane attack complex (MAC) of complement; (this resemblance includes immunological cross-reactivity between perforin and MAC). The perforin pore induces a rapid increase in cytosolic calcium. The co-secreted serine protease **granzyme B** enters the target cell within a secretory vesicle by receptor-mediated endocytosis. The internalized perforin protein frees granzyme B from its vesicle. Granzyme B now rapidly activates procaspase-8; this is followed by cleavage of procaspase-3 and other effector caspases with subsequent DNA fragmentation and apoptosis. A second secretory-granule protease, **granzyme A**, also acts synergistically with perforin in the apoptotic process.

Fas/FasL and TNFR/TNF (Figure 4-3)

The alternative non-secretory mechanism of apoptosis is through activation of the "death receptors" expressed on the cell membrane. **Fas** (CD95), a cell-surface receptor and a member of the tumor necrosis factor receptor (TNF-R) family, is a transducer of the apoptotic signal; it is expressed in a wide range of somatic cells and some tumor cells. Fas ligand (**FasL**) is a member of the TNF family; its expression is more restricted: it is found on cytotoxic T cells and natural killer (NK) cells. FasL, by binding, crosslinking and aggregating the Fas receptor, sets the apoptotic process in motion. This mechanism plays a significant role in: removal of activated T cells at the end of an immune response, deletion of virus-infected target cells, killing of tumor cells, and destruction of cells in numerous other pathological states.

Fas ligand and tumor necrosis factor (**TNF**) produce apoptosis in an analogous fashion – FasL through the Fas receptor protein, and TNF by binding to the TNF receptor (**TNFR-1**). Upon binding of their respective ligands, these receptors assemble into trimeric complexes. The cytoplasmic tail of each contains a so-called death domain (DD) that interacts with a cytoplasmic adapter protein: the cytoplasmic portions of the Fas trimer interacts with FADD (Fas associating protein with a death domain); the cytoplasmic tails of TNFR-1 interact with TRADD (TNFR associated death domain protein) and RIP (receptor-interacting protein). These latter proteins also contain death domains; they have a direct pathway to apoptosis through recruitment, oligomerization, and activation of procaspase-8. Aggregation of procaspase-8 molecules leads to autocatalytic activation with production of caspase-8. Caspase-8, subsequently, activates downstream effector caspases including procaspase-3. An additional receptor of the TNF family, **TRAIL** (**T**NF **r**elated **a**poptosis **i**nducing **l**igand), signals through FADD to caspase-8.

Two routes for the death-receptor pathway downstream of the activated receptor have

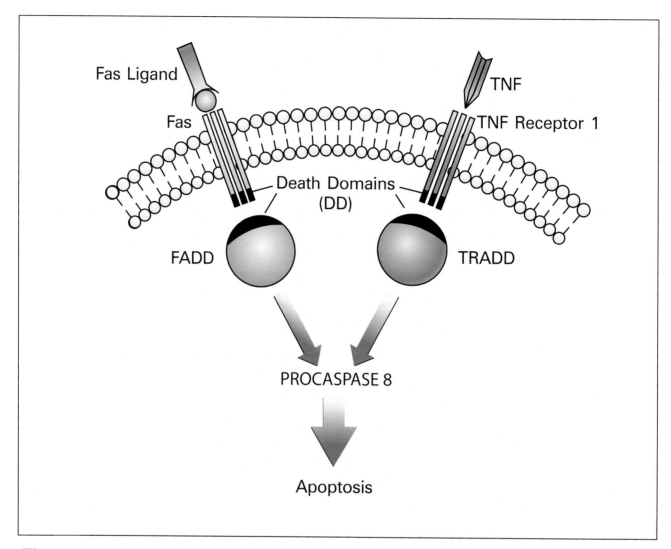

Figure 4-3 Fas Ligand and TNF Mediated Apoptosis

been described. In so-called Type I cells, the death signal is propagated as described. In Type II cells, insufficient caspase-8 is formed to activate the effector caspases – amplification is required. The small amount of caspase-8 that is formed cleaves the pro-apoptotic Bax-2 family member Bid. Truncated Bid translocates to the mitochondrial membrane and induces release of the pro-apoptotic proteins including cytochrome c and Smac/DIABLO. Subsequent formation of the apoptosome (cytochrome c, Apaf-1, and procaspase-9) results in activation of procaspase-9.

Removal of Apoptotic Bodies

Phospholipid (PL) asymmetry in the lipid bilayer is a feature of cell membranes. The phospholipids are distributed asymmetrically, with phosphatidylserine (PS) and phosphatidylethanolamine (PE), the anionic PLs, largely confined to the inner bilayer, and phosphatidylcholine (PC) to the outer bilayer. In normal cells, this asymmetry is maintained by the activity of an ATP-dependent **translocase**. During apoptosis, either failure of the translocase or activation of the enzyme **scramblase**, results in PS relocation to the surface bilayer. The presence of PS on the outer leaflet of the apoptotic body provides a signal for phagocytic uptake by macrophages and neighboring "non-professional" phagocytic cells, cells with membrane phosphatidylserine receptors. Cell removal is rapid, usually requiring less than 24 hours. For this reason, apoptotic cells are rarely seen in normal tissue.

Dendritic cells engulf and degrade apoptotic bodies and, in a process termed cross-priming, the peptides complexed with MHC class I molecules are presented on the surface membrane (Section 21). They are ignored by T-cells (as self) because there is no co-stimulatory ligand – therefore, there is no immune response. The possibility of an inflammatory response also is dampened by the release of anti-inflammatory cytokines (TGF-β1).

CLINICAL CORRELATES

Apoptosis in the Hematopoietic System

Both hematopoietic cell production and elimination are regulated by apoptosis. The maintenance of the erythropoietic stem cells (BFU-Es and CFU-Es) is dependent on the presence of erythropoietin (EPO); withdrawal of EPO results in apoptosis of these red cell precursors. A second apoptotic pathway also is operative: Fas is present on both early and late erythroid precursors – however its activating ligand FasL appears only on late erythroblasts. Within the erythropoietic islands, binding of FasL to Fas on early erythroid precursors activates the caspase system, inducing apoptosis – thus regulating red cell production.

Endogenously-mediated apoptosis is exemplified by the neutrophil. Following development and maturation in the marrow, this cell is resident in the blood stream for approximately 12 hours. Some disappear into the lung and gastrointestinal tract and are lost from mucosal surfaces. Many enter the tissue spaces – within one to two days, in the absence of an inflammatory focus, these cells spontaneously undergo apoptosis and are taken up by macrophages.

Lymphocyte death, in contrast, is mediated by exogenous events. These include removal of growth factors and activation of the FasL/Fas or TNF/TNFR death-receptor pathways. FasL/Fas initiation of apoptosis plays a major role in the deletion of T cells at termination of an immune response, and in the removal of non-functional or self-reactive T and B cells.

Apoptosis and Malignant Disease

An inappropriate increase in cell number is one of the hallmarks of malignant cell transformation. It may be due to either increased proliferation or decreased cell death. Decreased apoptosis may result from an absent or mutated form of the tumor suppressor gene *p53* or *Rb* (present in 50% and 40% of human tumors, respectively), from increased expression of Bcl-2, or a decrease in Bax. Deregulation and overexpression of Bcl-2 occurs with the translocation of the *bcl-2* gene from chromosome 18 into the Ig locus on chromosome 14. This translocation is associated with low grade follicular non-Hodgkin's lymphoma – a disease characterized, not by a rapidly proliferating tumor cell population, but by the gradual accumulation of slow growing lymphoma cells. The *bcl-2* gene was first identified in this **B-cell lymphoma** (Section18).

Overproduction of Bcl-2 protein also is associated with drug resistance in non-Hodgkin's lymphomas and chronic lymphocytic leukemia (CLL). In addition, the low apoptotic rate in CLL, with accumulation of lymphoid cells, has been attributed to the weak expression of Fas receptor on the cell membrane. Inhibitors of apoptosis (IAPs) inhibit effector caspases and may play a role in both tumor growth and drug resistance. Caspase-8 is deleted in some childhood neuroblastomas. Many chemotherapeutic and cytotoxic agents used in the treatment of malignant disease function by activating apoptosis – some by direct procaspase activation, others by DNA damage and p53 upregulation (Section 23). Newer experimental anti-tumor agents induce tumor-targetted caspase activation or Bcl-2 inhibition.

Autoimmune Lymphoproliferative Syndrome (ALPS)

Families have been identified with mutations in the Fas-encoding gene resulting in a dysfunctional Fas/FasL system. The region of the gene most frequently mutated encodes the death domain in the cytoplasmic tail of Fas. As a result of defects in functional Fas, there is a non-malignant accumulation of T lymphocytes with lymphadenopathy, splenomegaly, hepatomegaly, and associated autoimmune hemolytic anemia and thrombocytopenia (**ALPS I**). A clinically similar syndrome, **ALPS II**, is due to a mutation in procaspase-10; the Fas receptor is normal.

Apoptosis and Infectious Disease

An imperative in the evolutionary process of survival for viruses and some obligate bacterial pathogens is the preservation of the host cell. It is to be expected that these organisms will inhibit apoptosis. This interference or abrogation of the apoptotic process is realized in a number of ways – eg, by organisms that: (1) encode a protein similar to Bcl-2 (adenovirus), (2) promote expression of Bcl-2 (Epstein-Barr virus), (3) encode a protease inhibitor that inactivates procaspases 1 and 8 (cowpox), and (4) interfere with mitochondrial cytochrome c release into the cytosol (chlamydia).

Diseases Mediated by Increased Apoptosis

Disappearance of cells by apoptosis is central to a number of diseases as illustrated by:

1) AIDS which is characterized by depletion of $CD4^+$ T cells; these cells may die in the absence of intracellular infection by virus. Both virus and the viral protein gp120 have a high affinity for CD4 antigen; apoptosis is triggered when the virus or its gp120 protein bind to CD4 helper cells without the simultaneous engagement of the MHC class-II complex. 2) Disappearance of neurons in Alzheimer's disease, motor neuron disease and Parkinson's disease. 3) Death of cells in proximity to an area of acute infarction in brain or in heart. Tissue damage in myocardial infarction or in stroke extends beyond the infarcted area of initial cellular destruction as adjacent cells undergo apoptosis. It is postulated that therapeutic use of inhibitors of apoptosis (Bcl-2 or caspase inhibitors) might confine and reduce the amount of tissue loss in proximity to the infarct. 4) Overexpression of Fas in hepatocytes infected with hepatitis C renders these cells vulnerable to destruction by FasL-expressing cytotoxic T lymphocytes. 5) In Hashimoto's thyroiditis, the thyroid cells express both Fas and Fas ligand – as a result, they may destroy one another via the stimulus of an IL-1-induced increase in Fas expression. 6) Tumor cells that constitutively express FasL on their membrane or secrete FasL may escape cytotoxic T cell destruction. The tumor cell FasL activates the T-cell Fas pathway, destroying T cells that have infiltrated the tumor, thus eliminating these anti-tumor cytotoxic lymphocytes.

SUGGESTED READING

Alnemri ES. Mammalian cell death proteases: A family of highly conserved aspartate specific cysteine proteases. J Cell Biochem 64:33-42, 1997.

Berke G. The CTL's kiss of death. Cell 81:9-12, 1995.

Chin L, Pomerantz J, DePinho RA. The INK4a/ARF tumor suppressor: One gene – two products – two pathways. Trends Biochem Sci 23:291-296, 1998.

Grana X, Garriga J, Mayol X. Role of the retinoblastoma protein family, pRB, p107 and p130 in the negative control of cell death. Oncogene 17:3365-3383, 1998.

Green DG, Reed JL. Mitochondria and apoptosis. Science 281: 1309-1312, 1998.

Green DR. Apoptotic pathways: paper wraps stone blunts scissors. Cell 102:1-4. 2000.

Kasten MM, Giordano A. pRb and the CDKs in apoptosis and the cell cycle. Cell Death Differ 5:132-140, 1998.

Kroemer G, Zamzami N, Susin SA. Mitochondrial control of apoptosis. Immunol Today 18:44-51,1997.

Kumar S. The Bcl-2 family of proteins and activation of ICE-CED-3 family of proteases: A balancing act in apoptosis? Cell Death Differ 4:2-3, 1997.

LaCasse EC, Baird S, Korneluk RG, Mackenzie AE. The inhibitors of apoptosis (IAPs) and their emerging role in cancer. Oncogene 17:3247-3259, 1998.

Le Deist F, Emile JF, Rieux-Laucat F, et al. Clinical, immunological, and pathological consequences of Fas-deficient conditions. Lancet 348:719-723, 1996.

Liu C-C, Walsh CM, Young JD-E. Perforin: structure and function. Immunol Today 16:194-201, 1995.

Nagata S, Golstein P. The Fas death factor. Science 267:1449-1456, 1995.

Nunez G, Benedict MA, Hu Y, Inohara N. Caspases: The proteases of the apoptotic pathway. Oncogene 17:3237-3245, 1998.

Prives C. Signaling by p53: breaking the MDM2-p53 circuit. Cell 95: 5-8, 1998.

Raff M. Cell suicide for beginners. Nature 396: 119-122, 1998.

Reed JC. Cytochrome C: Can't live with it; can't live without it. Cell 91:559-562, 1997.

Reed JC. Bcl-2 family proteins. Oncogene 17:3225-3236, 1998.

Rudin CM, Thompson CB. Apoptosis and disease: regulation and clinical relevance of programmed cell death. Annu Rev Med 48:267-281, 1997.

Salvesen GS, Dixit VM. Caspases: intracellular signaling by proteolysis. Cell 91: 443-446, 1997.

Smyth MJ, Trapani JA. Granzymes: exogenous proteinases that induce target cell apoptosis. Immunol Today 16:202-206, 1995.

Straus SE (moderator). An inherited disorder of lymphocyte apoptosis: The autoimmune lymphoproliferative syndrome. Ann Int Med 130:592-601, 1999.

Thornberry NA, Lazebnik. Caspases: enemies within. Science 281: 1312-1316, 1998.

Wang J, Zheng L, Labito A, Chan FK, et al. Inherited human caspase 10 mutations underlie defective lymphocyte and dendritic cell apoptosis in autoimmune lymphoproliferative syndrome type II. Cell 98:47-58, 1999.

THE REGULATION OF HEMATOPOIESIS

"Thy bones are marrowless, thy blood is cold."
Macbeth, Act III Scene IV

The turnover of the hematopoietic cell pool in a 70 kg adult has been estimated to approach one trillion cells per day. Cell production is maintained by a small number of progenitor stem cells constituting approximately 0.1% of the nucleated cells in the marrow; only about 5% of these stem cells are in cycle at any one time. Stem cells are capable of both self-renewal and multilineage differentiation; they are responsible for maintenance and regeneration of the hematopoietic system. Marrow response to the demand of specific external stimuli is met by one or more of the cell lineages: hypoxia up-regulates red cell production, bacterial infection increases granulocyte production, parasitic invasion increases circulating eosinophils and, similarly, monocytes and megakaryocytes may increase with relatively minor impact on the other cell series. These responses are mediated by a series of cytokines that act, individually and in concert, to stimulate proliferation, differentiation, and function at various stages of cell development. As cytokines act singly, in unison, and by feedback mechanisms, their inter-relationships are complex; the schema in Figure 5-2 is a simplified view of these processes.

STEM CELLS

The stem cell pool maintains itself, with little if any depletion, by asymmetric division into a committed colony forming unit (CFU) and another stem cell. The stem cell pool is not reduced significantly during ageing. The quiescent stem cell resides in a G_0 state that provides protection from genotoxic events and allows extended time for DNA repair. This totipotent primitive stem cell is moved into its activated state by intrinsic controls and by cytokine binding to cell surface receptors. The early CFUs have a higher proliferative rate but more limited self-renewal than the progenitor stem cell; their proliferation and differentiation produce cells again regulated by both intrinsic mechanisms and external growth factors that, eventually, convert the dividing cells into a population of terminally differentiated functional cells. The progeny of pluripotent CFUs are heterogeneous, the result of a stochastic process with the possibility of more than one cell type evolving from early CFU progenitors. The lineage is defined by the cell, but proliferation and survival are regulated by growth factors. Most stem cells carry the surface marker CD34 (CD34+); some are probably CD34-. Although most hematopoietic stem cells reside in the marrow, some circulate in the peripheral blood along with early CFU cells.

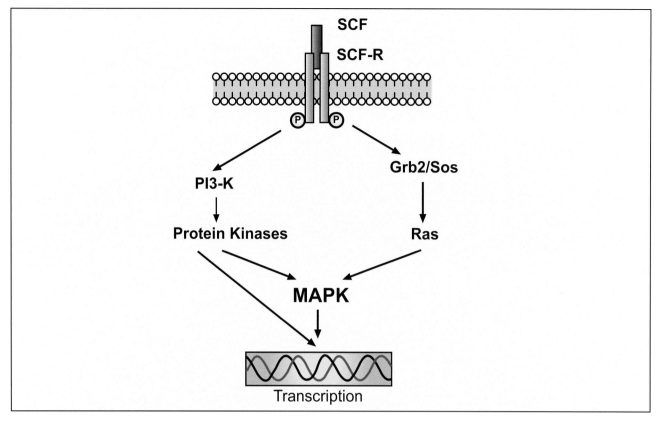

Figure 5-1   Stem Cell Factor Signaling

The hematopoietic cells replicate and evolve within the microenvironment of the bone marrow located in trabecular bone. The marrow consists of a network of sinusoidal venous channels with hematopoietic cells, fat cells and stromal cells in the spaces between the venous sinuses. The extensive vascular channels consist of endothelial cells supported by a layer of reticular cells with extending reticulin fibres. The hematopoietic cells, sequestered in specific sites, are "nursed" by stromal cells that provide the cytokines required for their development. The stromal cells include fibroblasts, macrophages, dendritic cells, T-cells and osteoblasts. The extracellular matrix (ECM) provides a support grid and an adhesive substrate; it consists of such proteins as collagen, fibronectin, reticulin, thrombospondin, proteoglycans and laminin. A number of adhesion molecules, including integrins and selectins, are expressed on the surface of hematopoietic cells; their density changes as the cell matures. Adhesive interactions between the cells and the ECM may govern both retention of the precursors within the marrow and release of the maturing cells into the peripheral circulation, and may have a role in stem cell homing following bone marrow transplant.

Stem Cell to Product

The G_0 stem cell is moved into its activated proliferative state by **Stem Cell Factor**

(SCF), also referred to as Steel factor or c-kit ligand. (The term Steel factor originates from studies in mice with a mutation or loss of the SCF gene that leads to defective melanocyte formation resulting in a steel-coloured coat; the gene product affects not only melanocyte development but also hematopoiesis, mast cell production and gametogenesis). SCF is produced by stromal cells in the local marrow environment. It binds to a receptor (SCF-R) expressed on hematopoietic progenitor cells; this receptor is the product of a proto-oncogene known as c-kit (c-kit is related to a feline sarcoma virus oncogene); thus SCF is also known as c-kit ligand.

SCF-R belongs to the superfamily of tyrosine kinase receptors that regulate cell survival, proliferation and differentiation. When activated by ligand binding, SCF-R undergoes autophosphorylation. The phosphorylated receptor transmits a message through its SH2-recognition domains to the adapter protein complex Grb2/Sos which, in turn, activates Ras. The message continues through the Ras-MAPK pathway to the nucleus. MAPK activates the early response genes (jun, fos and myc); these, in turn, activate the late response genes that encode the cyclins and cyclin-dependent kinases (CDKs), resulting in cell proliferation. In addition, SCF-R activation of PI3-kinase recruits the phosphotidylinositol-derived signaling pathway (Section 1, Figure 5-1).

The various cytokine regulators function at three levels of hematopoietic cell formation: early (on primitive stem cells), intermediate (lineage non-specific), and late (lineage specific). Cytokines that govern terminal differentiation also can stimulate cell function (eg, G-CSF, GMCSF).

Synergy and amplification of the SCF-R activation pathway are provided by the early acting cytokines: interleukins (IL-3, IL-6, IL-9), G-CSF (Granulocyte-Colony Stimulating Factor), and GM-CSF (Granulocyte Macrophage-Colony Stimulating Factor). The cell product derived from the stem cell in response to these stimuli is the multipotent CFU-GEMM (Colony Forming Unit-Granulocyte, Erythrocyte, Macrophage, Megakaryocyte). Although **CFU-GEMM** has a limited capacity for self renewal, it is the progenitor of the myeloid, monocyte, megakaryocyte and erythroid cells (Figure 5-2).

The next series of cytokines are also lineage non-specific. These are IL-3, G-CSF and GM-CSF that govern the formation of **CFU-GM** (Colony Forming Unit Granulocyte/Macrophage) – the precursor of granulocytes and monocytes. The addition of IL-11 and IGF-1 stimulates production of the Burst Forming Unit-Erythroid (**BFU-E**) for red cell production, and IL-11 stimulates the Colony Forming Unit (**CFU-Meg**) for megakaryocytes. The BFU-E colonies are further expanded by GM-CSF, IL-9, insulin-like growth factor 1 (IGF-1), and erythropoietin (EPO) to form **CFU-Es** – the colony forming units for erythrocyte precursors. In general, as precursor cells become more differentiated, their ability for self-renewal decreases. The late acting cytokines carry the process to completion: G-CSF, IL3 and GM-CSF stimulate granulocyte production, M-CSF stimulates monocyte formation, IL-3 regulates basophil production, and IL-5 and GM-CSF stimulate eosinophil formation. Cytokines

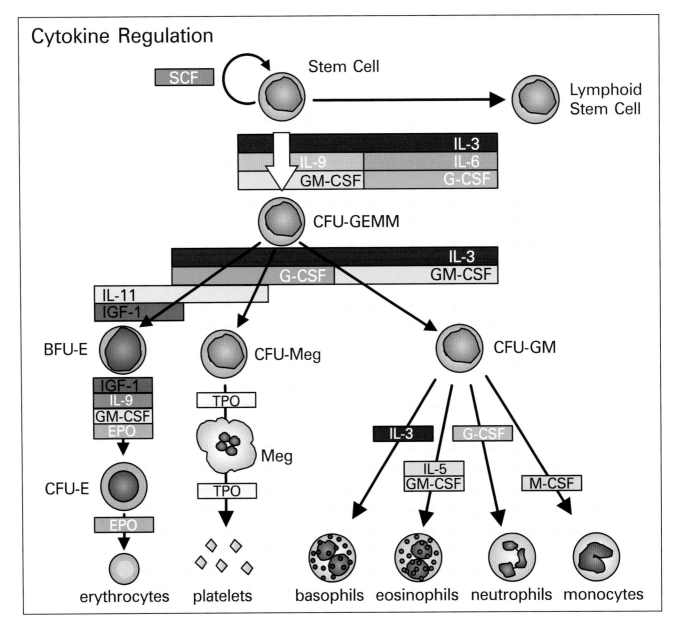

Figure 5-2 Hematopoiesis

also enhance the function of the end-stage cells (eg, GM-CSF and G-CSF activation of mature neutrophils). The production of erythrocytes from CFU-E is under erythropoietin (EPO) control. Thrombopoietin (TPO), a cytokine produced in the liver, regulates platelet production through interaction with a specific receptor, designated c-Mpl or Mpl. (The receptor was identified by isolation of the murine myeloproliferative leukemia virus (MPLV) which contains a truncated form of the proto-oncogene *c-mpl*). *c-mpl* encodes the cytokine receptor Mpl. TPO binding to Mpl results in proliferation of megakaryocyte progenitors, megakaryocyte maturation, and platelet production. TPO synthesis, for the most part, is regulated by circulating platelet levels (Section 30).

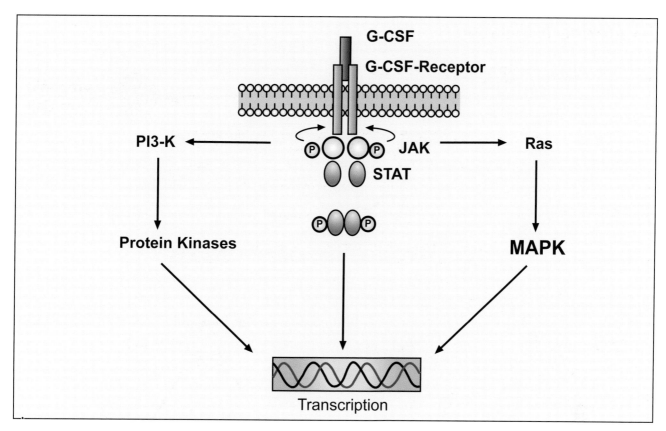

Figure 5-3 G-CSF Signaling

The Role of the Integrins

The integrins are cell surface glycoproteins that interact with complementary adhesion molecules. They are heterodimers of non-covalently associated α and β subunits, with a large extracellular binding domain, a transmembrane segment and a short cytoplasmic domain (Section 3). Integrins are bidirectional signaling molecules: activation signals can be conveyed from the outside of the cell to the interior, or from the inside of the cell to the integrin receptor. The engagement of ligand (outside-in signaling) triggers dynamic conformational changes in the integrin, activating intracellular transduction cascades and transcriptional events that ultimately result in cell adhesion and cell cycle progression. Activation of the cell by agonists that bind to a variety of other receptors conveys a message to the cytoplasmic region of the integrin that triggers increased ligand recognition (inside-out signaling).

The β_1 integrin family are receptors for fibronectin, collagen, thrombospondin and VCAM (vascular cell adhesion molecules); they may be responsible for the localization of the hematopoietic cells to "nurse" areas within the marrow that govern their survival and proliferation. Members of the β_2 integrin (CD11/18) family interact with intercellular adhesion molecules (ICAMS-1, 2, and 3) and with fibrinogen to regulate the exit of mature cells from the bone marrow.

The Role of the Cytokines and Their Receptors (Figure 5-3)

The hematopoietic cytokines include the growth and differentiation factors: G-CSF, GM-CSF, several interleukins (eg, IL-3 and IL-5), EPO and TPO. Their receptors are members of the cytokine-receptor superfamily. These receptors lack intrinsic kinase activity; on ligand binding they dimerize and transduce signals to various cytoplasmic kinases including the JAK kinases that, in turn, phosphorylate the receptor and increase its avidity for ligand and for STAT (signal transducer and activator of transcription); STAT dimerizes and moves as a transcription factor to the nucleus. The signal also is transmitted via Ras and PI3-kinase to a series of downstream kinases, resulting in nuclear activation (Section 1). EPO, G-CSF and GM-CSF are necessary, not only as stimuli to cell activation and proliferation, but also for cell survival – withdrawal of these cytokines results in apoptosis (Section 4).

The negative regulators of hematopoiesis, including prostaglandins, interferon, and transforming growth factor β (TGFβ), inhibit stem cell proliferation. TNFα can both stimulate and inhibit: its primary effect on granulopoiesis is stimulatory, while it is inhibitory to erythropoiesis.

CLINICAL CORRELATES

Disorders of hematopoiesis with marrow failure may occur at various levels of cell replication and involve one or more or all of the formed elements.

Aplastic Anemia

This is a syndrome marked by failure of hematopoietic progenitor cells and stem cells that results in pancytopenia and an "empty marrow" on aspirate and biopsy. A paucity of CD34+ stem cells can be demonstrated by *in vitro* marrow culture. The marrow stromal cells are intact and produce normal or increased amounts of stimulatory cytokines. Serum levels of EPO, G-CSF, GM-CSF and TPO are normal or increased. The response to therapeutic growth factor replacement is poor, with failure to increase hematopoietic cell production.

Fanconi anemia (FA) is a familial autosomal recessive aplastic anemia associated with multiple developmental anomalies. Increased susceptibility to DNA damage and impaired DNA repair results in loss of the stem cell compartment. FA cells are abnormally sensitive to bifunctional alkylating agents, manifest by DNA cross-linking and chromosomal-breakage. An increase in the number of chromosomal breaks in peripheral white cells following *in vitro* incubation with mitomycin C (a DNA cross-linking agent) is a marker for this disease.

FA is genetically heterogeneous – eight separate genes have been identified, subclassified A to H. FA gene products have been found to assemble in a multiprotein complex that localizes to the cell nucleus, suggesting that it may have a role in maintaining genomic integrity. Fanconi anemia type A accounts for 65% of clinical cases. The FA-C gene has been mapped to chromosome 9. The binding of the normal FA-C protein to CDK1 appears to be required for normal G_2/M progression – cells lacking this protein have a prolonged cell cycle with arrest at the G_2/M interface (Section 2). The absence of normal FA-C also is associated with increased apoptosis of stem and progenitor cells – related to the increased display of Fas on these cells (Section 4). Approximately 15% of these patients develop leukemia, myelodysplasia, or various solid tumors. The response to growth factors is poor. Early transplant from sibling matched donors offers the best therapeutic option.

Acquired aplastic anemia results from the destruction or impaired replication of stem cells, with concomitant or preceding damage to CFU-GEMM, CFU-GM, BFU-E and CFU-E. The result is pancytopenia. Direct marrow injury may result from radiation or cytotoxic drugs such as alkylating agents, antimetabolites, and other cancer chemotherapeutic agents. Additional agents capable of producing marrow aplasia or hypoplasia include gold and other heavy metals, sulfonamides, chloramphenicol, and phenylbutazone. Also, industrial compounds such as benzene, and insecticides (chlordane, lindane and DDT) have been implicated. Pancytopenia progressing to bone marrow aplasia may follow viral infections such as infectious mononucleosis or hepatitis.

Most frequently, acquired aplastic anemia is immune-mediated. The immune mechanism may encompass the aplasia associated with some of the agents cited above; drugs and viruses may function as the triggering antigen. Support for this etiology is provided by bone marrow recovery in response to immunosuppression with antithymocytic globulin or cyclosporin. Immune destruction of hematopoietic cells may stem from an antigenic stimulus to T-cells with overproduction of TNF and INFγ. There are two possible mechanisms: direct suppression of hematopoietic cell reproduction by these cytokines, or increased production of Fas ligand and TNF by cytotoxic T-cells culminating in stem cell apoptosis. Although the aplasia may respond to immunosuppressive therapy, in 10-15% of patients there is a second delayed (10-15 years) manifestation of stem cell damage: paroxysmal nocturnal hemoglobinuria, myelodysplasia, or acute myeloblastic leukemia.

Myeloproliferative Disorders

These closely linked and clinically related diseases include polycythemia vera, chronic myelocytic leukemia (CML), thrombocythemia, and myelofibrosis. A stem cell or CFU disorder results in proliferation of bone marrow precursors directed primarily toward a single cell line: erythropoiesis (polycythemia), myelopoiesis (CML), thrombopoiesis, or marrow fibrosis. There is often overlap in these proliferative cell lines, eg, polycythemia vera frequently is associated with high neutrophil and platelet counts and may terminate in myelofibrosis.

Myelodysplastic Syndrome (MDS)

This is a heterogeneous group of clonal hematological disorders that frequently evolve into a leukemia-like or frankly leukemic picture. It is characterized by ineffective hematopoiesis rather than a lack of hematopoietic activity. Impaired cellular maturity is the basic abnormalty. The bone marrow is often cellular and the cell lines dysplastic. The nature and site of the cell injury is ill-defined; some cases follow the use of alkylating agents or other chemotherapeutic drugs for treatment of pre-existing malignant disease. Clinically, MDS is divided into: (1) refractory anemia, (2) refractory anemia with ringed sideroblasts, (3) refractory anemia with excess blasts, (4) chronic myelomonocytic leukemia, (5) transformation to acute leukemia.

Stem Cell Transplantation

Stem cell transplant may be used to repopulate the bone marrow in aplastic anemia or after clearing the marrow of malignant cells by chemotherapy and radiation. This procedure depends upon the ability of stem cells, infused into the peripheral venous system, to home (locate to their proliferative niche), repopulate the marrow and produce peripheral blood cells. The source of stem cells may be an identical twin (syngeneic), the patient's own stem cells (autologous), or a related or unrelated donor (allogeneic). Stem cells may be obtained from bone marrow, peripheral blood or umbilical cord blood. A conditioning regimen, chemotherapy or radiotherapy, is used to eradicate the primary disease (eg, leukemia, lymphoma), to suppress the immune response against the foreign (allogeneic) cells, and to create a marrow environment more spacious and hospitable to these cells. This regimen also may alter endothelial permeabity and allow easier access to marrow spaces and niches for seeding and growth. Post-transplant treatment with G-CSF and GM-CSF accelerates granulocyte recovery.

In normal subjects, administration of G-CSF increases the number of circulating neutrophils and enhances their respiratory burst metabolism and superoxide release. It also produces an increase in circulating CD34+ cells as well as colony forming units (CFU-GM) and erythroid burst forming units (BFU-E). Mobilization of progenitor cells prior to leukopheresis increases the yield in the peripheral blood of donors for bone marrow repopulation.

───── •••●◉●••• ─────

SUGGESTED READING

D'Andrea AD, Grompe M. Molecular biology of Fanconi anemia: implications for diagnosis and treatment Blood 90:1725-1736, 1997.

de Koning JP, Touw IP. Advances in understanding the biology and function of the G-CSF receptor. Curr Opin Hematol 3:180-184, 1996.

Duarte RF, Frank DA. SCF and G-CSF lead to the synergistic induction of proliferation and gene expression through complementary signaling pathways. Blood 96:3422-3430, 2000.

Garcia-Higuera I, Kuang Y, D'Andrea AD. The molecular and cellular biology of Fanconi anemia. Curr Opin Hematol 6:83-88, 1999.

Heaney ML, Golde DW. Myelodysplasia. N Engl J Med 340:1649-1660, 1999.

Kaushansky K. Thrombopoietin and the hematopoietic stem cell. Blood 92:1-3, 1998.

Metcalf D. Haemopoietic growth factors 1. Lancet 1:825-827, 1989.

Metcalf D. Haemopoietic growth factors 2: clinical applications. Lancet 1:885-886, 1989.

Metcalf D. The colony stimulating factors: discovery, developments and clinical applications. Cancer 65:2185-2195,1990.

Morrison SJ, Uchida N, Weissman IL. The biology of hematopoietic stem cells. Annu Rev Cell Dev Biol 11:35-71, 1995.

Ogawa M. Differentiation and proliferation of hematopoietic stem cells. Blood 81:2844-2853, 1993.

Sieff CA, Nisbet-Brown E, Nathan DG. Congenital bone marrow failure syndromes. Br J Haematol 111:30-42, 2000.

Stead RB, Harker LA. Preclinical studies and potential clinical applications of c-mpl ligand. Curr. Opin. Hematol. 3:197-202, 1996.

Wendling F, Vainchenker W. Thrombopoietin and its receptor, the proto-oncogene c-mpl. Curr Opin Hematol 2:331-338, 1995.

Whetton AD, Graham GJ. Homing and mobilization in the stem cell niche. Trends in Cell Biol 9:233-238, 1999.

Witte ON. Steel locus defines new multipotent growth factor. Cell 63:5-6, 1990.

Young NS, Maciejewski J. The pathophysiology of acquired aplastic anemia. N Engl J Med 336:1365-1372, 1997.

Youssouifian H, Longmore G, Neumann D, Yoshimure, A and Lodish HF. Structure, function, and activation of the erythropoietin receptor. Blood 81:2223-2236, 1993.

GRANULOPOIESIS

Bonnie Cham
Lyonel Israels

"Eat and drink for tomorrow we shall die."
Isaiah 22:13

Under physiological conditions, a stable equilibrium exists between the number of neutrophils produced in the marrow and the number present in the circulation and in the tissues. Normal granulopoiesis maintains peripheral neutrophil counts in the circulation at 1.8 to 9.0 x 10^9/L; in the marrow, production proceeds at a baseline rate of 1.6 x 10^9 cells/kg/day. Proliferation of precursors and release of mature cells into the circulation can be increased significantly under conditions of physiological or pathological stress.

Neutrophil precursors in the bone marrow can be divided into two pools: mitotic and post-mitotic. The cells in the mitotic pool are the myeloblast, promyelocyte and myelocyte; the metamyelocyte, young and mature neutrophils are non-proliferating. Under basal physiologcal conditions, transit time through the mitotic pool approximates 6 days. The post-mitotic cells are retained in the bone marrow another 6 to 7 days before the mature neutrophils enter the peripheral circulation. The post-mitotic pool in the bone marrow exceeds the number of circulating neutrophils six to seven fold. Circulating neutrophils spend six to twelve hours in the peripheral blood – approximately 50% in the axial stream and 50% in the marginated pool. They then migrate into extravascular sites where they survive another 1 to 2 days before undergoing apoptosis. With an increase in Granulocyte Colony-Stimulating Factor (G-CSF), generated by an infectious or inflammatory process or subsequent to exogenous administration, there is a decrease in the transit time through the mitotic pool as large numbers of band and segmented neutrophils are released into the circulation (Figure 6-1).

The earliest identifiable granulocyte precursor is the myeloblast – a round or oval cell of 10-18 μm with a large nucleus and little cytoplasm; the nucleus contains 2-4 nucleoli; cytoplasmic granules are absent. The promyelocyte is larger (> 20 μm) with a coarser nuclear chromatin pattern, and nucleoli are present; the cytoplasm is relatively more abundant and contains azurophil granules. The myelocyte is smaller (12-18 μm) with a more dense eccentric nucleus; nucleoli still may be seen but they are not prominent; there are secondary granules in the cytoplasm. In the metamyelocyte, there is increased chromatin condensation, nucleoli are absent, and the nucleus is indented; primary, secondary and tertiary granules and secretory vesicles are now present. Further indentation of the nucleus produces the young (band) form, then the mature neutrophil with a segmented nucleus containing highly condensed chromatin; these cells have a full complement of granules and secretory vesicles.

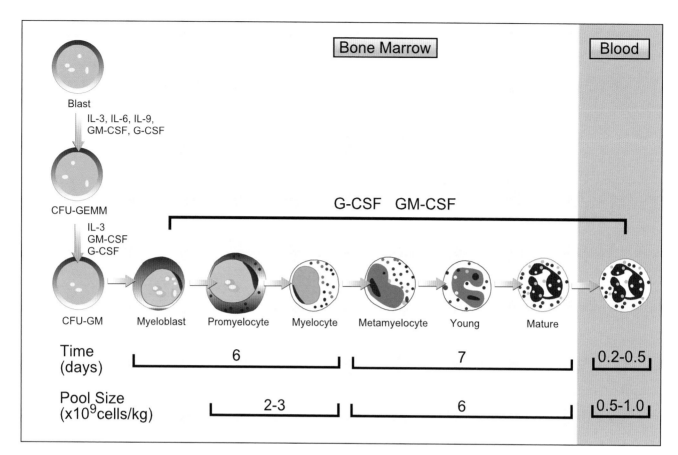

Figure 6-1   Granulopoiesis

Neutrophil Granules and Secretory Vesicles (Figure 6-2)

Neutrophils contain four types of cytoplasmic inclusions: primary (azurophil), secondary (specific), and tertiary (gelatinase) granules, and secretory vesicles. Formation of granules during neutrophil maturation begins at the transition from myeloblast to promyelocyte and continues during the further developmental stages. Proteolytic and bactericidal proteins are contained in the storage organelles (granules and secretory vesicles), and a variety of signaling proteins are present in their membranes. In response to the appropriate stimulus, the membrane of the organelle fuses with the plasma membrane of the cell, followed by exocytosis of the contents to the outside of the cell or into a phagocytic vacuole. In addition, the membrane receptor/proteins (eg, integrins) of the organelles become incorporated into the plasma membrane of the cell, where they enhance the interaction of the neutrophil with its environment.

Based on their content of myeloperoxidase (MPO), the granules originally were classified as either peroxidase-negative or peroxidase-positive; now they are subdivided according to the content of major marker proteins. The divisions are arbitrary as the granules form a continuum – many of the same proteins are present in both the matrix and the membranes of these organelles. The earliest to appear are the azurophil (primary) granules in the promyelocyte;

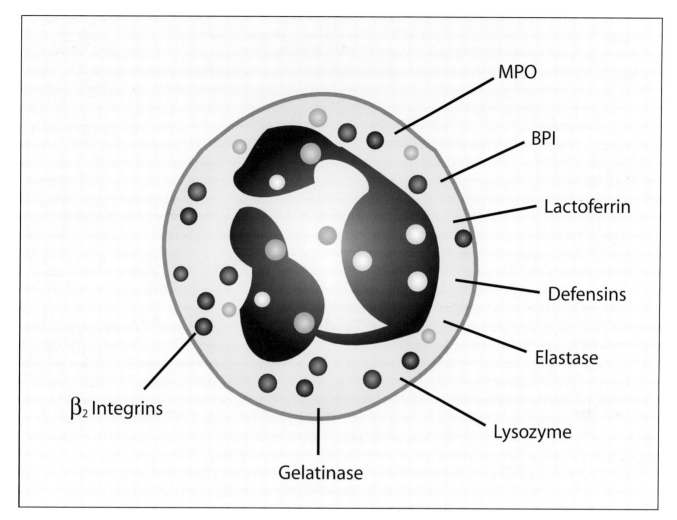

Figure 6-2 Neutrophil Granules and Secretory Vesicles

they contain MPO and therefore are peroxidase positive – MPO is exclusive to these granules. Specific secondary granules are identified by their content of lactoferrin; the tertiary granules containing gelatinase appear as the cell matures.

The antimicrobial proteins are confined largely to primary and secondary granules. In addition to MPO, primary granules contain bactericidal/ permeability-increasing proteins (BPI), the defensins, and a family of serine proteases that includes elastase. BPI functions by permeabilizing bacterial membranes, neutralizing endotoxin, and opsonizing bacteria for phagocytosis. The defensins, small (4 kD) cationic proteins, form pores that permeabilize cellular membranes – they are capable of cytotoxic activity against a broad spectrum of organisms: bacteria, fungi, parasites and viruses. The antimicrobial effect of lactoferrin in secondary granules is due to its high affinity for iron, depriving bacteria of this essential element. Lysozyme, capable of lyzing the bacterial cell wall, is present in both primary and secondary granules.

Secretory vesicles are distinct organelles, originating from a different cellular site than the granules. A significant number of receptors are present in the vesicle membrane. When the neutrophil is exposed to inflammatory stimuli and begins to roll along the endothelial surface, there is rapid mobilization of the secretory vesicles. The vesicles fuse with the surface membrane of the cell; incorporation of its β_2 integrins (CD11b/CD18) into the plasma membrane enhances neutrophil adhesion to the endothelium.

Gelatinase released from tertiary granules is essential for extravascular migration – its substrates are collagen IV of the basement membrane and collagen V of the interstitial tissues. The subsequent exocytosis of the granular contents (myeloperoxidase, lysozyme, BPI, defensins) into the phagosome and the surrounding tissues are important for bacterial kill and the inflammatory response.

Regulation of Granulopoiesis

Granulopoiesis maintains the resting basal level of neutrophils and has the capacity to respond rapidly in the event of infection or inflammation. A series of cytokines regulate granulopoiesis under physiological conditions. Inflammation-associated chemokines and cytokines stimulate increased granulopoiesis.

G-CSF (Granulocyte Colony-Stimulating Factor)

The G-CSF cytokine is produced by a variety of cells, including neutrophils, endothelial cells, fibroblasts and bone marrow stromal cells. Its production follows stimulation by tumor necrosis factor, IL-1, GM-CSF, and by endotoxin. Under basal conditions, circulating levels of G-CSF range from 20 to 50 pg/ml; during bacteremic events, levels may exceed 2000 pg/ml. G-CSF receptors are present on promyelocytes, myelocytes, metamyelocytes and mature neutrophils (Figure 5-2).

G-CSF acts on both precursor cells and mature terminally-differentiated neutrophils. It stimulates the proliferation of committed granulocyte progenitors (promyelocytes and myelocytes), decreases apoptosis, and reduces the maturation time from precursor to neutrophil. In addition, it modulates the function of mature neutrophils: migration and phagocytosis are enhanced, and the cell is primed for the respiratory burst. Therapeutic or prophylactic administration of G-CSF increases the number of circulating mature neutrophils by augmenting the mitotic pool, reducing the maturation time, and releasing the bone marrow storage pool.

The G-CSF receptor belongs to the same cytokine receptor superfamily as the eryrthropoietin receptor. It is a single chain receptor without intrinsic tyrosine kinase activity. G-CSF binding to the receptor induces a series of intracellular events beginning with the phosphorylation of the non-receptor adjacent tyrosine kinases JAK-2 and JAK-1. These, in turn, phosphorylate the cytoplasmic region of the receptor and induce its dimerization – the result is an increased avidity of the receptor for its G-CSF ligand and activation of intracellular signaling through the JAK/STAT, Ras/MAPK and phosphoinositide pathways (Section 5).

GM-CSF (Granulocyte-Macrophage Colony-Stimulating Factor)

GM-CSF augments the proliferation of neutrophil, basophil, eosinophil and macrophage progenitor cells and stimulates the functional activity of these terminally differentiated cells. GM-CSF receptors are present on immature granulocyte precursors, mature neutrophils, eosinophils, and basophils. *In vitro*, GM-CSF is produced by a variety of cells: lymphoid cells, endothelial cells, and cells of the extracellular matrix. Unlike G-CSF, GM-CSF is not detectable in serum under physiological conditions, suggesting that it may function as a paracrine stimulus.

GM-CSF stimulates proliferation of the Colony Forming Unit-Granulocyte/Macrophage (CFU-GM). It has a more profound influence (than G-CSF) on effector function of the terminally differentiated neutrophils, eosinophils, and basophils: it directly enhances neutrophil expression of adhesion molecules, locomotion, responsiveness to chemotactic factors, biosynthetic function, and phagocytic activities – all critical to the inflammatory response.

The receptor for GM-CSF belongs to a family of cytokine receptors, shared with IL-3 and IL-5; these receptors have a common β chain but unique α chains – this may account for the overlap in signaling by these three ligands. Dimerization of the receptor precedes signaling which is transmitted through the β chain. In parallel with the G-CSF receptor, this receptor also lacks intrinsic tyrosine kinase activity; phosphorylation of the cytoplasmic tail of the receptor depends on the JAK kinases and, similarly, signaling is transmitted through STATs, Ras-MAPK and the PI3-K pathways (Section 5).

CLINICAL CORRELATES

NEUTROPHILIA

Neutrophilia refers to an excess of mature neutrophils in the peripheral circulation. It can result from three different mechanisms, functioning alone or in combination: (1) increased mobilization of neutrophils from the bone marrow or the marginated pool; (2) expansion of the progenitor pool or shortening of the mitotic cycle; (3) failure to exit the circulation.

Physiological Neutrophilia. In response to the stimulus of vigorous exercise or epinephrine, mobilization of the marginated pool occurs within minutes. Leukocytosis is present in normal pregnancy, commonly with 1 to 2% myelocytes and metamyelocytes in the peripheral blood.

Acute Responsive Neutrophilia. Acute infectious or inflammatory disease produces a rapid and sustained neutrophilia. This response typically is associated with local or systemic bacterial invasion, tissue necrosis (eg, myocardial infarction), gout, acute hemorrhage, or hemolysis.

Chronic neutrophilia may be associated with prolonged administration of corticosteroids, persistent inflammatory reactions, or low-grade infections. Leukemoid reactions, with early granulocyte precursors in the circulation, is common in myeloproliferative disease, sepsis, metastatic malignancy, and may follow the administration of G-CSF. Post-splenectomy transient neutrophilia may be due to delayed removal of neutrophils from the peripheral circulation.

Neutrophilia Associated with Disorders in Neutrophil Migration. The leukocyte adhesion deficiency syndrome (LAD-I) is due to genetic mutations of the integrin β_2 subunit CD18, resulting in decreased endothelial adhesion and migration; infected tissues generally are devoid of extravascular neutrophils. LAD-II is due to a genetic defect in the selectin ligands required for leukocyte margination and vascular egress (Section 3).

NEUTROPENIA

Neutropenia may result from: (1) decreased production, (2) increased utilization, (3) peripheral destruction, or (4) increased vascular margination.

Pseudo-Neutropenia is manifest by low normal counts in patients with no history of infectious episodes. Most are due to increased neutrophil margination along the vessel wall; these cells are excluded in routine blood counts that sample only the axial stream. There is rapid mobilization of the marginated neutrophils in response to acute infections, moderate exercise, or epinephrine. Neutrophil entry into the circulation and exit from the vascular pool are normal.

Infection-Induced Neutropenia is common in acute viral illness during the peak viremic phase, and is usually transient. Protracted neutropenia may accompany infectious mononucleosis, hepatitis B and HIV-1. Neutropenia associated with bacterial septicemia and endotoxemia may be due to the production of the complement component C5a (with resultant upregulation of the neutrophil/endothelial adhesion molecules and increased tissue migration), direct marrow toxicity, or shortened life span.

Drug-Induced Neutropenia. Exposure to toxic drugs and chemicals is a common cause of neutropenia. Anecdotal reports have implicated over 100 drugs. The mechanism may be immune-mediated drug toxicity or direct destruction of granulocyte precursors. Chemotherapy for malignant disease is associated with various grades of neutropenia; it is dose dependent, and related to precursor cell kill at the levels of the various CFUs – recovery usually is complete, indicating no permanent impairment of the stem cell pool. Treatment with GM-CSF or G-CSF accelerates recovery.

Immune Neutropenia due to antibody directed against neutrophils or their immediate precursors may be associated with: (1) other immune cytopenias (hemolytic anemia and immune thrombocytopenia), (2) autoimmune diseases such as systemic lupus, rheumatoid arthritis, or scleroderma. In drug-induced neutropenia, antibodies produced in response to the drug or its metabolite form antigen-antibody complexes that fix to neutrophils or their precursors, resulting in rapid removal of the cells from both blood and bone marrow.

Chronic Benign Neutropenia may occur in children or in adults. Infections are infrequent although the clinical spectrum is broad. The bone marrow shows maturation arrest at the myelocyte stage despite an otherwise normal appearing or hypercellular marrow. Although G-CSF levels are normal, the peripheral counts do increase in response to administration of this cytokine.

Congenital Neutropenia

Many of the chronic benign neutropenias present in childhood – the majority resolve spontaneously within the first four years of life. Most patients have few clinical problems and require no treatment; others have recurring bacterial infections that respond clinically to G-CSF. Because the number of CFU-GM in the marrow (demonstrated by in vitro culture) is normal, it has been suggested that the disorder may be due to an inhibitor of CFU-GM maturation or an absence of local cytokine production.

Cyclic Neutropenia is an autosomal dominant disorder manifest by regularly recurring episodes of marked neutropenia at approximately 21 day intervals; the nadir lasts three to seven days. The marrow shows maturation arrest at the level of the promyelocyte. Sporadic cases have been described. Patients are subject to recurrent severe infections. DNA analysis has located a defect in the neutrophil elastase (ELA2) gene on chromosome 19; the mutations are clustered around the active site of the enzyme. Elastase is a serine protease synthesized by promyelocytes and present in cytoplasmic granules of mature neutrophils. The neutropenia responds to the administration of G-CSF. (A similar autosomal recessive cyclic neutropenia occurs in gray collie dogs – the genetic defect has not been determined.)

Severe Congenital Neutropenia, previously referred to as Kostmann syndrome, is present at birth. Absolute neutrophil counts may be less than 200/μL. Neutrophil production is arrested at the level of the promyelocyte; in the marrow, there is a relative deficiency of more mature cells. The mode of inheritance is variable, although many cases are autosomal dominant. In Kostmann's original families, the inheritance was autosomal recessive. Sporadic cases have been described. Defects in the elastase gene (ELA2) have been identified in most of the patients but, in contrast to cyclic neutropenia, the mutations do not map to the active site of the enzyme. Increased apoptosis of the neutrophil progenitors may account for the neutropenia. Neutrophil counts increase in response to G-CSF administration. Many of these children go on to develop acute myeloblastic leukemia or myelodysplasia.

The **Shwachman-Diamond Syndrome** is a rare autosomal recessive disorder with varying cytopenias and a marked tendency for malignant myeloid transformation (in the order of 20-35%). It is associated with exocrine pancreatic dysfunction and with growth and developmental abnormalities. The elastase gene is normal. The recurrent infections in these patients are due to bone marrow myeloid hypoplasia. Administration of G-CSF increases granulopoiesis.

The Role of the Cytokines in Neutropenia

When adequate numbers of stem cells and myeloid precursors persist, as in chemotherapy-induced neutropenia, recovery is accelerated by G-CSF. G-CSF is also of therapeutic use in the congenital neutropenias: severe congenital neutropenias, the chronic more benign granulocytopenia of childhood associated with episodes of infection, and cyclic neutropenia.

In normal subjects, G-CSF increases the number of circulating neutrophils and enhances the respiratory burst and superoxide release. There is also an increase in circulating CD34+ cells, colony forming units (CFUs), and erythroid burst forming units (BFU-E). This mobilization of progenitor cells to enhance the yield of donor peripheral blood stem cells may be of value prior to leukopheresis for bone marrow repopulation.

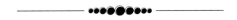

SUGGESTED READING

Borregaard N, Cowland JB. Granules of the human neutrophilic polymorphonuclear leukocyte. Blood 89:3503-3521, 1997.

Dale DC, Person RE, Bolyard AA, Aprikyan AG, et al. Mutations in the gene encoding neutrophil elastase in congenital and cyclic neutropenia. Blood 96:2317-2322, 2000.

Dror Y, Freedman MH. Shwachman-Diamond Syndrome: An inherited preleukemic bone marrow failure disorder with aberrant hematopoietic progenitors and faulty marrow microenvironment. Blood 94:3048-3054, 1999.

Evans T. Developmental biology of hematopoiesis. Hemato/Onco Clin of North Am 11:1116-1147, 1997.

Freedman MH, Bonilla MA, Fier C, et al. Myelodysplasia syndrome and acute myeloid leukemia in patients with congenital neutropenia receiving G-CSF therapy. Blood 96:429-436, 2000.

Gabrilove J. Granulopoiesis. In Scientific Basis of Transfusion Medicine. Anderson KC, Ness PM (eds): W.B. Saunders Company, 13-29, 2000.

Levy O. Antimicrobial proteins and peptides of blood: templates for novel antimicrobial agents. Blood 96:2664-2672, 2000.

Tidow N, Pilz C, Teichmann B, et al. Clinical relevance of point mutations in the cytoplasmic domain of the granulocyte colony-stimulating factor receptor gene in patients with severe congenital neutropenia. Blood 89:2369-2375, 1997.

Welte K, Boxer LA. Severe chronic neutropenia: pathophysiology and therapy. Semin Hematol 34:267-278, 1997.

NEUTROPHIL FUNCTION

"There is at bottom only one scientific treatment for all diseases,
and that is to stimulate the phagocytes."
The Doctor's Dilemma – George Bernard Shaw – 1906

Neutrophils continuously patrol the vasculature, scanning for signals of bacterial infection or inflammation. When such signals are received, neutrophils leave the circulation, migrate to the focus of infection, phagocytose and, through release of packaged microbicidal systems, kill the invading organisms. In the absence of specific signals, neutrophils move into the tissues, are disarmed quietly and disappear by apoptosis.

Neutrophils arise from bone marrow mitotic stem cells, evolve through the identifiable sequence of dividing cells (myeloblasts, promyelocytes and myelocytes) and through the post-mitotic maturation pool of metamyelocytes and band forms; the total process takes approximately two weeks. After entering the peripheral blood, the intravascular life-span of the neutrophil is short (5-12 hours) as compared with platelets (8-12 days) and red cells (100-120 days). Maintenance of this peripheral pool in a 70 kg adult requires the entrance (and exit) of about 100 billion neutrophils per day. The circulating neutrophils are divided almost equally between two intravascular pools – half riding the central axial stream and the remainder marginated along the endothelial walls or sequestered in lung and spleen; there is a continuous interchange of cells between these two pools. Leukocyte counts obtained from venous blood measure only cells in the axial flow. Neutrophils may be lost from mucosal surfaces, or disappear into the extravascular tissue space in areas of infection or inflammation, or migrate into normal extravascular sites where they undergo apoptosis. Apoptosis depends on a cellular clock set for timed self-destruction – the cell, though packed with potentially reactive inflammation-inducing elements, is defused, shrinks, and is taken up by macrophages (Section 4).

Rolling/Selectins (Figure 7-1)

As they approach the post-capillary venules in areas of subendothelial inflammation, patrolling neutrophils slow and begin to roll along the vessel wall. The initial contact is random but, where the endothelium has undergone some inflammatory perturbation, neutrophil contact evolves into rolling along the endothelial wall. This rolling motion, which keeps the cells in juxtaposition to the surface, is due to the shear forces of vascular flow and to the adhesive action between endothelium and neutrophils mediated by a series of carbohydrate-binding membrane proteins. These glycoproteins, the **L-selectins** of the neutrophils, and the **P- and E-selectins** of the endothelial cells, share a similar structure with a characteristic free N-terminal lectin domain. As the neutrophils travel along the vessel wall, the earliest event is the alternating

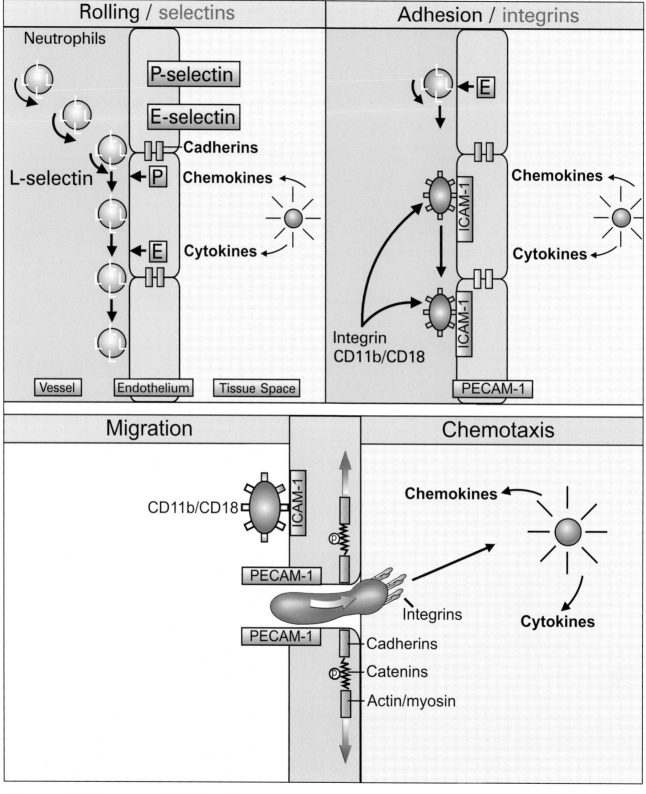

Figure 7-1 Neutrophil Migration

interaction and release between the L-selectins and their corresponding counter-structural carbohydrate ligands. Neutrophils constitutively express both L-selectin and ligands for P- and E-selectins; the high-affinity P-selectin ligand (PSGL-1) has been well characterized. L-selectin is present on the microvilli of neutrophils, lymphocytes and monocytes. P-selectin is stored in the endothelial cell Weibel-Palade bodies and in platelet alpha-granules; E-selectin is found only in endothelial cells, its production dependent on inflammatory stimuli. When endothelial cells are stimulated by cytokines or chemokines from an adjacent subendothelial inflammatory site, preformed P-selectin and induced newly-synthesized E-selectin move to the vascular surface of the cell, augmenting leukocyte rolling. At sites of vascular injury, platelet aggregation and release of platelet P-selectin augments neutrophil accumulation. In mice genetically engineered to produce neither P- nor E-selectin, there is an absence of both leukocyte rolling and extravasation into areas of infection; this results in increased numbers of circulating neutrophils unable to migrate, while the animals die of bacterial infection.

Neutrophil Activation

As the neutrophil enters the vessels within the inflammatory radius, it is exposed to a variety of stimuli: 1) **Chemoattractants** – C5a (an activated component of complement) and the bacterial N-formyl oligopeptides; 2) **Cytokines**–IL-1, GM-CSF; 3) **Chemokines** – 8 to 10 kD protein molecules with both chemoattractant and cytokine properties (eg, IL-8). The α chemokines are chemotactic for neutrophils – they are characterized by a C-X-C (cysteine-other amino acid-cysteine) sequence adjacent to the N-terminus. (The β chemokines, with a C-C sequence near the N-terminus, are selective for lymphocytes and macrophages). Chemokines are produced by a variety of cells including endothelial cells. They have a strong affinity for proteoglycans (heparans) present on the endothelial surface. Chemokines bind and activate G protein-coupled receptors on the neutrophil surface to stimulate protein kinase and phosphoinositide signaling pathways (Section 1); this upregulates neutrophil expression of the CD11b/CD18 integrin leading to endothelial adhesion and subsequent diapedesis. Chemokines also prime the neutrophil for migration through the tissues and the microbicidal response.

Adhesion/Integrins (Figure 7-1)

In concert with cell activation, L-selectin is shed from the leukocyte membrane as the increased expression of the neutrophil cell surface integrin **CD11b/CD18** mediates more stable adhesion. Stimulated endothelial cells release platelet activating factor (PAF) that further induces the display of CD11b/CD18 on the tethered neutrophil. Bacterial endotoxin (lipopolysaccharide) and cytokines (IL-1, interferon, and tumor necrosis factor – TNF α), produced by macrophages and neutrophils at the inflammatory site, stimulate expression of the **intercellular adhesion molecule (ICAM-1)** by the adjacent endothelial cells. ICAM-1 is a strong ligand for the neutrophil integrin CD11b/CD18, inducing tight binding to the endothelial surface.

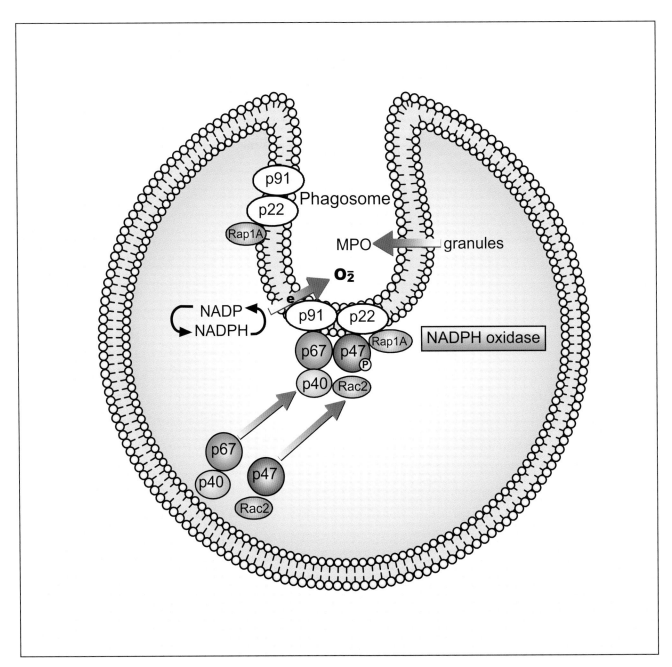

Figure 7-2   Neutrophil Microbicidal Respiratory Burst

Diapedesis/Migration (Figure 7-1)

The chemoattractants, chemokines and cytokines also induce increased endothelial cell surface-expression of **PECAM-1** (platelet-endothelial cell adhesion molecule) located primarily at the inter-endothelial cell junctions. PECAM-1, a 130 kD member of the immunoglobulin superfamily, is expressed on platelets, neutrophils, monocytes and endothelial cells. The neutrophils, rendered tightly adherent through their CD11b/CD18 integrin, crawl along the endothelial surface; on reaching the intercellular junction, they interact with PECAM-1 to move through the junction into the subendothelial space. Neutrophil and monocyte migration from the circulation through the inter-endothelial cell junctions is mediated by PECAM-1 recognition of its leukocyte homologue, PECAM-1.

The inter-endothelial adherens junction must open to allow the passage of activated neutrophils into the subendothelial space. The adherens junction consists of clusters of cadherin molecules. Cadherin is a single-pass membrane protein; its extracellular region binds to a twin protein on the adjacent cell (homophilic binding); the intracellular tail associates with cytoplasmic proteins (catenins) which, in turn, link it to the actin/myosin cytoskelton. Various agonists, including activated neutrophils, induce phosphorylation of the catenin proteins resulting in disruption of the inter-cadherin bonds – the endothelial cells then separate to allow passage of the leukocyte out of the vascular channel.

Having breached the endothelial barrier, the cell must move through the basement membrane and subendothelial space. This is facilitated by a series of proteases including collagenase, gelatinase, elastase, and plasminogen activators (Section 6). Guided by its activated integrins, the neutrophil crawls along fibrillar structures towards the focus of opsonized microbes—the nucleus to the rear of the cell and the extended cytoplasm in front. This crawling motion represents a complex assembly of cytoplasmic filamentous actin interacting with myosin filaments in an alternating sol-gel medium. On reaching the inflammatory focus, the pseudopodia engulf the bacteria that have been primed by coating with opsonins. The opsonins ('to prepare for dining' - Greek) are immunoglobulins and products of complement (C3b). The cell membrane encloses the microorganisms, trapping them inside a phagocytic vacuole. This engulfment is followed by the release of lysozymes and proteases from the cytoplasmic granules into the phagosome and the triggering of the respiratory burst.

Microbicidal Systems (Figure 7-2)

Respiratory Burst Pathway. The metabolism of the unstimulated neutrophil is dependent primarily on anaerobic glycolysis – glycogen stores provide the glycolytic substrate for the anaerobic maintenance of ATP. However, within seconds after ingesting bacteria, oxygen consumption is increased 100-fold; most of the extra oxygen consumed is converted to reactive oxygen species. This "respiratory burst" is mediated through the membrane-bound **NADPH oxidase**. In the resting cell, the components of this oxidase are separated in two subcellular compartments, the membrane and the cytosol; the oxidase is inactive. Assembly of the components occurs when neutrophil activation is triggered – by chemokines, immune complexes, C5a, or by the N-formyl oligopeptides released from microorganisms. The oxidase is a multicomponent complex assembled from five proteins, two on the plasma membrane and three in the cytoplasm, each group associated with a monomeric GTP-binding (G) protein. The two membrane proteins p22^{phox} and gp91^{phox} (glycoprotein 91 <u>p</u>hagocytic <u>ox</u>idase) are the α and β subunits of the flavocytochrome b$_{558}$; the α and β subunits each contain a heme group that can bind NADPH. The Ras-related protein Rap1A is tightly associated on the membrane with cytochrome b$_{558}$. The cytoplasmic components are p47^{phox}, p67^{phox} and p40^{phox} accompanied by the small GTP-binding protein Rac2. On neutrophil activation, phosphorylation of the cytosolic proteins, in particular the highly phosphorylated p47^{phox}, triggers translocation of the cytoplasmic complex to the membrane. The assembly of the cytosolic proteins with the membrane gp91^{phox} and p22^{phox} generates the enzymatic activity of the oxidase. The NADPH oxidase now transfers electrons across the plasma membrane from cytosolic NADPH to oxygen to generate the oxygen radical O$^-_2$. (An oxidase-associated H$^+$ channel leads to the efflux of H$^+$ ions). The superoxide anion (O$^-_2$) is formed both in the phagosome and in the extracellular space. H$_2$O$_2$ is produced from O$^-_2$ in a reaction catalyzed by superoxide dismutase. H$_2$O$_2$ reacts with a halide to generate hypochlorous acid; HOCl kills both ingested bacteria and extracellular organisms adjacent to the cell. The NADPH in this reaction is made available through the hexose-monophosphate shunt of the glycolytic pathway (Section 10).

The generation of the microbicidal oxidants, superoxide anion (O$^-_2$), hydrogen peroxide (H$_2$O$_2$,) and hydrochlorous acid (HOCl), occurs through the following sequential reactions:

Reaction	Enzyme
1) $2O_2 + NADPH \rightarrow 2\,O^-_2 + NADP + H^+$	NADPH oxidase
2) $2H^+ + 2\,O^-_2 \rightarrow H_2O_2 + O_2$	superoxide dismutase
3) $H_2O_2 + Cl^- \rightarrow HOCl + OH^-$	myeloperoxidase

The neutrophils themselves are protected from these oxidative agents by catalase (which destroys H$_2$O$_2$), and by the antioxidant activity of reduced glutathione (GSH).

Myeloperoxidase is a heme-containing enzyme confined to the azurophil granules. Following phagocytosis, the membranes of the granules fuse with the membrane of the phagosome and the granule contents enter the phagosome. MPO catalyzes the reaction of hydrogen peroxide with a halide (Cl$^-$) to produce hypochlorous acid.

The Inflammatory Response

Cells at the inflammatory focus include neutrophils, macrophages and bacteria. The macrophages release a number of chemotactic and regulatory molecules including interleukins, interferons and tumor necrosis factor; bacteria contribute endotoxin and N-formyl oligopeptides. In the stimulated neutrophils and macrophages, arachidonic acid is cleaved from membrane phospholipids through the action of phospholipase A_2. Arachidonic acid (AA) is converted to a series of eicosanoids through two enzyme pathways initiated by cyclooxygenase-2 (Cox-2) and lipoxygenase. Cox-2 converts AA to prostaglandins responsible for the pain, vasodilation, erythema and fever that accompany the inflammatory reaction. Through the lipoxygenase pathway, AA is converted to the leukotrienes, potent chemoattractants.

Cox-2, induced in phagocytes during the inflammatory response, differs structurally from the constitutive enzyme cyclooxygenase-1 (Cox-1) expressed in platelets, endothelium, gastric mucosa, and most other cell systems. The constitutive enzyme Cox-1 responds to physiological stimuli, while Cox-2 is an inducible enzyme that can be upregulated by cytokines involved in inflammation. A number of anti-inflammatory drugs (aspirin) inhibit both Cox-1 and Cox-2. Corticosteroids and specific Cox-2 inhibitors target primarily Cox-2 and therefore do not interfere with platelet function or other physiological processes mediated by Cox-1 (Section 30). Corticosteroids also reduce endothelial expression of E-selectin and ICAM-1 – this may explain, in part, the observation that glucocorticoids induce leukocytosis (reduced vascular adhesion) and increased susceptability to infection (reduced leukocyte recruitment). The non-steroidal anti-inflammatory drugs (NSAIDS), including aspirin, exhibit differential effects on neutrophil function that depends on the structure and dosage of the agent. In addition to inhibition of eicosanoid metabolism, some NSAIDS have other anti-inflammatory effects: inhibition of neutrophil adherence mediated through CD11b/CD18, inhibition of neutrophil activation, and inhibition of O^-_2 generation.

CLINICAL CORRELATES

Defects in Neutrophil Function

Defects in Adhesion - *Leukocyte Adhesion Defect-1* (**LAD**-1) is a rare congenital autosomal recessive abnormality associated with severe and sometimes fatal bacterial infections. The defect is the inability to synthesize the integrin subunit CD18; this is responsible for partial or total deficiency of the CD11/CD18 integrin at the cell surface with failure of integrin-mediated adhesion and chemotaxis. The number of circulating neutrophils is increased as they are unable to migrate outside the vascular compartment. Adherence to opsonized bacteria also is compromised, thus limiting both phagocytosis and stimulation of the respiratory burst. **LAD-2**, a clinically similar but less severe disease, is due to the congenital absence of the ligands for the selectins. Although the selectins are present, the absence of their ligands results in impaired leukocyte recruitment (Section 3).

Defects in the Hexose-Monophosphate Shunt - As in the red cell, the neutrophil generates NADPH by glycolysis. Congenital deficiencies in this pathway (**G6PD deficiency**) result in the inability to generate sufficient NADPH to produce the respiratory burst necessary for O_2^- formation. Neutrophil function, however, is compromised only in the most severe forms of G6PD deficiency as the neutrophils are less vulnerable than are red cells. In the red cell, the supply of G6PD decays over its life span of many weeks leaving the older cells sensitive to oxidative injury. In contrast, the short-lived neutrophils carry their assigned complement of G6PD for only the few hours of their active life-span and, unless the defect is major, the enzyme activity is sufficient to provide the NADPH required for the generation of O_2^-.

Defects in the Generation of NADPH Oxidase (*Chronic Granulomatous Disease*). The term **chronic granulomatous disease (CGD)** embraces a variety of congenital disorders in which there is failure to express the respiratory burst. This disease is characterized by recurrent suppurative infections and chronic abscess formation due to bacterial and fungal organisms of usually low pathogenicity (eg, catalase-positive staphylococcus aureus, serratia, and fungal aspergillus). The failure of functional NADPH oxidase activity and the related deficit in O_2^- production results from genetic defects in this multicomponent system: mutations of gp91^{phox} or p22^{phox} of the membrane cytochrome b_{558} complex, or of cytosolic p47^{phox} or p67^{phox}. The majority of patients (over 60%) have an X-linked form of the disease due to mutations of the gp91^{phox} gene located on this chromosome. This phenotype, accordingly, occurs only in males; defects in the other three proteins occur equally in males and females – inheritance is autosomal recessive. Recently, an analogous clinical syndrome due to a mutation in Rac2 has been described. The failure to produce the respiratory burst, common to all of these molecular defects, can be detected by a simple qualitative *in vitro* assay, the nitroblue tetrazolium (NBT) test. Neutrophil phagocytosis of formazan particles tagged with pale yellow NBT that results in the appearance of reduced (blue-black) NBT particles within the cell is indicative of normal oxidase activity; this reaction is absent in the enzyme-deficient cell.

Myeloperoxidase (MPO) Deficiency – The green MPO lysosomal protein is present in very high concentrations in neutrophil azurophil granules (it is responsible for the green colour of pus). MPO deficiency is the commonest inherited neutrophil defect. Inheritance is autosomal recessive. The MPO gene on chromosome 17 is near the breakpoint in the 15-17 translocation of promyelocytic leukemia. MPO deficiency may be congenital or appear as an acquired defect in promyelocytic (M3) leukemia. Clinical manifestations are relatively minor as reactions catalyzed by NADPH oxidase and superoxide dismutase (with production of O_2^- and H_2O_2) are sufficient to bring about bacterial kill, although some patients with MPO deficiency are more prone to fungal infections. Neutrophils are peroxidase negative.

Neutrophil Granule Dysfunction (*Chediak-Higashi Syndrome - CHS*) is a rare autosomal recessive disorder affecting intracellular granules. The LYST gene encodes a cytosolic protein, the lysosomal-trafficking regulator; mutations in this gene are responsible for defective molecular sorting in the Golgi apparatus or endosomes. Dysmorphic large lysosomal granules compromise cell function in neutrophils, platelets, macrophages, and lymphocytes; the defect in melanocytes results in oculo-cutaneous albinism. The neutrophils are characterized by giant granules with defective lysosomal activity, chemotaxis and phagosome formation. Recurring bacterial infections are the result of deficient neutrophil function associated with defective T cell and NK cell activity. Other manifestations of CHS include progressive peripheral neuropathy, a lymphoma-like syndrome with histiocytic infiltration of liver, spleen and lymph nodes, and platelet dysfunction (Section 30).

Increased Neutrophil - Endothelial Interaction

Avid neutrophil-endothelial interaction is a normal response within an inflammatory locus. However, inappropriate or excessive adhesion, leukocyte pooling, plugging of the vasculature with neutrophils, their activation and degranulation, results in endothelial damage that may initiate or promote the disease process. Systemic vasculitides, such as the vasculitis present in collagen-vascular disease, polyarteritis, and temporal arteritis, are associated with upregulation of E-selectin and ICAM-1. The pooling of neutrophils in areas of ischemia and reperfusion, as in frost-bite, adult respiratory disease syndrome, and graft rejection, are also examples of increased expression of E-selectin and ICAM-1 that results in major tissue damage. Experimentally induced vascular disease in laboratory animals demonstrates that blocking antibodies to P- and E- selectin, ICAM-1, or CD11, can reduce neutrophil accumulation and tissue injury.

———— •••●●●●•• ————

SUGGESTED READING

Albelda SM, Smith CW, Ward PA. Adhesion molecules and inflammatory injury. FASEB J 8:504-512, 1994.

Babior BM. NADPH oxidase: an update. Blood 93:1464-1476, 1999.

Bevilacqua MP, Nelson RM, Mannori G, Cecconi O. Endothelial-leukocyte adhesion molecules in human disease. Annu Rev Med 45:361-378, 1994.

Bokoch GM. Chemoattractant signaling and leukocyte activation. Blood 86:1649-1660, 1995.

Certain S, Barrat F. Pastural E, et al. Protein truncation test of LYST reveals heterogeneous mutations in patients with Chediak-Higashi syndrome. Blood 95:979-983, 2000.

Carlos TM, Harlan JM. Leukocyte-endothelial adhesion molecules. Blood 84:2068-2101, 1994.

Clark RA. Activation of the neutrophil respiratory burst oxidase. J Inf Dis 179(Suppl 2):S309-S317, 1999.

Cronstein BN, Weissmann G. Targets for antinflammatory drugs. Annu Rev Pharmacol Toxicol 35:449-46, 1995.

Dell'Angelica EC, Mullins C, Caplan S, Bonifacino JS. Lysosome-related organelles. FASEB J 14:1265-1278, 2000.

Ganz T, Lehrer RI. Antimicrobial peptides of leukocytes. Curr Opin Hematol 4:53-58, 1997.

Klebanoff SJ. Myeloperoxidase. Proc Assoc Am Phys 111:383-389, 1999.

Luster AD. Chemokines-chemotactic cytokines that mediate inflammation. N Engl J Med 338:436-445, 1998.

Malech HL, Nauseef WM. Primary inherited defects in neutrophil function: Etiology and treatment. Semin Hematol 34:279-290, 1997.

Mollinedo F, Borregaard N, Boxer LA. Novel trends in neutrophil structure, function and development. Immunol Today 20:535-537, 1999.

Murphy PM. Neutrophil receptors for interleukin-8 and related CXC chemokines. Semin Hematol 34:311-318, 1997.

Nauseef WM. The NADPH-dependent oxidase of phagocytes. Proc Assoc Am Physicians III:373-382, 1999.

Olkkonen VM, Ikonen E. Genetic defects of intracellular-membrane transport. N Engl J Med 343:1095-1104, 2000.

Roos D, de Boer M, et al. Mutations in the X-linked and autosomal recessive forms of chronic granulomatous disease. Blood 87:1663-1681, 1996.

Smith WL, DeWitt DL, Garavito M. Cyclooxygenases: structural, cellular, and molecular biology. Annu Rev Biochem 69:145-182, 2000.

Stossel TP. The machinery of blood cell movements. Blood 84:367-379, 1994.

Vane JR, Botting RM. New insights into the mode of action of anti-inflammatory drugs. Inflamm Res 44:1-10, 1995.

EOSINOPHILS, BASOPHILS & MAST CELLS

"Better red than dead"
Slogan of the 50's

Eosinophils, basophils, and mast cells have tightly linked effector roles in the allergic response. They share key membrane receptors, and produce and respond to some of the same cytokines and chemokines. Activation of one often is followed by secondary activation of the other two. Although there are many instances of selective recruitment and localization, in general their responses to antigenic stimuli are sufficiently interwoven that they may be considered a functional unit. All three cells are components of the innate immune system, that is they do not require immunological memory to activate their immune response.

EOSINOPHILS

The eosinophil is a bilobed terminally differentiated cell containing large refractile cytoplasmic granules that stain intensely with eosin. The mature cells largely reside outside the blood vessels in submucosal and subepithelial tissues.

Origin

Eosinophils arise from bone marrow $CD34^+$ stem cells, their early lineage shared with neutrophils and basophils (Figure 5-1). As they mature beyond the CFU-GEMM stage, eosinophils and basophils probably develop through a common progenitor as evidenced by some cells that contain both eosinophilic and basophilic granules. Eosinophil development is governed primarily by IL-5, GM-CSF and IL-3, cytokines that share a common β chain but have unique α chains. **IL-5** is key to eosinophil production and differentiation: it is the major promoter of the terminal stages of maturation; it stimulates release from the bone marrow and migration into tissues, enhances cell function, and prolongs survival.

The Granules

Four distinct types of cytoplasmic inclusions have been identified: specific granules, small granules, primary granules (Charcot-Leyden crystal protein), and lipid bodies (Figure 8-1). The large **specific granules** consist of an electron dense core surrounded by a less dense matrix; these granules contain four dominant cationic proteins: (1) major basic protein, (2) eosinophil cationic protein, (3) eosinophil peroxidase, and (4) eosinophil derived neurotoxin. The **small granules** contain a number of enzymes, including acid phosphatase and arylsulfatase. **Lipid bodies** are sites for storage and metabolism of arachidonic acid; they contain cyclooxygenase and

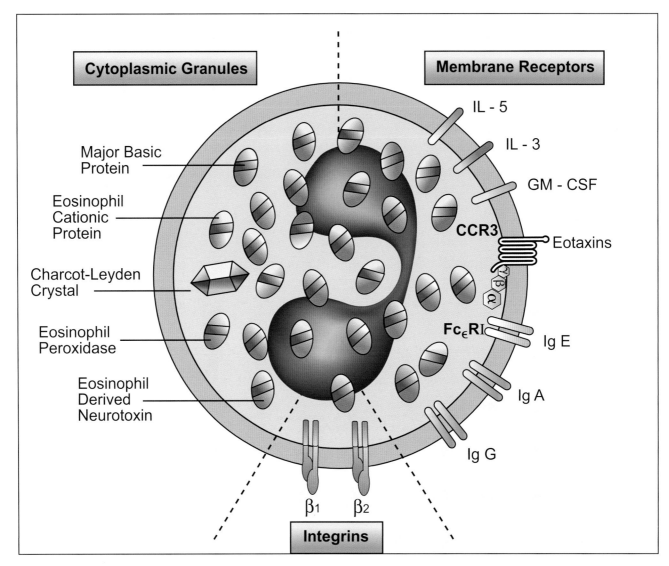

Figure 8-1 The Eosinophil

lipoxygenase, enzymes that catalyze the synthesis of arachidonic acid-derived mediators (eg, prostaglandins and leukotrienes). The protein comprising the **Charcot-Leyden crystals** has lysophospholipase activity.

Major basic protein (MBP) is an arginine-rich polypeptide composed of 117 amino acids, localized in the core of the eosinophilic granule. MBP is translated as a more neutral protein due to the association with a 90 amino acid pro-portion – pro-MBP may protect the cell from the toxic effects of MBP as it is transported from the Golgi apparatus to the storage granule. Pro-MBP is converted into mature MBP within the granules during eosinophil differentiation. Secreted MBP stimulates histamine release from basophils and mast cells. It is highly toxic to neighboring host cells as well as to adjacent helminths, protozoa, or bacteria. MBP damages target cells and parasites by increasing membrane permeability through surface charge interactions—binding to anionic domains results in perturbation of the membrane lipid bilayer.

Eosinophil cationic protein is a ribonuclease located in the granule matrix. It promotes degranulation of mast cells. It is toxic to helminths, protozoa, bacteria and adjacent host cells.

Eosinophil peroxidase, located in the granule matrix, is a two-chain peroxidase with a major resemblance to myeloperoxidase. In the absence of H_2O_2, it functions as a cationic toxin that is destructive to parasites and tissue cells. In the presence of H_2O_2, it functions as a peroxidase, catalyzing peroxidative oxidation of halides to generate toxic hypohalous acids, HOCl and HOBr.

Eosinophil derived neurotoxin is a ribonuclease present in the granule matrix. The designation is based on its intense neurotoxic action in experimental animals. It is only weakly toxic to parasites.

Charcot-Leyden Crystals – The protein comprising these hexagonal crystals is a distinctive lysophospholipase. The enzyme may be harmful to host tissues: when released in lung (as in asthmatics), it degrades lysophosphatidylcholine in pulmonary surfactant.

The Membrane Receptors

Eosinophil migration and activity are determined by interactions that involve membrane receptors. The cytokine receptors for IL-5, IL-3, and GM-CSF have an important role in cell activation; they do not possess intrinsic tyrosine kinase activity but signal through a JAK/STAT pathway with links to the Ras-MAPK system (Section 1), inducing granule release and leukotriene, prostaglandin, and cytokine synthesis. A number of G protein-coupled receptors (GPCRs) have been identified; their ligands include potent effector proteins: platelet activating factor (PAF), leukotrienes, chemokines (eotaxin), and complement components (C3a, C4a, and C5a). There are Fc receptors for the immunoglobulins IgG, IgA, IgE, and non-GPCR receptors for other complement components (C1q, C4b). Membrane expression of the β_2 integrin CDIIb/CD18 and the β_1 integrin **VLA-4 (very late antigen-4)** mediates adhesion to the endothelium. Receptors for glucocorticoids are key to their therapeutic interruption of the allergic response.

Migration

After exiting the marrow, the eosinophil moves through the peripheral blood with an average transit time of 26 hours. Migration into extravascular tissues involves a series of adhesive interactions similar to that of the neutrophil (Section 7). Eosinophil-endothelial cell interactions are stimulated by the release of mediators from inflammatory sites. Interaction of eosinophil L-selectin with the endothelial adhesion molecules and the display of P- and E-selectins on the endothelium initiate rolling along the vessel wall. This is followed by eosinophil surface display of the β_2 integrin CD11b/CD18 and tight adherence to ICAM-1 on the endothelial cell. (The expression of surface CD11b/CD18 is induced by chemokine binding and eosinophil activation). Significantly, and unlike the neutrophil, eosinophils express the $\beta_1$integrin **VLA-4**. VLA-4 mediates adhesion of eosinophils to endothelial **VCAM-1 (vascular cell adhesion molecule-**1), an interaction that results in selective homing of eosinophils to allergic and parasitic subendothelial sites. The expression of endothelial cell VCAM-1 is induced by IL-4 secreted by basophils. Migration of eosinophils into subendothelial tissues is facilitated by endothelial PECAM-1 (the same interaction responsible for neutrophil migration). Chemoattractants include the leukotrienes and the eotaxin chemokines secreted by both basophils and eosinophils in the subendothelial allergenic focus.

The eosinophil exits the circulation primarily into surface-associated connective tissue spaces (eg, gut, bronchi, and skin). Eosinophil binding to secretory IgA aids in concentrating these cells in submucosal spaces in the respiratory and gastrointestinal tract (Section 17). The eosinophil is essentially a tissue resident; the extravascular population is some 100 – 500 fold that of the circulation.

Unlike the neutrophil, eosinophils can survive extravascularly for prolonged periods of time (weeks) when stimulated by IL-5, IL-3 and GM-CSF. The cytokine IL-5 is most prominent in promoting eosinophil function and survival. Thus, eosinophils are in part under the control of the IL-5 producing $CD4^+$ Th2 T cells (Section 19). On withdrawal of these cytokines, eosinophils undergo apoptosis and are removed by macrophages.

Eotaxins

Leukocytes are recruited to inflammatory sites by a number of chemokines; eosinophils are significant targets for the eotaxins. Eotaxins belong to the CC family of chemokines (defined by the two adjacent cysteine residues near the N-terminus of the peptide); they are recognized by a G protein-coupled seven transmembrane receptor (CCR3) on eosinophils, basophils, mast cells, and Th2 T-cells, but are not found on neutrophils. (Neutrophils recognize CXC chemokines – two cysteine residues separated by one other amino acid, eg, IL-8). Eotaxin recruits CCR3-bearing cells to the allergenic or inflammatory site, with a particular specificity for eosinophils. (It also has chemotactic activity for basophils, mast cells and Th2 cells). It stimulates production and release of eosinophils from marrow, increases eosinophil margination and migration by upregulating the integrin CD11b/CD18, and recruits eosinophils to submucosal sites. It also regulates eosinophil motility and chemotaxis, and is an initiator of degranulation and of the respiratory burst. Eotaxin is expressed constitutively by epithelial cells of small bowel, colon, and lung; its production is increased by chronic inflammatory disease at these sites; eotaxin also has been identified in eosinophils. Eotaxin maintains and sustains the eosinophil population by stimulating Th2 T-cells to release IL-3, IL-5 and GM-CSF; these cytokines in turn inhibit eosinophil apoptosis and increase eosinophil production in the bone marrow.

The Inflammatory Response

The eosinophils located in tissue spaces adjacent to surfaces occupy ideal defensive sites for the interception of invading organisms from the gut or lung. They kill parasites by releasing cationic proteins and reactive oxygen metabolites into the extracellular fluid; they are only weakly phagocytic. Peripheral eosinophils represent two functionally and physically distinct phenotypes (identification is based on in vitro density gradient separation). Normodense eosinophils are present in the circulation of healthy subjects. Hypodense cells are found in the circulation and biological fluids (eg, bronchoalveolar lavage fluids) in patients with eosinophil-mediated disease. The hypodense cells are primed for an immediate inflammatory response – probably the result of cytokine and chemokine stimulation. Hypodense eosinophils, compared to the normodense phenotype, are functionally more active: oxygen consumption and leukotriene production are increased, and the generation of superoxide and cytotoxic activity are enhanced.

Eosinophils are involved in the pathogenesis of numerous inflammatory processes, modulating the response through a variety of mechanisms: (1) degranulation releases the cytotoxic cationic proteins, (2) activation of NADPH oxidase (the respiratory burst) generates the highly toxic oxygen metabolite superoxide O^-_2 (Section 7), (3) generation and release of lipid-derived mediators such as leukotriene C_4 (LTC_4), increases vascular permeability and attracts additional eosinophils to the site, (4) production of chemokines, such as eotaxin and PAF, augment eosinophil recruitment, (5) elaboration and release of a wide range of cytokines, eg, interleukins, tissue necrosis factor α (TNFα), and interferon γ (IFNγ), enhance the inflammatory response.

BASOPHILS

Basophils represent approximately 0.5 percent of the total circulating leukocyte population. They are identified by their bilobed nucleus and round or oval cytoplasmic granules that stain intensely blue-black in the routine blood film. The granules closely resemble those of the tissue mast cell.

Origin and Migration

The basophil originates and matures in the bone marrow, progeny of the CD34$^+$ stem cell. During its evolution, it probably shares a common ancestor with the eosinophil; in patients with chronic myelocytic leukemia it is not uncommon to find myelocytes, metamyelocytes and

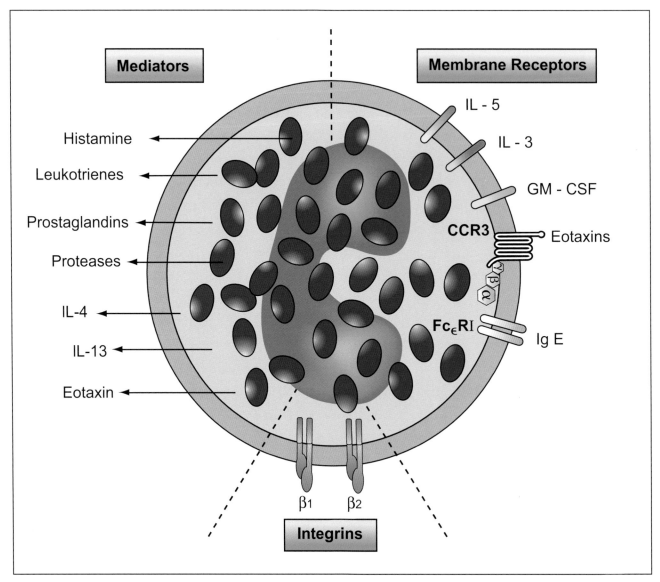

Figure 8-2 The Basophil

mature cells with both eosinophilic and basophilic granules. Growth and differentiation are promoted primarily by **IL-3**; other growth factors for basophils are IL-5 and GM-CSF. Basophils are mature terminally differentiated granulocytes that do not reproduce. Compared to the eosinophil, there are fewer basophils in peripheral tissues and their distribution is more limited. They are recruited selectively to sites of immunologic or inflammatory processes. The eotaxin receptor (CCR3) is expressed on basophils (as well as on eosinophils, Th2 cells, and mast cells); eotaxin recruits basophils to areas of IgE-mediated allergic reactions. Upon challenge by allergens, there is rapid recruitment of basophils to the allergenic site, most frequently lung, nose, gut, or skin. Basophil migration from blood to tissue is dependent upon IL-3 upregulation of the β_2 integrin CD11b/CD18.

Granules and Intracellular Mediators

The basophils contain a large number of biologically active mediators, some present in the resting cell, others elaborated on cell stimulation. The preformed mediators include: histamine, proteoglycans, proteases, elastase, lysophospholipase (Charcot-Leyden crystal protein), and major basic protein – the latter two molecules also are present in eosinophils. On stimulation, there is activation of the cyclooxygenase and lipoxygenase pathways of arachidonic acid metabolism with production of prostaglandins and leukotrienes. Activation also induces the production of the cytokines IL-4 and IL-13 that augment the inflammatory response.

Basophils possess high affinity IgE receptors ($Fc_{\varepsilon}RI$). Multivalent allergens cross-link the IgE molecules bound to $Fc_{\varepsilon}RI$, inducing intracellular signaling events that result in secretion of inflammatory mediators. IL-3 in conjunction with C5a can induce mediator release directly, independent of IgE-receptor cross-linking; this suggests that basophils have a role in nonallergic inflammatory disease. C5a by itself is a potent inducer of histamine release from basophils.

MAST CELLS

As mast cells morphologically resemble basophils and participate in similar allergic and inflammatory reactions, they have been referred to as "tissue basophils". Mast cells, however, are a distinct entity and are not basophil derived. Cytoplasmic granules that stain with basic dyes are a prominent feature of both cells. Mast cell granules are smaller and more numerous.

Origin and Migration

Mast cells originate from pluripotent $CD34^+$ progenitors in the bone marrow. Growth and differentiation of mast cell precursors are controlled primarily by stem cell factor (SCF) produced by marrow stromal cells: the **SCF receptor** (c-kit) is expressed on mast cells at every stage including the mature cell. Early in their development, they migrate to extravascular sites. Migration and tissue localization are influenced by local production of chemokines. Mature mast cells are not identifiable in the blood; early precursors enter the circulation in small numbers. As they move through the peripheral blood, their hypogranular transit morphology frequently misidentifies them as monocytes. Chemokine binding to membrane receptors induce mast cell adhesion to the endothelial surface and migration into peripheral tissues. A variety of adhesive interactions control this process: initiation of rolling depends on cytokine-induced expression of P-selectin on endothelial cells; tight adhesion develops through the interaction of VLA-4 on the mast cell with endothelial surface VCAM-1. In the tissues, differentiation into mature mast cells is regulated by SCF, IL-3, and other cytokines. Mature tissue mast cells retain their SCF receptors and their proliferative potential; their life span is measured in months or even years. With selective migration into subepithelial connective tissue spaces in skin, lung and

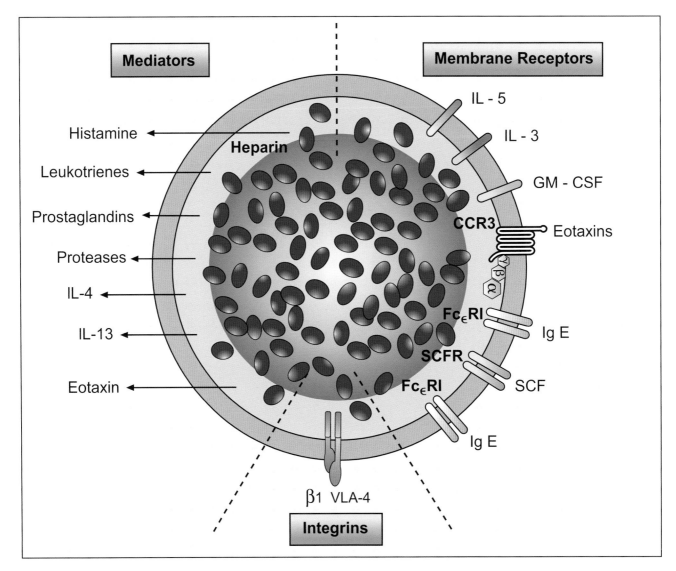

Figure 8-3 The Mast Cell

gastrointestinal tract, mast cells are strategically positioned to monitor the external environment. They have a key role in the early phase of IgE-mediated allergic reactions.

Granules and Mediators

Cytoplasmic granules contain preformed histamine, proteoglycans (heparin and chondroitin sulfate), neutral proteases and acid hydrolases. Mast cells are the major source of heparin; it is sequestered inside resting mast cells and is not present in circulating blood. Heparin regulates the amount of the other biologically active mediators in the cytoplasmic granules; because of its negative charge, heparin may be the storage site for the positively charged histamine.

Activation of mast cells initiates release of granule contents and generation of a heterogeneous group of mediators. Multivalent allergens bind to specific IgE antibodies fixed to the high affinity $Fc_\varepsilon RI$ receptors on the mast cell; cross-linking of IgE results in the formation of receptor dimers, triggering intracellular protein phosphorylation (eg, PLC, PIP3) to initiate signaling (Section 1). Mediators released from the activated mast cells fall into three categories: (1) preformed granule-associated mediators, (2) lipid-derived mediators (the arachidonic acid metabolites – leukotrienes and prostaglandins), (3) cytokines and chemokines. The selective release of histamine may be induced by a number of initiators, including the neuropeptide substance P, PAF, and cytokines (eg, IL-1 and IL-3). The bee venom mellitin can trigger selective and specific histamine release without perturbation of mast cell structure.

Role in Host Defense

Mast cells have a critical role in the innate immune response to invading bacteria. Mast cell recognition of bacteria triggers slow selective release of granule contents; this bactericidal process is not toxic to host cells, in contrast to allergen-triggered immediate and complete degranulation. Release of the chemoattractants, leukotrienes and TNF-α, are important to the subsequent recruitment of neutrophils to the site. Mast cells phagocytose and process adherent bacteria then, as antigen-presenting cells, interact with neighboring T-cells to engage the immune response.

THE ALLERGIC RESPONSE

Mast cells, basophils, and eosinophils are the primary effector cells in the allergic and inflammatory response triggered by inciting antigens and amplified by a series of feedback loops. Because of their tissue location, mast cells have a key role in the immediate IgE-mediated allergic reaction as they make the initial contact with the provoking allergen. All three cells express $Fc_\varepsilon RI$, the high affinity IgE receptor (although the expression in eosinophils is relatively low). The Fc region of the IgE molecule binds to the receptor (Section 17). Allergen cross-linking of the specific IgE antibodies bound to $Fc_\varepsilon RIs$ results in receptor aggregation, cell activation and degranulation. The immediate allergic response usually occurs within minutes. A second late phase reaction (LPR) may begin 2-4 hours after the original challenge and peaks between 6 and 12 hours.

The **immediate allergic reaction** is the result of the interaction of mast cell mediators with the surrounding tissues. Explosive degranulation and release of preformed mediators, including histamine, proteases and chemokines, is complete in minutes. This is followed closely by release of arachidonic acid metabolites, leukotrienes and prostaglandins, and, subsequently, by release of newly synthesized cytokines. The nature of the response is determined by the local environment. Histamine, leukotrienes, PAF, and prostaglandins induce a microvascular

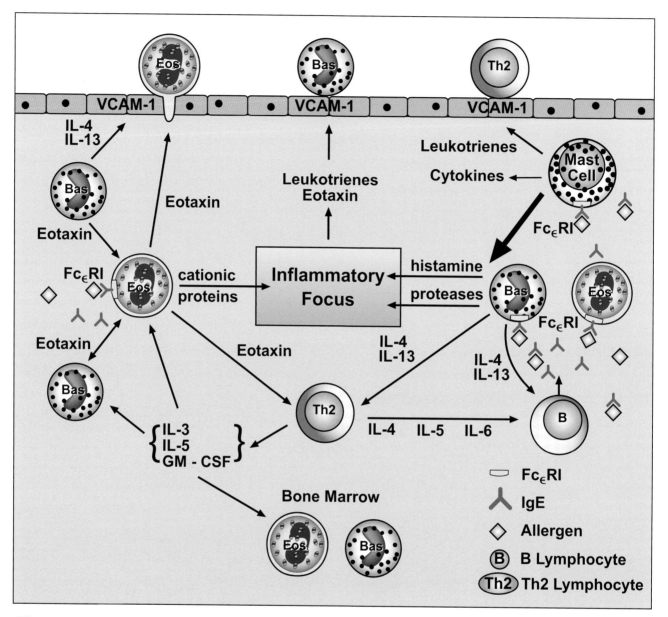

Figure 8-4   The Allergic Response

response: increased vascular permeability, leukocyte adhesion, and vasodilatation. In the lungs, there may be pulmonary vasoconstriction and bronchoconstriction.

The **late phase reaction (LPR)** develops as a consequence of the recruitment of basophils, eosinophils, and Th2 cells into the area. Vessel dilatation, upregulation of endothelial adhesion molecules, cytokines, and chemokines contribute to leukocyte migration to the site of allergen challenge.

Recruitment of **eosinophils** to the allergic focus is the result of enhanced eotaxin production by the adjacent epithelial cells,. Other chemokines augment migration into the site. The eosinophils are primed for their inflammatory response by IL-5 generated by the local Th2 population. Allergen binding to specific IgE antibodies on the $Fc_\epsilon RI$ receptors results in cell activation; degranulation with release of cationic proteins amplifies the allergic and inflammatory response.

Recruited basophils are stimulated by allergen cross-linking of IgE molecules bound to the $Fc_\epsilon RI$ receptors. Basophil activation results in granule fusion with the cell membrane and discharge of the mediators including histamine and leukotrienes. IL-3, IL-5, and GM-CSF augment the IgE-mediated release. The activated basophils synthesize and release the immunomodulatory cytokines IL-4 and IL-13. These cytokines: (1) induce the expression of VCAM-1 on endothelial cells thus increasing eosinophil margination and migration to the inflammatory site; (2) induce eotaxin synthesis in the adjacent epithelial cells; (3) stimulate Th2 T-cell production and differentiation – resulting in the release of cytokines, IL-5, IL-3 and GM-CSF, that increase eosinophil production, prime their reactivity, and prolong their life span; (4) induce class switch in B cells for IgE production independent of T cell regulation, thereby increasing IgE synthesis. As IgE levels increase, there is increased expression of IgE receptors ($Fc_\epsilon RI$) on basophils and mast cells, further amplifying the IgE response.

The **Th2 lymphocytes** within the inflammatory focus are stimulated by IL-4 and IL-13 derived from the basophils and mast cells. Th2 cells in turn promote local B cell proliferation and IgE synthesis. The size of the Th2 population increases as a result of local expansion and through recruitment by eotaxin. These cells also produce IL-3, IL-5 and GM-CSF that stimulate eosinophil and basophil production in the marrow and prolong eosinophil life span in the tissues.

CLINICAL CORRELATES

Eosinophilia

Eosinophils normally make up less than 0.5% of circulating leukocytes. The storage pool of eosinophils in the bone marrow is approximately five times the total circulating population. The eosinophil spends approximately 24 hours in the circulation before taking up residence in extravascular tissues. The peripheral blood eosinophil count is a poor index of the extent of tissue eosinophilia as it only monitors the traffic from production in the bone marrow to extravascular migration. (There are a few exceptions, eg, eosinophilic leukemia). Eosinophilia frequently is associated with an expansion of the eosinophil regulatory CD4[+] Th2 lymphocytes.

Peripheral blood eosinophilia characteristically is observed in allergic disease, parasitic infections, inflammatory bowel disease, hypersensitivity diseases, and some neoplasms. The allergic reaction, initiated by multivalent allergen binding to specific cell-bound IgE antibodies, results from the linked responses of mast cells, basophils, Th2 cells, and eosinophils. The commonest sites of allergic manifestations are the lung (asthma), nose (allergic rhinitis and polyps), and skin (urticaria and atopic dermatitis).

The parasitic diseases include those due to intestinal parasites, particularly the helminths. Eosinophils located in the intestinal submucosa are in an optimal position to intercept these invaders. As these parasites are too large to be phagocytosed, the eosinophils kill the invaders through degranulation and extracellular release of the cationic proteins and the products of the respiratory burst. Eosinophils also attack parasites in deeper tissues such as muscle (eg, trichinosis).

Eosinophilic gastroenteritis, esophagitis, and inflammatory bowel disease are chronic debilitating disorders that are the result of allergic hypersensitivity reactions. They are manifest by elevated IgE, eosinophilia, and eosinophil infiltration in various segments of the gastrointestinal tract. Inflammation and tissue damage are due to release of cationic proteins and other mediators from eosinophil granules.

Eosinophilia may occur in collagen vascular disease, hypersensitivity vasculitis, and eosinophilic fasciitis. Neoplastic diseases with eosinophilia include the lymphomas, Hodgkin's disease, and eosinophilic leukemia. Toxic drug or chemical reactions associated with eosinophilia have been responsible for severe illness affecting large numbers of the exposed population. The L-tryptophan-induced eosinophilic myalgia syndrome and the toxic cooking oil syndrome have both been linked to toxic contaminants.

Glucocorticoids are effective in terminating or reducing the allergic response and reducing eosinophil levels. By suppressing transcription of the genes for IL-5, IL-3, IL-4, IL-13, and GM-CSF, they probably induce eosinophil apoptosis.

Idiopathic Hypereosinophilic Syndrome

This disease of unknown etiology is marked by persistent hypereosinophilia associated with major end organ damage. Tissue damage may manifest as endomyocardial fibrosis, pulmonary infiltrates, central nervous system involvement either by vasculitis or microemboli, urticaria or cutaneous skin nodules. The pathogenesis of this syndrome cannot be explained solely on the basis of the increased number of eosinophils because other forms of hypereosinophilia, frequently with higher sustained eosinophil counts, do not lead to this type of organ damage. The release of eosinophil cationic proteins can produce major local tissue damage, but the degree of end organ damage in this syndrome suggests that other factors are involved. This may be a disease of the regulatory T cells, with the eosinophil as a secondary participant. Corticosteroid therapy may result in a long term clinical response; sometimes improvement is transient. Interferon-α can produce remissions in some patients refractory to steroids.

Systemic Mast Cell Disease

Two important features distinguish mast cells: they express stem cell factor receptors, and have the capacity for self-renewal. Systemic mastocytosis may result from an activating mutation (816 Asp→Val) in the SCF receptor (c-kit). This mutation is associated with ligand-independent cell activation and growth. Mast cell proliferation is most marked in skin, bone marrow, and gastrointestinal tract. Secondary involvement of liver, spleen, and lymph nodes is due to mast cell infiltration; cytokines and chemokines produced by the mast cells attract major infiltration by eosinophils and lymphocytes. The release of histamine and proteases by these cells produces a local inflammatory reaction.

The clinical manifestations include attacks of flushing, syncope, nausea, and diarrhea, probably related to histamine release. Cutaneous manifestations (urticaria pigmentosa, mast cell tumors, and diffuse erythroderma) may be present at birth or develop in early childhood. Histamine-induced gastric hypersecretion may be responsible for peptic ulceration. Infiltration of lymphoid organs and bone marrow manifests as lymphadenopathy, splenomegaly, myelofibrosis, or a myelodysplastic syndrome. Anemia and peripheral blood eosinophilia are common.

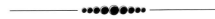

SUGGESTED READING

Bochner BS, Schleimer RP. Mast cells, basophils, and eosinophils: distinct but overlapping pathways for recruitment. Immunol Rev 179:5-15, 2001.

Boyce JA. The pathobiology of eosinophilic inflammation. Allergy Asthma Proc 18:293-300, 1997.

Broide D, Sriramaras P. Eosinophils trafficking to sites of allergic inflammation. Immunol Rev 179:163-172, 2001.

Costa JJ, Weller PF, Galli SJ. The cells of the allergic response: mast cells, basophils, and eosinophils. JAMA 278:1815-1822, 1997.

Falcone FH, Haas H, Gibbs BF. The human basophil: a new appreciation of its role in immune responses. Blood 96:4028-4038, 2000.

Giembyczi MA, Lindsay MA. Pharmacology of the eosinophil. Pharmacol Rev 51:213-339, 1999.

Gleich GJ, Adolphson CR, Leiferman KM. The biology of the eosinophilic leukocyte. Annu Rev Med 44:85-101, 1993.

Gutierrez-Ramoz JC, Lloyd C, Gonzalo JA. Eotaxin: from an eosinophilic chemokine to a major regulator of allergic reactions. Immunology Today 20:477-534, 1999.

Hirai K, Miyamasu M, Takaishi T, Morita Y. Regulation of the function of eosinophils and basophils. Crit Rev Immunol 17:325-352, 1997.

Lui F-T. Truly MASTerful cells: mast cells command B cell IgE synthesis. J Clin Invest 99:1465-1466, 1997.

Malaviya R, Abraham SN. Mast cell modulation of immune responses to bacteria. Immunol Rev 179:16-24, 2001.

Metcalfe DD, Baram D, Mekori YA. Mast cells. Physiol Rev 77:1033-1079, 1997.

Rankin SM, Conroy DM, Williams TJ. Eotaxin and eosinophil recruitment: implications for human disease. Mol Med Today 6:20-27, 2000.

Rothenberg ME. Eosinophilia. N Eng J Med 338:1592-1600, 1998.

Rothenberg ME, Mishra A, Brandt EB, Hogan SP. Gastrointestinal eosinophils. Immunol Rev 179:139-155, 2001.

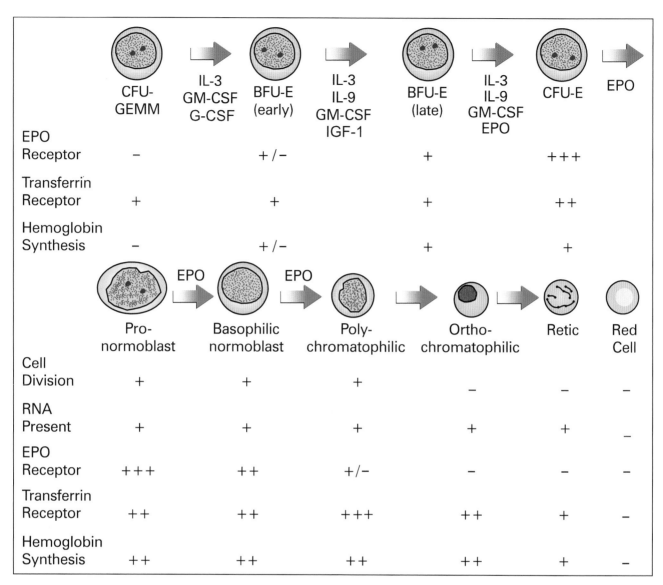

Figure 9-1 Erythropoiesis

contribute to local cytokine production; T cells are a source of IL-3, the most important of these cytokines. The presence of these "accessory" cells in vivo probably accounts for the much more rapid progression of the erythroid cells through BFU-E and CFU-E than occurs in *in vitro* culture. At the CFU-E stage, definitive membrane and cytoskeletal proteins begin to assemble with expression of some of the mature red cell antigens. The developing erythroid cells also express surface adhesion molecules that interact with the extracellular matrix. These include ICAM-1, a member of the immunoglobulin superfamily (also expressed on endothelium), and $\alpha_4\beta_1$ integrin (that interacts with fibronectin). These adhesion molecules are lost as maturation proceeds, freeing the cell to exit the bone marrow.

The first morphologically identifiable red cell precursor in bone marrow aspirates is the pronormoblast, a moderately large cell (15-20 μm in diameter) with basophilic cytoplasm and a

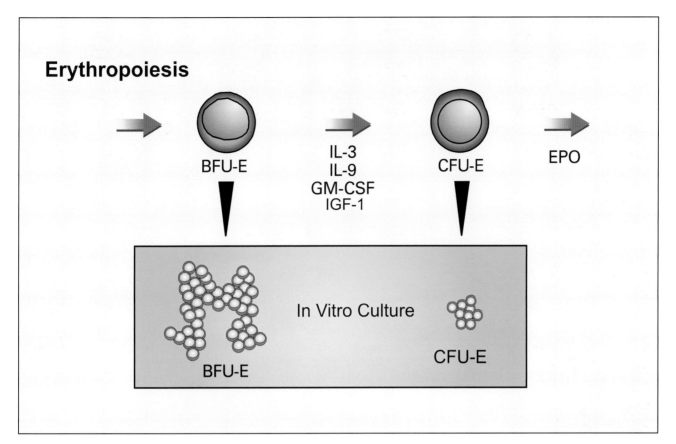

Figure 9-2 BFU-E and CFU-E

large nucleus containing multiple nucleoli. Cell division continues through the next two stages, the basophilic and the polychromatophilic normoblasts, with decreasing cell size. Due to alterations in chromosomal structure the nucleus becomes smaller and more dense and finally is extruded from the orthochromatophilic normoblast, leaving the reticulocyte with some residual strands of RNA. After a residence of 24-48 hours in the bone marrow, the reticulocyte emerges into the peripheral circulation where, within 24-48 hours with a further decrease in size and loss of the reticulin, it becomes a mature circulating red cell. During much of this first 48 hour period outside the bone marrow, the cells are retained in the spleen where surface adhesion molecules and residual RNA (reticulin) are removed. The elapsed time from pronormoblast to mature red cell approximates 7 days. When there is need for increased red cell production, the time to maturity can be shortened by reducing the inter-mitotic interval or by skipping some mitotic divisions.

It is postulated that the hemoglobin content of the cell is a negative regulator of cell division. When hemoglobin synthesis is delayed or reduced, as in iron deficiency anemia, the cells undergo an extra division yielding smaller microcytic red cells. Alternately, when hemoglobin synthesis exceeds DNA synthesis as in the megaloblastic anemias, the cells skip a division, nuclear extrusion occurs earlier, and macrocytic red cells result.

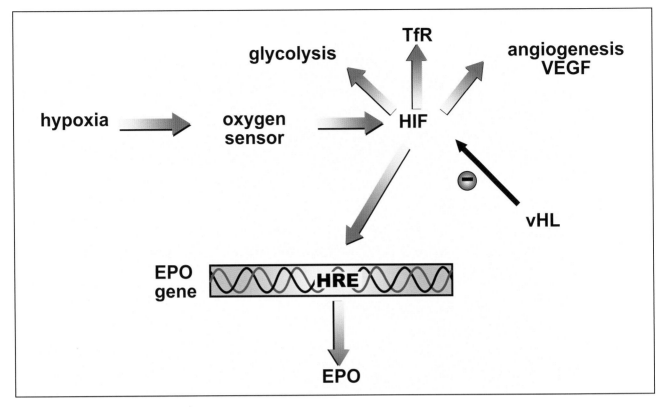

Figure 9-3 Control of Erythropoietin Synthesis

Regulation of Erythropoiesis

Erythropoietin (EPO), a 35kD glycoprotein, is the primary humoral regulator of erythropoiesis – promoting both proliferation and survival of erythroid precursors. Approximately 90% of EPO is synthesized in renal peritubular interstitial cells that respond to an O_2-sensing mechanism. As in other cells, the oxygen sensor in renal cells probably is a ferrous iron prolyl hydroxylase that requires molecular O_2 as a cosubstrate to hydroxylate specific proline residue(s) in the **hypoxia inducible factor (HIF)**. The transcription factor HIF targets a number of erythropoietic genes, including erythropoietin, transferrin, the transferrin receptor (TfR), and the vascular-endothelial growth factor (VEGF). When HIF binds to the **hypoxia-response element (HRE)** on the EPO gene, enhanced transcription results in increased EPO synthesis (Figure 9-3). In response to a hypoxic stimulus, recruitment of additional EPO-producing peritubular cells supplements the cells that constitutively synthesize EPO; when the hypoxic stimulus is removed, the recruited cells return to their non-secretory state.

HIF is the key regulator of the cellular response to hypoxia. It is a heterodimeric transcription factor consisting of two subunits: the β subunit is expressed constitutively, independent of tissue oxygenation; the α subunit (the target of prolyl hydroxylase) is undetectable until cells are exposed to hypoxic stimuli. In **hypoxic states**, the level of HIFα increases as a result of reduced prolyl hydroxylase activity. The consequent formation of the

HIFαβ dimers leads to transcriptional activation of the target genes, upregulating EPO, VEGF, anaerobic glycolysis for ATP production, and other factors that engage in maintaining O_2 homeostasis.

In **normoxic states**, HIF is downregulated as proline residues on the α subunit are hydroxylated. This renders HIFα a target for ubiquitination and proteasomal destruction by the **vHL (von Hippel-Lindau)** protein complexed with an E3 ligase (Section 1). When vHL is absent or mutated, HIFα degradation is decreased and the HIFαβ dimer continues to stimulate gene transcription. In the von Hippel-Lindau syndrome, the functional loss of vHL protein is associated with multiple vascular tumors (due to unregulated VEGF production) and, in some patients, erythrocytosis (due to increased EPO synthesis). The tumor suppressor protein p53 also is a regulator of HIFα. p53 recruits the E3 ligase MDM2 to promote ubiquitin-mediated degradation of HIFα (Section 4). Loss of p53 function may result in HIFα over-expression and the increased VEGF synthesis associated with highly vascular tumors.

CFU-Es probably represent the focal point for EPO regulation of red cell production. When circulating EPO increases, the existing CFU-Es quickly respond by proliferation and differentiation; when EPO levels fall, the CFU-Es undergo apoptosis. A stable constitutive EPO level is required to maintain CFU-E production at a rate appropriate to physiological requirements. EPO stimulates red cell production, differentiation and maturation, and prevents apoptosis.

The **erythropoietin receptor** is a member of the cytokine receptor superfamily (Figure 9-4). It consists of extracellular, transmembrane and cytoplasmic domains. The receptor first appears in small numbers in early BFU-Es, increases in CFU-Es and pronormoblasts, and declines in the later erythropoietic cells. The binding of EPO results in dimerization of the receptor, transmission of signal to the intracellular domain, and initiation of signal transduction pathways. Although the receptor lacks intrinsic growth-promoting kinase activity, it does induce secondary tyrosine kinase activity in a number of EPO receptor-associated cytoplasmic proteins. Phosphorylation and activation of the cytoplasmic tyrosine kinase JAK2 leads to JAK2 phosphorylation of the EPO receptor and the latent cytoplasmic transcription factor STAT (signal transducer and activator of transcription); STAT dimerizes and migrates to the nucleus where it activates gene transcription. Phosphorylation of other cytoplasmic effector proteins, including PI3-kinase and Ras, induce additional signaling pathways that contribute to gene response and cell activation (Section 1).

The EPO-initiated signal transduction pathway is highly regulated – molecules in the signaling pathway are activated within minutes of EPO binding, and the signal is terminated within a few hours. The rate at which the signal is turned off is determined by the net effect of several factors: (1) deprivation of EPO, (2) specific phosphatase (SHP-1) dephosphorylation of the EPO receptor cytoplasmic domain and JAK kinase, (3) activation of negative-regulators of

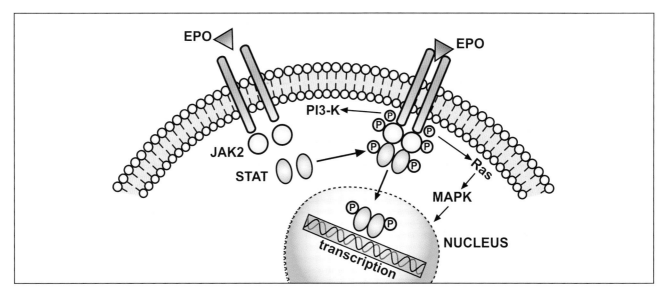

Figure 9-4 Erythropoietin Signaling

JAK kinase and STAT transcription.

In addition to extracellular signals, there is an internal program that is central to erythroid differentiation. The transcription factor **GATA-1**, expressed in erythroid precursors, is essential for the development and survival of these cells. GATA-1 recognizes conserved DNA-GATA (guanine, adenine, thymine, adenine) motifs in the regulatory regions of many erythroid-expressed genes. GATA-1 transcription activity regulates the levels of heme synthetic enzymes, globin, membrane proteins, and other red cell components. Both EPO and GATA-1 strongly upregulate expression of the anti-apoptotic gene $bcl-X_L$, thus ensuring erythroblast survival (Figure 9-5).

Other Erythropoietic Signaling Pathways

Angiotensin II regulates renal hemodynamics and blood pressure. It is also a ligand for receptors on red cell precursors and can stimulate erythropoiesis. The angiotensin II receptor articulates with a JAK-2 kinase, suggesting the possibility of a shared intracellular signaling pathway with EPO. Ten to twenty percent of renal transplant patients develop erythrocytosis although EPO levels are within the normal range. The erythrocytosis decreases following the administration of angiotensin converting enzyme (ACE) inhibitors.

The role of **insulin-like growth factor-1 (IGF-1)** is unclear. In *in vitro* cell culture systems, IGF-1 can substitute for EPO, and it appears that its signaling pathway is independent of EPO. It may substitute for EPO as an erythropoietic stimulus in anephric patients. Erythroid cultures from patients with polycythemia vera (PV) are hyper-responsive to IGF-1, suggesting it may have a role in the increased erythropoiesis in PV.

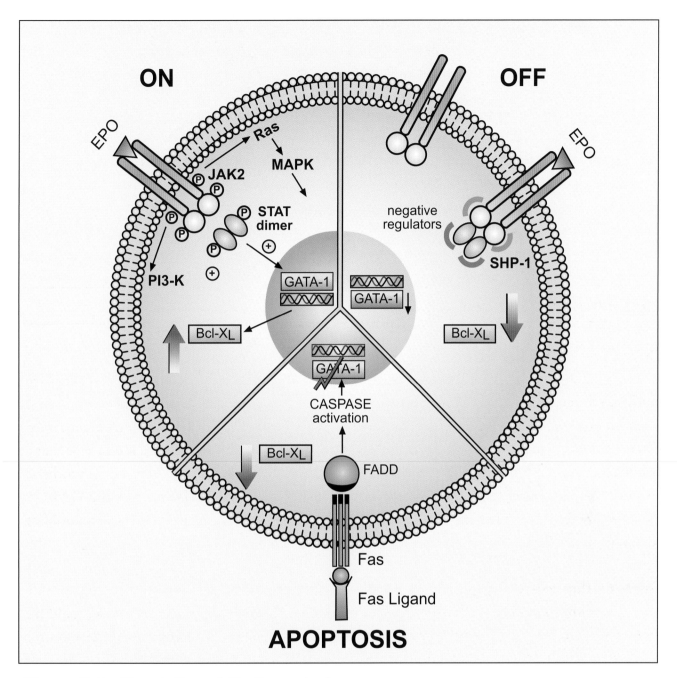

Figure 9-5 Regulation of Erythropoiesis

Apoptosis (Figure 9-5)

Apoptosis of the erythroid precursors may be induced by loss of Bcl-X$_L$, by absence of EPO signaling with concomitant loss of GATA-1, or by activation of the death signal through the Fas receptor. Fas is present on both early and late erythroid precursors, however, its activating ligand (Fas L) appears only on late erythroblasts. Binding of Fas L to Fas activates the proteolytic caspases (Section 4) that cleave a number of intracellular proteins, including

GATA-1 with the subsequent loss of Bcl-X$_L$. This negative regulation of erythropoiesis takes place within the erythropoietic islands of the bone marrow where the mature erythroblasts can control the expansion and differentiation of their immature precursors.

The Transferrin Receptor (TfR)

Cell membrane transferrin receptors are common to most cells; the receptor on red cell precursors is an immunologically distinct isoform. The receptor provides access to the cell for transferrin-bound iron required for the synthesis of heme and other iron-containing proteins. There are large numbers of these receptors on hemoglobin-synthesizing cells, reaching a peak of some 800,000 per cell on the polychromatophilic normoblasts, and falling to 100,000 on reticulocytes. They are absent on mature red cells as there is no hemoglobin synthesis and therefore no further requirement for iron. The receptor is a transmembrane protein that can bind either monoferric or diferric transferrin. With the binding of the iron-bearing transferrin, the complex is internalized by receptor-mediated endocytosis and the iron is released into the cytoplasm for intracellular synthesis of heme. The receptor-transferrin complex then returns to the membrane, the transferrin is released to the plasma and the receptor again becomes available (Section 15). The transferrin receptor is up-regulated in hypoxia under the control of HIF.

CLINICAL CORRELATES

ANEMIA

Anemias classically are divided into two categories, due either to decreased red cell production or to increased red cell destruction. Some of the disorders that result in precursor failure, loss of EPO production, or cytokine suppression of erythropoiesis are discussed.

Red Cell Aplasia

Failure of red cell production may occur as a component of complete bone marrow aplasia due to stem cell failure, or appear as an isolated defect – a "pure" red cell aplasia. The latter presents as a severe anemia with no reticulocyte response; the leukocytes and platelets are normal. The bone marrow is cellular but contains few red cell precursors.

Congenital red cell aplasia (Diamond-Blackfan Syndrome) is an anemia frequently associated with multiple congenital anomalies. It usually presents within six months of birth; it is sometimes familial. The defect is probably the result of a prenatal mutation at a critical time in developmental erythropoiesis. The clinical entity likely encompasses a number of molecular defects; *in vitro* studies have described defects at the level of CFU-E, BFU-E, and CFU-GEMM. In most cases, the bone marrow is cellular but there is a paucity of red cell precursors – the anemia is severe but white cells and platelets are not decreased; plasma EPO levels are high. A number of patients may go on to bone marrow aplasia indicative of a trilineage hematopoietic defect. In some cases, a defect in the EPO receptor has been demonstrated; these patients do not respond to EPO, although IL-3 can promote erythropoiesis. A high level of circulating Fas ligand has been identified in some cases; the binding of the ligand to the Fas receptor on the membrane of the erythropoietic cells activates the caspase system and induces apoptosis. The good clinical response to prednisone, often at a low dose, remains unexplained. In unresponsive cases, bone marrow transplant has been successful.

Acquired red cell aplasia usually results from immunological blockade of erythropoiesis at the level of BFU-E and CFU-E by either antibody or T cells. IgG antibodies capable of inhibiting the growth of BFU-E or CFU-E colony formation can be demonstrated in about half of these patients. Aplasia may occur in association with thymomas or lymphomas as well as with some non-hematological tumours; the production of α-interferon by the tumor cells may induce increased expression of Fas on erythroid precursor cells resulting in apoptosis. Anecdotal reports of drug-associated pure red cell aplasia have been recorded. A number of patients with immunologically mediated aplasia respond to immunosuppressive therapy (antithymocytic globulin and/or cyclosporin). Patients unresponsive to immunosuppressive therapy may be considered for bone marrow transplantation.

Parvovirus B19, a single stranded DNA virus, is the etiological agent of the childhood exanthem fifth disease. B19 has a high affinity for, and replicates only in, erythroid progenitor cells, and it is directly cytotoxic to CFU-Es. The receptor for the virus is the red cell blood group P antigen: individuals who do not express P antigen are naturally resistant to B19 infection. Suppression of erythropoiesis persists for 1-2 weeks until the viremia is cleared by the immune response. This transient red cell aplasia is of little clinical importance in the presence of a normal red cell life span. In patients with a compensated hemolytic process and a short red cell life span, however, the drop in hemoglobin can be precipitous - in this "aplastic crisis", the reticulocytes disappear and the hemoglobin level plummets. Persistent parvovirus infection with red cell aplasia and anemia may occur in immunosuppressed patients.

Anemia of Chronic Disease

This common anemia is seen most typically in patients with chronic infections, chronic non-infectious inflammatory disease or malignant disease. Inflammatory cytokines may play a role in decreasing EPO gene expression and may interfere with iron mobilization from macrophages (Section 15).

Anemia of Chronic Renal Failure

The primary cause of this anemia is loss of EPO production as the renal synthetic cells disappear. In addition, there is often a significant reduction in red cell life span and some bone marrow suppression due to retained toxic products. Inflammatory cytokines may further reduce

EPO expression. The increased incidence reflects the increased number of patients maintained on dialysis. In most patients, the anemia responds to replacement therapy with recombinant human erythropoietin (rHu EPO).

POLYCYTHEMIA

Polcythemia or erythrocytosis can be separated into three main categories: (1) associated with high erythropoietin levels, (2) associated with normal or low erythropoietin levels, and (3) a myeloproliferative disease due to a somatic mutation of hematopoietic stem cells (polycythemia vera).

Erythrocytosis With High Plasma Erythropoietin Levels

Erythrocytosis is associated most commonly with hypoxemia related to residence at high altitude, chronic lung disease, sleep apnea, supine hypoventilation, or cyanotic congenital heart disease with right to left shunt. All induce EPO synthesis and increased erythropoiesis. A more subtle cause is the chronic CO intoxication present in cigarette smokers. The affinity of hemoglobin for CO is more than 200 times that for oxygen. CO slowly displaces O_2 and, in addition, suppresses red cell 2,3-BPG production – the O_2 dissociation curve is shifted to the left (the p50 is decreased) resulting in reduced peripheral O_2 release and tissue hypoxia (Section 13).

The congenital familial polycythemias are the result of tissue hypoxia related to: (1) decreased O_2 release by high-affinity hemoglobins – the result of amino acid substitutions in the globin chains that govern heme-O_2 interaction or compromise 2,3 BPG binding (Section 13), (2) congenital methemoglobinemia associated with HbM, or failure of methemoglobin reduction due to mutant or absent NADH-cytochrome b_5 reductase (methemoglobin reductase), or a mutant cytochrome b_5 (Section 10), (3) congenital deficiency of 2,3-BPG (due to deficiency of the mutase that converts 1,3-BPG to 2,3 BPG). 2,3 BPG is a major regulator of O_2 release in the tissues – with decreased levels, the oxygen dissociation curve is shifted to the left, the p50 is decreased, and there is reduced O_2 release in peripheral tissues (Section 13), (4) an abnormal renal oxygen sensor or dysregulation of HIF resulting in inappropriate EPO synthesis – this is probably the cause of the familial erythrocytosis described in the Chuvash region of Russia.

von Hippel Lindau (vHL) disease is a hereditary cancer syndrome due to the functional loss of the vHL tumor suppresser gene. The vHL syndrome develops when both copies of the gene are inactivated. In the "two-hit model" (similar to retinoblastoma), one mutated gene is inherited (a germline mutation); disease develops when a somatic mutation inactivates the second gene. Sporadic cases are the result of somatic mutations in both copies of the gene. The genetic lesions include deletions, missense and frame-shift mutations. The vHL protein regulates HIF by binding and targeting the HIFα subunit for ubiquitination and proteasomal destruction.

Loss of vHL results in inappropriate overexpression of HIF and, consequently, increased angiogenesis (VEGF); there may be an associated erythrocytosis due to EPO overproduction. vHL disease is characterized by vascular tumors, including hemangioblastomas of the cerebellum, retina, and spinal cord. Most clear cell renal carcinomas have a somatic mutation of the vHL gene; there may be an associated erythrocytosis. The erythrocytosis that is associated with other tumors as a "paraneoplastic syndrome" may be due to a similar molecular lesion.

Erythrocytosis With Normal Erythropoietin Levels

Primary familial erythrocytosis is an autosomal dominant disease due to a mutated EPO receptor gene; the defect may be the result of missense or frameshift mutations. The abnormal truncated EPO receptor is hypersensitive to the EPO ligand because the cytoplasmic negative-regulator of the receptor is absent or insensitive to the phosphatase (SHP-1) that normally turns off the EPO signal (Figure 9-5). As a result, the EPO proliferative response is maintained in the presence of a minimal EPO stimulus. Patients are reported to have early cardiovascular disease (although one propositus of a Finnish family won three Olympic gold medals in cross-country skiing – the advantage of the elevated hematocrit in this cardiovascular demanding sport).

Polycythemia Vera (PV) is a myeloproliferative disease. It is due to a clonal somatic mutation in hematopoietic precursor cells, leading to red cell overproduction independent of EPO regulation. The level of circulating EPO may be either normal or low. The increased red cell production, frequently associated with concomitant increases in platelets and granulocytes, represents a clonal proliferation at the level of the stem cell or CFU-GEMM.

In cultures of normal erythropoietic precursors, the absence of erythropoietin leads to apoptosis. In contrast, in polycythemia vera, the *in vitro* growth of erythroid colonies takes place in the presence of low concentrations or in the absence of erythropoietin. A deregulated increase in the expression of the apoptosis inhibitor Bcl-X_L may allow these cells to escape normal apoptotic regulation; the result is red cell overproduction. The PV clone is exquisitely sensitive to EPO and to IGF-1, possibly due to a functional deletion of the negative-regulatory mechanism of signal transduction. In these patients, initially, there is a mixed population of red cell precursors. Over time, the hyper-responsive clone increases and dominates, exhibiting a survival advantage compared to normal red cell precursors.

—————— ••••◉••• ——————

SUGGESTED READING

Allen DA, Breen C, Yaqoob MM, MacDougal IC. Inhibition of CFU-E colony formation in uremic patients with inflammatory disease: Role of IFN-gamma and TFN-alpha. J Investig Med 47:204-211, 1999.

Carper E, Kurtzmann GJ. Human parvovirus B19 infection. Curr Opin Hematol 3:111-117, 1996.

DeMaria R, Zeuner A, Eramo A, Domenichelli C, Bonci D, Grignani F, et al. Negative regulation of erythropoiesis by caspase-mediated cleavage of GATA-1. Nature 401:489-493, 1999.

Ebert BL, Bunn HF. Regulation of the erythropoietin gene. Blood 94:1864-1877, 1999.

Erslev AJ, Soltan A. Pure red cell aplasia: a review. Blood Rev 10:20-28, 1996.

Friedrich, CA. Von Hippel-Lindau Syndrome. Cancer 86:2478-2482, 1999.

Gregg XT, Prchal JT. Erythropoietin receptor mutations and human disease. Semin Hematol 34: 70-76, 1997.

Gregory T, Yu C, Ma A, Orkin SH, Blobel GA, Weiss MJ. GATA-1 and erythropoietin cooperate to promote erythroid cell survival by regulating bcl-XL expression. Blood 94:87-96, 1999.

Hanspal M. Importance of cell-cell interactions in regulation of erythropoiesis. Curr Opin Hematol 4:142-147, 1997.

Ihle JN. Cytokine receptor signalling. Nature 377:591-594, 1995.

Juvonen E, Ikkala E, Fyhrquist F, Ruutu T. Autosomal dominant erythrocytosis caused by increased sensitivity to erythropoietin. Blood 78:3066-3069, 1991.

Kaelin WG Jr, Maher EA. The VHL tumour-suppressor gene paradigm. Trends in Genetics 14:423-426, 1998.

Klingmuller U, Lorenz U, Cantley LC, Neel BG, Lodish HF. Specific recruitment of SH-PTP1 to the erythropoietin receptor causes inactivation of JAK2 and termination of proliferative signals. Cell 80:729-738, 1995.

Means RT Jr. Advances in the anemia of chronic disease. Int J Hematol 70:7-12, 1999.

Ohh M, Park CW, Ivan M, Hoffman MA, et al. Ubiquitination of hypoxia-inducible factor requires direct binding to the β-domain of the von Hippel-Lindau protein. Nat Cell Biol 2:423-427, 2000.

Prchal JF, Prchal JT. Molecular basis of polycythemia. Curr Opin Hematol 6: 100-109, 1999.

Semenza GL. HIF-1 and mechanisms in hypoxia sensing. Curr Opin Cell Biol 13:167-171, 2001.

Silva M, Richard C, Benito A, Sanz C, Olalla I, Fernandez-Luna J. Expression of bcl-XL in erythroid precursors from patients with polycythemia vera. N Engl J Med 338:564-571, 1998.

Starr R, Hilton DJ. Negative regulation of the JAK/STAT pathway. Bioessays 21:47-52, 1999.

Zhu H, Gunn HF. How do cells sense oxygen? Science 292:449-451, 2001.

THE RED CELL

"The red particles of blood in the human subject have been so generally allowed to be spherical that in almost all books they are denominated as red globules...I found that these particles of the blood were as flat as a guinea."
William Hewson – 1773

Although devoid of a nucleus and intracellular organelles, the red cell, squeezed through small capillary beds, buffeted by high shear forces in the heart, and subjected to sequestration, stasis, and substrate deprivation in the spleen, has a life-span approximating four months. It maintains its shape, pH, ionic equilibrium, and protects hemoglobin integrity and function by virtue of its membrane-cytoskeletal structure and its metabolic activity.

STRUCTURE (Figure10-1)

The mature red cell is a biconcave disc with a diameter of 7.5 µm and a circumferential thickness of 2.5 µm. This shape provides a surface area of about 140 µm², 50% greater than that of a sphere of the same volume, thereby providing an efficient transport vehicle for oxygen exchange. The shape also allows for deformability as the erythrocytes move through capillaries of less than half their diameter. This pliability is provided by a cell membrane attached to an underlying cytoskeleton that is adaptable to shape change, elongation and deformation.

The membrane constituents are 50% protein, 40% lipid and 10% carbohydrate. The lipid bilayer provides the membrane continuity of the cell; it consists, primarily, of cholesterol and phospholipid in equal proportions. The phospholipids are arranged asymmetrically in the bilayer with the uncharged phosphatidylcholine (PC) and sphingomyelin (SM) in the outer leaf, and the negatively charged phosphatidylethanolamine (PE) and phosphatidylserine (PS) in the inner leaf. This phospholipid asymmetry, common to most eukaryotic cell membranes, is maintained by an active process requiring ATP and a translocase enzyme. Cholesterol moves freely in and out of the bilayer, and to and from the surrounding plasma.

Transmembrane Proteins

Band 3 is the anion exchange channel that maintains Cl^-/HCO_3^- eqiulibrium. It traverses the phospholipid membrane multiple times (probably 12) and displays the ABO blood group antigens as well as antigens I and i on its extracellular domains. It is anchored intracellularly to ankyrin (band 2.1) which in turn binds to spectrin – the major cytoskeletal protein.

Glycophorins are glycoproteins. They provide most of the negative surface charge that prevents red cells from sticking to the endothelium and to each other. Glycophorin A carries the

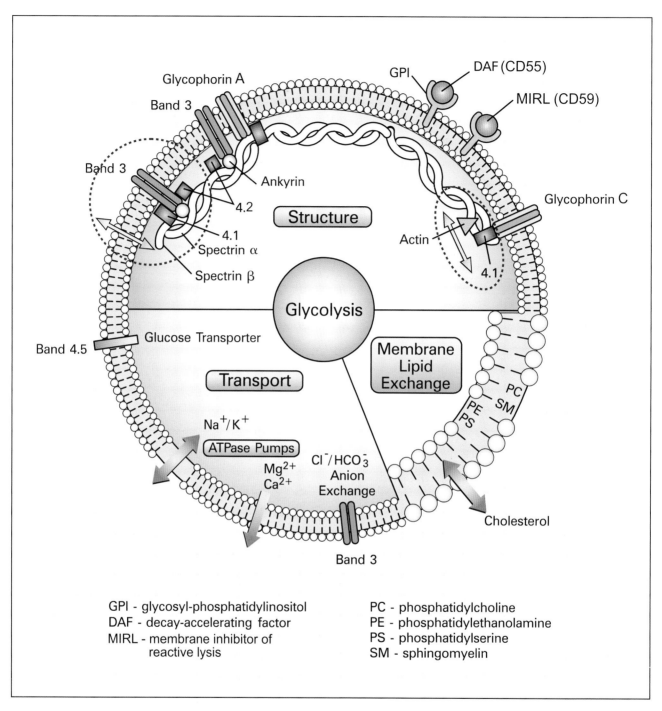

Figure 10-1 The Red Cell - Structure and Function

red cell antigens M and N; glycophorin B carries the antigens S, s and U. Glycophorin C binds intracellularly to the cytoskeletal protein band 4.1. Glycophorin A is a binding site for the malarial parasite Plasmodium falciparum. A surface glycoprotein bearing the Duffy blood group antigen is the receptor for Plasmodium vivax. Individuals negative for the Duffy antigens, Fy (a⁻b⁻), are resistant to P. vivax infection (Section 11).

Rh proteins are also integral membrane proteins. Their absence, the Rh null phenotype, is associated with a shortened red cell life span (Section 11).

Cytoskeletal Proteins

The cytoskeleton forms a lattice at the inner surface of the membrane; it consists of five principal proteins – the spectrins, actin, ankyrin and bands 4.1 and 4.2. The α and β spectrins (bands 1 and 2) are two similar rod-like proteins that closely intertwine with each other as heterodimers which come together head to head to form tetramers. The tails of the spectrin tetramers are associated with band 4.1 and with actin (band 5); proteins tropomyosin, tropomodulin and adducin also interact at this site. The vertical stability of the membrane is provided by the spectrins, band 3, ankyrin and protein 4.2. The horizontal interactions that contribute to red cell shape include the spectrins, actin and protein 4.1.

Other membrane proteins serve transport functions. Non-polar substances enter the red cell by diffusion; polar solutes enter at special transport sites (band 3, cation transporters, glucose and water transit sites). An active water channel protein, aquaporin-1, contributes up to 85% of the osmotic water permeability pathway. Glucose enters the cell by facilitated diffusion mediated by the glucose transporter (band 4.5). Because the glucose transporter can supply much more glucose than is required by the glycolytic pathway, glucose is not rate-limiting in normal red cell metabolism. The concentrations of Na^+ and K^+ within the cell are regulated by the Na^+/K^+ ATPase pump. The intracellular concentrations of these cations approximate 130 mM of K^+ and 8 mM of Na^+; plasma contains about 140 mM of Na^+ and 4 mM of K^+. Passive diffusion ("leak") of the cations is countered by the active transport mechanism; the cell must continuously move Na^+ out and K^+ in by way of the Na/K ATPase powered pump. Ca^{2+} and Mg^{2+} concentrations are regulated by the Ca^{2+}/Mg^{2+} ATPase pump. Band 3 both links the lipid bilayer to the cytoskeleton and functions as an anion exchanger for chloride-bicarbonate exchange.

Glycosylphosphatidylinositol (GPI) embedded in the outer leaflet of the bilayer is a phospholipid anchor for a number of externally exposed hydrophilic proteins. Two complement-regulatory proteins are clinically important: **decay accelerating factor DAF (CD55)** and **membrane inhibitor of reactive lysis MIRL (CD59)**. DAF protects the cell against complement-induced lysis by accelerating the dissociation of the membrane-assembled enzyme complexes that constitute complement C3 convertase. MIRL protects against complement-mediated lysis by binding to C8, thereby blocking the binding and polymerization of C9 and the formation of the membrane attack complex. Paroxysmal nocturnal hemoglobinuria (PNH) is an acquired somatic mutation in a totipotent hematopoietic stem cell resulting in a defect in GPI synthesis; with defective anchoring and loss of DAF and MIRL the red cell becomes vulnerable to complement-induced lysis (Section 20).

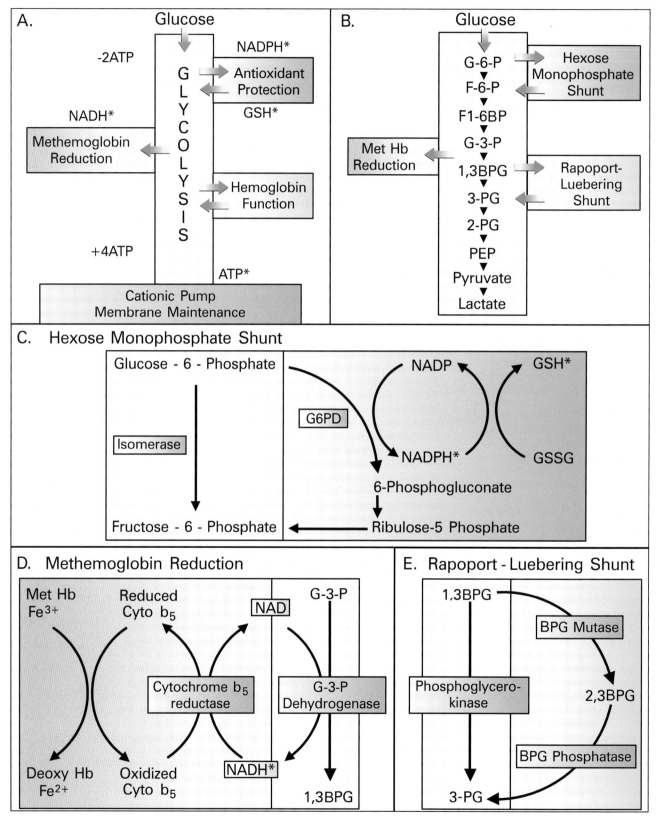

Figure 10-2 Red Cell Metabolism

METABOLISM (Figure 10-2)

The red cell is dependent upon a continuous supply of glucose for its energy requirements. These energy needs are supplied by glycolysis; the pathway begins with the facilitated, insulin-independent, uptake of glucose and ends with the production of lactate. In Figure 10-2, Panel A indicates the role of glycolysis in supporting the energy-requiring housekeeping duties of membrane maintenance and osmotic stability, and the metabolic offshoots which provide for antioxidant protection, methemoglobin reduction and regulation of hemoglobin function; Panel B describes anaerobic glycolysis in more detail; Panels C, D and E examine the associated metabolic pathways. In the normal red cell, 90% of glucose follows the anaerobic pathway to lactate and 10% flows through the aerobic hexose monophosphate shunt. The energy generated is required to: (1) maintain cationic balance, cell shape and membrane integrity, (2) prevent oxidative damage, (3) maintain hemoglobin in its unoxidized functional deoxy-form, and (4) provide 2,3 BPG – a facilitator of hemoglobin function. These four functions are made possible through: (1) generation of energy in the form of ATP, (2) generation of NADPH and reduced glutathione (GSH) in the hexose monophosphate shunt, (3) the methemoglobin reduction NADH system, and (4) the Rapoport-Luebering shunt that produces 2,3 BPG.

Anaerobic Glycolysis

The first step in the glycolytic (Embden-Meyerhof) pathway is the phosphorylation of glucose to glucose-6-PO_4 (G-6-P) catalyzed by **hexokinase**. **Phosphoglucose isomerase** converts G-6-P to fructose 6-PO_4 (F-6-P). F-6-P then is converted by **phosphofructokinase** to fructose 1-6 bisphosphate (F-1-6BP) at the expense of 2 mols of ATP. F-1-6BP is split by aldolase to yield the triose glyceraldehyde-3-PO_4 (G-3-P). The addition of inorganic phosphate by **G-3-P dehydrogenase** produces 1,3-bisphosphoglyceric acid (1,3-BPG); in this step NAD is reduced to NADH which functions as the cofactor for cytochrome b_5 reductase. 1,3-BPG either may enter the Rapoport-Luebering shunt to produce 2,3-BPG, or proceed directly to 3-phosphoglycerate (3-PG). This junction regulates the distribution of flow to either lactate with ATP production, or to the formation of 2,3-BPG with no attendant production of ATP.

Glycolysis continues through 2-phosphoglycerate (2-PG), phosphoenolpyruvate (PEP), and thence to pyruvate, the latter reaction mediated by the enzyme **pyruvate kinase (PK)**. The enzyme **lactic dehydrogenase** (LDH) finally converts pyruvate to lactate.

In the first phase of glycolysis, 2 mols of ATP are utilized and, subsequently, with the sequence proceeding through to lactate production, 4 mols of ATP are generated, yielding a net gain of 2 mols of ATP per mol of glucose consumed.

The Hexose Monophosphate Shunt (Aerobic Glycolysis)

The red cell, as a carrier of reactive O_2, must have a mechanism for maintaining its key functional moieties in a reduced state. The hexose monophosphate shunt serves this function. Normally, less than 10% of glycolysis passes through this aerobic cycle the products of which are NADPH and reduced glutathione (GSH). Under conditions of oxidant stress, to protect the cell membrane and cell contents against oxidative damage, there may be up to a ten-fold increase in the production of NADPH. The key enzyme is **glucose 6-PO_4 dehydrogenase (G6PD)**; it converts G-6-P to 6-phosphogluconate (6-PG), generating the NADPH necessary for the reduction of oxidized glutathione (GSSG) to its reduced form (GSH). GSH is an essential intracellular reducing agent that protects cells against oxidant injury.

Rapoport-Luebering Shunt

The enzyme **BPG mutase** converts 1,3 BPG to 2,3 BPG. **BPG phosphatase** removes the phosphate at the 2 position of 2,3 BPG, and returns 3-PG to the glycolytic pathway. This shunt has two primary roles: (1) it produces 2,3-BPG which is a regulator of hemoglobin oxygenation-deoxygenation (Section 13), and (2) it modulates ATP synthesis. When 1,3-BPG is converted directly to 3-PG (in the glycolytic pathway) the high energy phosphate from the 1 position generates ATP. In the conversion of 1,3-BPG to the lower energy 2,3-BPG through the action of **BPG mutase**, no ATP is formed.

Methemoglobin Reduction

Methemoglobin is formed under conditions which allow the oxidation of heme Fe^{2+} to Fe^{3+}. Because methemoglobin cannot transport O_2, the return of methemoglobin to functional deoxyhemoglobin is essential. This is mediated through the transfer of an electron from NADH to the iron atom of heme via cytochrome b_5 and **cytochrome b_5 reductase**. The NADH required for this reaction is generated in the conversion of G-3-P to 1,3 BPG by **G-3-P dehydrogenase.**

CLINICAL CORRELATES

Defects in Red Cell Membrane

Changes in lipid content or cholesterol/phospholipid ratios, with expansion of the lipid bilayer relative to cell volume, are reflected in changes of red cell morphology (stomatocytes and target cells) frequently present in patients with liver disease. Target cells due to decreased cell volume relative to surface membrane are present in iron deficiency anemia and thalassemia.

Hereditary Spherocytosis (HS). The sphering of red cells results from a primary defect in the cytoskeleton with secondary changes in the lipid membrane. It is the commonest non-immune hemolytic anemia in Caucasians. Seventy-five percent of cases demonstrate an autosomal dominant pattern of inheritance; the remainder occur sporadically – some of these are new mutations but many are due to a recessive form of HS.

This is a heterogeneous syndrome due to over 100 genetic defects associated with reduced or abnormal synthesis of those proteins governing the vertical axis of the cytoskeleton – α or β spectrin, ankyrin, band 3 or band 4.2 (Figure 10-1). The result is defective cytoskeletal binding to the membrane and loss of membrane surface area. The loss of surface membrane produces a more spherical cell with less deformability, resulting in increased splenic trapping; prolonged sequestration in the spleen leads to metabolic stress due to glucose deprivation. This cumulative stress injury results in increased loss of membrane, further sphering and, eventually, in premature red cell removal within the splenic cords (Section 16). Most patients have a combined deficiency of both spectrin and ankyrin. Because α spectrin is produced in excess of β spectrin, it is β spectrin that is rate limiting in the synthesis of the membrane skeleton and is the most common site of spectrin defects producing clinical disease. Defects in band 3 and band 4.2 occur either singly or in combination with other missense mutations or deletions. The heterogeneity of the molecular defects in HS is responsible for the wide variation in clinical severity and hereditary patterns leading to the production of spherocytes with shortened red cell life-span.

Hereditary Elliptocytosis (HE). HE is a heterogeneous disorder associated with a variety of molecular genetic cytoskeletal defects in α or β spectrin or band 4.1 – the proteins that stabilize the cytoskeletal horizontal axis (Figure 10-1). The severity of hemolysis in elliptocytosis is highly variable; most frequently, hemolysis is minimal and not clinically detectable – probably because the elliptocytic shape does not produce impedance to flow or splenic trapping. Some elliptocytic defects do produce mild hemolysis, and rarer forms are associated with major hemolysis.

Paroxysmal Nocturnal Hemoglobinuria. This is an acquired clonal disorder at the level of the stem cell that affects red cells, platelets, lymphocytes and myeloid cells. In each cell series, the percentage of affected cells is highly variable. Clinical manifestations include hemolysis with acute exacerbations, pancytopenia due to marrow failure, and thrombotic disease. PNH is due to a somatic mutation in the *PIG-A* gene located on the X chromosome; some 100 mutations have been identified. The *PIG-A* gene governs the synthesis of the phosphatidylinositol glycan-class A membrane glycolipid, the GPI anchor. GPI and the GPI-linked proteins are synthesized separately – a signal sequence directs attachment of the proteins to the GPI anchor; after transport through the Golgi apparatus the complex is integrated into the cell membrane. The lesion in PNH is a defect in GPI synthesis; as a result there is loss of surface expression of all 19 of the known GPI-anchored proteins including DAF (CD55) and MIRL (CD59). DAF accelerates decay of the complement C3 convertase formed through activation of both the classical and alternative complement pathways; MIRL inhibits the assembly of the components of the complement membrane attack complex. A defect in MIRL alone is sufficient to produce the hemolytic phenotype of PNH; a defect in DAF plays a lesser role. The increased sensitivity of the affected erythrocytes to complement-induced hemolysis can be demonstrated in vitro in acidified serum (Ham test) as the alternative pathway of complement is activated at a pH of 6.2: the defective red cells are up to 25-fold more sensitive to complement-mediated lysis than normal red cells. Flow cytometric analysis demonstrating absence of CD55 and CD59 on the red cell membrane is a more sensitive diagnostic index.

PNH has a close relationship to aplastic anemia: a significant number of PNH patients develop aplastic anemia; a number of patients presenting with aplastic anemia display the molecular defects of PNH and some evolve into clinical PNH. Although not well explained, the proliferating PNH cells appear to have a survival advantage. One explanation is that the loss of normal hematopoietic cells in aplastic anemia is due to external factors which are less destructive of stem cells with the PNH phenotype. Patients with PNH frequently exhibit more than one PNH clone (Section 20).

Defects in Red Cell Metabolism

Hereditary defects, manifest by structurally altered or unstable glycolytic enzymes, occur in both the anaerobic and the aerobic pathways. Many of these defects are of little or no clinical significance, others produce varying degrees of shortened red cell life-span – congenital non-spherocytic hemolytic anemias. The major clinical features of hemolysis are: anemia, jaundice, splenomegaly and cholelithiasis. The most common hereditary enzyme defects of red cells are PK and G6PD deficiencies.

Defects in Anaerobic Glycolysis. These are, with few exceptions, autosomal recessive enzymopathies manifest by chronic, often low grade hemolysis with a compensatory reticulocytosis. The red cells are not spherocytic. Splenomegaly is frequently present.

Pyruvate Kinase (PK) Deficiency. PK catalyzes the conversion of phosphoenolpyruvate (PEP) to pyruvate, converting ADP to ATP in the process. In PK deficiency, the deficit in ATP production produces a net energy loss; as a result there is decreased cationic pump activity, reduced Na^+/K^+ exchange, osmotic water loss, cell shrinkage, and distortion of the membrane with resultant hemolysis. More than eighty mutations have been identified. The block in endstage glycolysis increases the metabolic flow through the Rapoport-Luebering shunt, resulting in increased 2,3 BPG production which, by facilitating O_2 release from hemoglobin, partly compensates for the anemia. Most cases have been found in patients of Northern European ancestry; clinical symptoms are present in the homozygous or doubly heterozygous state.

Other less common enzymopathies in the glycolytic chain causing varying degrees of hemolysis include: hexokinase (G to G-6-P), phosphoglucose isomerase (G-6-P to F-6-P), phosphofructokinase (F-6-P to F-1-6BP), aldolase (F-1-6BP to G-3-P), and phosphoglycerate kinase (1,3-BPG to 3-BPG).

Defects in Aerobic Glycolysis. Defects in the hexose monophosphate shunt are many times more frequent than those of the glycolytic pathway. They are manifest by oxidative injury to red cell membrane and cell contents, resulting in hemolysis. Normally, the primary defence against oxidative injury is the tripeptide glutathione (glutamic acid-cysteine-glycine) in its reduced form (GSH). Various oxidants, including drugs as well as superoxide (O^-_2) and H_2O_2 produced by neutrophils or macrophages during infection, are inactivated by GSH. In response to oxidative stress, the normal red cell is able to mount a ten-fold increase in the activity of the hexose monophosphate shunt. Enzyme defects that render it impossible to maintain adequate GSH levels result in hemolysis.

Glucose-6-Phosphate Dehydrogenase (G6PD) Deficiency is the most common red cell enzymopathy, affecting more than 400 million people worldwide. Over 100 different G6PD X-linked isoenzyme anomalies have been described in various racial groups. Anemia may be low grade and chronic or acute and explosive, complicating infections or exposure to oxidant drugs such as antimalarials, sulfonamides and analgesics, or to fava beans. G6PD deficiency results in decreased NADPH synthesis with inability to maintain GSH levels. The oxidants damage the red cell membrane, oxidize heme to methemoglobin, and denature globin which precipitates on the membrane as Heinz bodies (visible in the peripheral blood smear by supravital staining with methyl violet). These membrane changes reduce deformability, increase cation leakage, and result in a fragile cell with a shortened lifespan and frequently intravascular hemolysis with hemoglobinuria.

Rare abnormalities in the production pathway of reduced glutathione include deficiencies of glutathione reductase and glutathione synthetase.

Methemoglobinemia may be congenital or acquired. Congenital methemoglobinemia is due to a deficiency of NADH-cytochrome b_5 reductase (methemoglobin reductase), very rarely to a mutant cytochrome b_5, or associated with abnormal hemoglobins (Hb M) in which an amino acid substitution allows oxidation of heme iron (Section 13). Acquired methemoglobinemia is due to ingestion or absorption of strong oxidants. Examples are the "blue babies" fed formula made with well-water containing high levels of nitrite. Historically, aniline dye workers have been a high-risk group.

———— •••◉◉◉••• ————

SUGGESTED READING

Bessler M, Hillman P. Somatic mutation and clonal selection in the pathogenesis and in the control of paroxysmal nocturnal hemoglobinuria. Semin Hematol 35:149-167, 1998.

Beutler E. G6PD deficiency. Blood 84:3613-3636, 1994.

Fujii H, Miwa S. Red blood cell enzymes and their clinical application. In Adv Clin Chem. HE Speigel (ed) 33: 1-54, 1999.

Hillman P, Richards SJ. Implications of recent insights into the pathophysiology of paroxysmal nocturnal haemoglobinuria. Br J Haematol 108:470-479, 2000.

Kinoshita T, Inoue N, Takeda J. Role of phosphatidylinositol - linked proteins in paroxysmal nocturnal hemoglobinuria pathogenesis. Annu Rev Med 47:1-10, 1996.

Liu S-C, Derick LH. Molecular anatomy of the red blood cell membrane skeleton: structure-function relationships. Semin Hematol 29:231-243, 1992.

Luzzato, L. Somatic mutation in paroxysmal nocturnal hemoglobinuria. Hosp Practice 32:125-140, 1997.

McMullin MF. The molecular basis of disorders of the red cell membrane. J Clin Path 52:245-248, 1999.

Nishimura JI, Murakami Y, Kinoshita T. Paroxysmal nocturnal hemoglobinuria: an acquired genetic disease. Amer J Hematol 62:175-182, 1999.

Tanaka KR, Zerez CR. Red cell enzymopathies of the glycolytic pathway. Semin Hematol 27:165-185, 1990.

Tse WT, Lux SE. Red blood cell membrane disorders. Brit J. Haemat 104:2-13, 1999.

Valentine WN, Paglia DE. Erythroenzymopathies and hemolytic anemia: the many faces of inherited variant enzymes. J Lab Clin Med 115:12-20, 1990.

Yeh ETH, Rosse WF. Paroxysmal nocturnal hemoglobinuria and the glycosylphosphatidylinositol anchor. J Clin Invest 93:2305-2310, 1994.

BLOOD CELL ANTIGENS

Marlis Schroeder

"Blut ist ein ganz besondrer Saft"
Blood is a very special fluid
Goethe, 1808

RED CELL ANTIGENS

The red cell membrane is home to a number of genetically determined structural components that confer antigenic specificity on the individual. Because of their physiological, pathological and clinical roles, they are grouped together as the red cell antigens. Most are glycosylated proteins. Although their functions remain largely unknown, some participate in membrane transport or in stabilization of the lipid membrane by articulation with the cytoskeletal proteins.

The ABO blood group system was first defined in 1900 by Karl Landsteiner. He described the reaction patterns that supported the identification of separate groups and their classification based on the presence of the "agglutinogens" termed A or B. In 1939, Levine described an antibody in a woman whose fetus had died with hemolytic disease of the newborn (HDN) and, in 1940, Landsteiner and Weiner demonstrated that rabbits, immunized with red cells from rhesus monkeys, produced an antibody that reacted with 85% of human red cells. This antibody was termed "Rh" (for rhesus); individuals were designated as Rh positive or Rh negative, depending on their reactivity with the antibody. This antibody was later termed anti-D, and the antigen in the Rh positive individual was designated D. Four additional antigens, C, c, E and e, were identified as members of the Rh blood group system. A total of 23 human blood group systems and over 300 antigens have been identified. Clinically, ABO is the most important. Determination of ABO compatibility between donor and recipient is the basis of all pretransfusion testing.

THE ABO AND HH BLOOD GROUP SYSTEMS

The A and B antigens are inherited in Mendelian fashion. The ABO group is determined by the presence of one (homozygous) or two (heterozygous) of the three alleles: *A*, *B* and *O* (Table 11-1).

H substance is the precursor of A and B antigens. The ***H,h* genes** govern the expression of the enzyme **H-fucosyltransferase** which converts the antecedent protein termed **precursor substance (PS)** to **H substance**. The products of the ***A* and *B* genes**, located on chromosome 9, are **glycosyltransferases**. The presence of the *A* or *B* allele dictates the structure of the corresponding A or B glycosyltransferase that converts H substance to either A or B antigen – the major alteration that distinguishes group A from group B red cells is the result of the structural difference between the two sugar molecules. **Group O** individuals carry only H

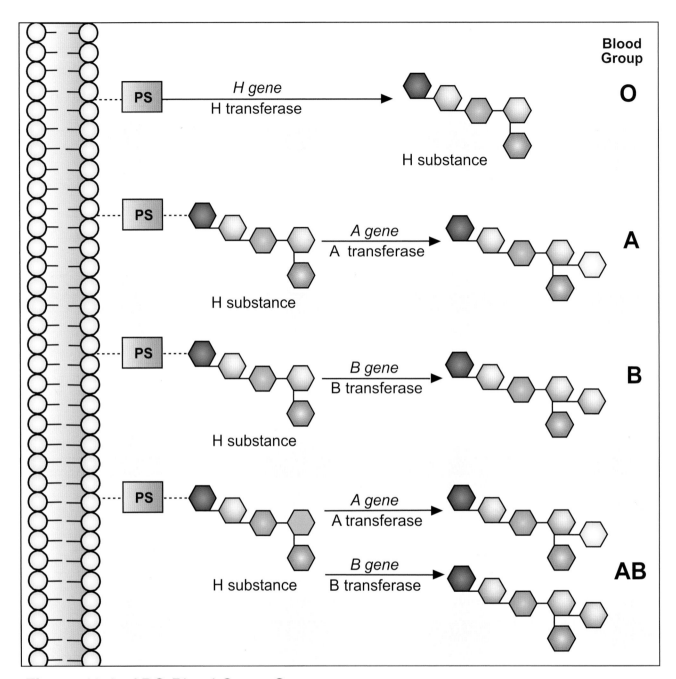

Figure 11-1   ABO Blood Group System

substance (Figure 11-1).

    A, B, and H substances are present on a wide variety of cells, including platelets, lymphocytes, endothelium and some epithelial cells. They also are found in soluble form in secretions, including saliva, milk, and urine. The secretion of A, B, and H substances is controlled by the secretor gene, *Se*. *Se* is the dominant gene (*Se, se*) and is inherited in a simple Mendelian pattern.

    A and B antigens are located on the outer surface of the red cell membrane. There are

Table 11-1   The ABO System

Phenotype	Genotype	Red Cell Antigens	Antibodies
O	00	(H)	Anti-A, Anti-B
A	OA or AA	A	Anti-B
B	OB or BB	B	Anti-A
AB	AB	A + B	None

some 1×10^6 antigenic sites on group A cells, 7×10^5 on group B, and 5×10^5 on group AB cells; all have some residual H substance. About 80% of group A individuals are group A_1 and 20% are A_2. Because of fewer antigenic sites or weak antigen expression, A_2 and other A variants react less strongly with anti-A typing sera than do A_1 red cells. A_1 can be distinguished by using specific anti-A_1 typing sera. The major significance of the A_2:A_1 distinction relates to the proper typing of donor red cells: because A_2 is a weak antigen, red cells may be typed incorrectly as group O. If an A_2 recipient is typed incorrectly and receives group O red cells, no hemolysis results. If group A_2 red cells are given to a group O recipient, an intravascular hemolytic transfusion reaction may develop as the recipient's anti-A destroys the A_2 cells. Subgroups of B are less frequent than those of A and can be differentiated by their serologic reactions.

Naturally occurring **IgM antibodies (isohemagglutinins)** are present in the plasma of individuals who lack the corresponding antigen. The presence of these antibodies permits ABO testing of serum as well as red cells. They are absent at birth, but develop over the first three to six months of life and gradually increase to adult levels. They arise as a result of exposure to ABO-like sugars that occur in a wide variety of exogenous sources such as bacteria, seeds and plants; they are absent in certain immune deficiency states. Individuals who type as group A or B make predominantly IgM isohemagglutinins, while group O individuals produce both IgM and IgG antibodies. IgG antibody, however, is produced as an immune response in group A or B individuals following sensitization by transfusion or fetomaternal bleeds. Because IgM does not cross the placenta, ABO incompatible newborns born to A or B mothers rarely have HDN unless the mother has been previously sensitized to produce IgG antibodies. The fetus of a group O mother is more likely to be affected because IgG anti-A and anti-B can cross the placenta to react with cells bearing the paternal A or B antigen. (Table 11-2)

THE RH BLOOD GROUP SYSTEM

The importance of the Rh blood group system is second only to ABO in transfusion practice. Although there are over 50 Rh antigens, only five are common. These are D, C, c, E and e. The term **Rh positive** indicates the presence of the D antigen and **Rh negative**, its

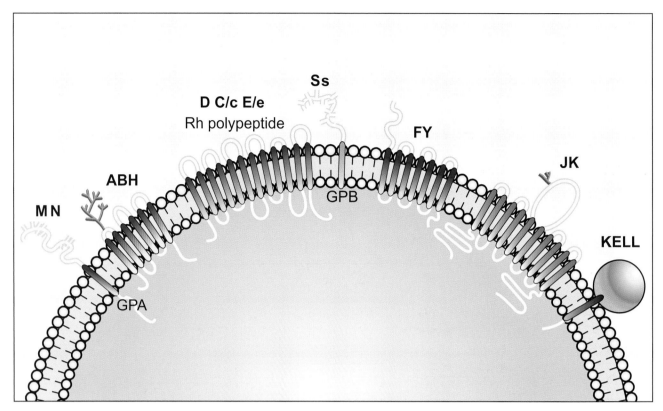

Figure 11-2 Red Cell Display of Blood Group Antigens

absence. Regardless of an individual's D status, other Rh antigens are present; these are C and c, E and e.

The two Rh genes, *RhD* and *RHCE,* are located on chromosome 1. *RhD* confers the D specificity on the red cell, while *RHCE* determines the presence of Cc and Ee antigens. Rh positive individuals express both genes, Rh negative individuals only *RHCE*. The tight linkage of the two loci dictates the simultaneous expression of these proteins – eg, *Dce, DcE, DCE*, and so on. There is no "d" – the notation of *dce, dCE*, etc., implies the absence of D.

The protein products of these genes are part of a large membrane complex. The Rh antigens are multipass membrane proteins that traverse the red cell membrane 12 times. Unlike other red cell antigens, they contain no sugar moieties (Figure11-2).

Weak D Phenotypes

The term weak D (D^U) denotes red cells that have a weak expression of D antigen due to decreased gene expression or epitope display. These individuals are Rh positive. Weak D is present in <1% of Caucasians and in higher frequency (3 - 4%) in Blacks. Blood banks test donor blood for weak D. If weak D donor blood is typed erroneously as Rh negative, it may sensitize the Rh negative recipient or result in a hemolytic transfusion reaction. Similarly, pregnant women are tested for weak D to confirm their Rh status, since those who type as weak D are Rh positive and do not require Rh immune globulin prophylaxis during their pregnancy.

Table 11-2   Significance of Some Blood Group Antibodies

Blood Group System	Antibody	Relative Frequency in Antibody Screening	Clinical Significance HTR*	HDN**
ABO	Anti-A	All group B and O	Yes	Yes
	Anti-B	All group A and O	Yes	Yes
Rhesus	Anti-D	Common	Yes	Yes
	Anti-c	Common	Yes	Yes
	Anti-E	Common	Yes	Yes
	Anti-C	Common	Yes	Yes
	Anti-e	Uncommon	Yes	Yes
Lewis	Anti-Le^a	Common	Rare	No
	Anti-Le^b	Uncommon	No	No
Kell	Anti-K	Common	Yes	Yes
	Anti-k	Rare	Yes	Yes
Duffy	Anti-Fy^a	Common	Yes	Yes
	Anti-Fy^b	Rare	Yes	Yes
Kidd	Anti-Jk^a	Common	Yes	Yes
	Anti-Jk^b	Rare	Yes	Yes
MN	Anti-M	Common	Rare	Rare
	Anti-N	Rare	Rare	Rare
SsU	Anti-S	Uncommon	Yes	Yes
	Anti-s	Rare	Yes	Yes
	Anti-U	Rare	Yes	Yes

*HTR   Hemolytic Transfusion Reaction
**HDN   Hemolytic Disease of the Newborn

Rh System Deletions – Rh_{NULL} and Rh_{MOD}

Rh_{null} individuals have no detectable Rh antigens on their red cells; Rh_{mod} red cells express low levels of Rh antigens. Because these antigens are intrinsic membrane proteins, their absence results in impaired membrane integrity and a shortened red cell life span.

Rh Antibodies

Antibodies to the Rh antigens usually develop after exposure of an Rh negative individual to Rh positive foreign red cells through transfusion or pregnancy. During pregnancy, small placental bleeds that allow fetal cells to enter the maternal circulation are common. Rh antibodies are usually IgG and are the most frequent antibodies encountered in pretransfusion testing. The D antigen is the most immunogenic followed by E and c antigens; in transfusion practice, donors and recipients are matched routinely only for the D antigen.

Anti-D causes hemolytic transfusion reactions (usually delayed), and severe HDN as the maternal IgG antibodies cross the placenta. Anti-c, which usually develops after transfusion, is also an important cause of HDN. Anti-E may occur naturally and may be IgM. Anti-e is a common autoantibody in autoimmune hemolytic anemia but rarely arises after transfusion (Table 11-2).

THE LEWIS BLOOD GROUP SYSTEM

Lewis antigens are not intrinsic to the red cell, but are adsorbed onto the red cell membrane from the plasma. The Lewis, H, and secretor genes interact to produce Lewis antigens (Table 11-3). The Lewis antigens are derived from the same precursor as H substances involved in the biosynthesis of the A and B antigens, and are formed by the addition of a sugar to the precursor. The product of the *Le* gene is a **fucosyltransferase** that transfers a sugar to the precursor substance (PS). The expression of Lewis antigens, Le^a and Le^b, is dependent upon the individual's *Se/se* and *H/h* alleles. All Le(a-b+) individuals are secretors while Le(a+b-) individuals are non-secretors of ABH. Le(a-b-) may be either, depending on the *Se/se* status.

Antibodies that react with Lewis system antigens are relatively common. They are acquired naturally and are usually IgM. The majority are reactive at room or cold temperature and are not clinically significant. Only the antibodies that react at temperatures above 30° C and cause *in vitro* hemolysis are considered clinically significant as they may result in a hemolytic transfusion reaction. They do not cause HDN (Table 11-2).

THE KELL BLOOD GROUP SYSTEM

The Kell antigens (K, k) are highly immunogenic. Anti-K usually arises after transfusion. Maternal alloimmunization may occur during pregnancy and is second in frequency only to the Rh system. The K antigens have approximately 10% of the immunogenicity of the D antigen. The antibodies are IgG, cross the placenta to produce HDN, and are capable of producing hemolytic transfusion reactions. Other Kell system antibodies, such as anti-k, also are clinically significant as they are associated, although less frequently, with both HDN and hemolytic transfusion reactions (Table 11-2).

THE DUFFY BLOOD GROUP SYSTEM

The Duffy blood group system has two major antigens, Fy^a and Fy^b. The antibodies to the Duffy system are produced either as a result of transfusion or pregnancy. They are clinically significant as they may cause delayed hemolytic transfusion reactions and HDN (Table 11-2).

Table 11-3 The Lewis System

| Genes Present | Blood Group Substances | | Red Cell |
	In Secretions	On Red Cells	Phenotype
H, Se, Le	H, Le^a, Le^b	H, Le^b	Le(a$^-$b$^+$)
H, sese, Le	Le^a	H, Le^a	Le(a$^-$b$^+$)
H, Se, lele	H	H	Le(a$^-$b$^+$)
H, sese, lele	–	–	Le(a$^-$b$^+$)

THE KIDD BLOOD GROUP SYSTEM

The Kidd blood group system (Jk^a/JK^b) was discovered during the investigation of a mother whose child had HDN. The antibodies, IgG or IgM, are generally of low titer and bind complement. This antibody may not be detectable by standard techniques, therefore, hemolytic transfusion reactions (delayed or immediate) may occur despite a negative antibody screen or crossmatch. HDN occasionally does occur but is rarely severe (Table 11-2).

I AND i ANTIGENS

These antigens are regulated developmentally: I is present on the red cells of virtually all adults (I+i-), while the i antigen is expressed (I-i+) on cord or neonatal red cells. The corresponding naturally occurring antibody is active at cold temperatures, and has no clinical significance. Anti-I may be present in chronic cold agglutinin disease and in some of the autoimmune hemolytic anemias. Cold agglutinins identified in Mycoplasma pneumoniae infections also have anti-I specificity, but rarely cause hemolysis. Autoantibody-i is less frequent but is seen in association with diseases such as the lymphomas and infectious mononucleosis.

THE P BLOOD GROUP SYSTEM

The P blood group system antigens are determined by oligosaccharide structures associated with glycolipids of the red cell membrane. The P antigen is present on most human red cells. P antigen is the receptor for parvovirus B19 (the causative agent for the childhood exanthem fifth disease). This DNA virus replicates only in erythroid progenitors bearing P antigen with resultant suppression of erythropoiesis. Individuals who do not express P antigen are naturally resistant to B19 infection (Section 9). Anti-P$_1$ is a naturally occurring IgM antibody that is usually of no clinical significance. The development of complement-fixing IgG anti-P$_1$ (classically present in syphilis) is associated with paroxysmal cold hemoglobinuria.

THE MNS SYSTEM

The MNS system antigens are associated with the red cell trans-membrane sialoglycoproteins known as glycophorins (Section 10). Two groups of closely associated antigens are M and N situated on glycophorin A (GPA), and S/s and U on glycophorin B (GPB). Approximately 84% of Blacks lack U antigen; 1% lack S and s. The antibodies to M and N are naturally occurring and not clinically significant. Anti-S, anti-s and anti-U are produced as a result of transfusion or pregnancy and can cause HTR and HDN. Anti-U is found only in Blacks with a history of prior transfusion or pregnancy (Table 11-2).

PLATELET ANTIGENS

Platelets express a variety of surface antigens including those shared with other cells, and some that are specific to platelets. The specific antigen systems have been defined mainly through the study of neonatal alloimmune thrombocytopenia (NATP) and post transfusion purpura (PTP) (Table 11-4).

SHARED ANTIGENS

Red Cell Antigens on Platelets. ABH blood group substance is found on the surface of platelets, however, the amount varies with the individual. The presence of red cell antigens on platelets is of importance in platelet transfusion because of the decreased survival of ABO incompatible platelets. Transfusion across the ABO blood group barrier is acceptable in adults if group compatible platelets are not available, although the recovery may be decreased. In infants with a small blood volume, the donor plasma should be compatible because of the risk of inducing hemolysis. ABO-incompatibility always must be considered as a possible cause of refractoriness in platelet transfusion therapy.

HLA Antigens. HLA class I antigens are the most important of the shared antigens expressed on platelets. They are an intrinsic platelet membrane protein but their expression on the platelet surface is variable. The number of HLA Class I molecules on the surface of a single platelet ranges from 15,000 to 120,000. Because the presence of antibodies to HLA class I antigens is of major significance in immune-mediated refractoriness to platelet transfusions, this variable expression of HLA antigens on platelets may be important in the selection of HLA compatible platelets for alloimmunized recipients.

PLATELET-SPECIFIC ANTIGENS

The platelet antigen systems previously were designated by letters, which usually referred to the name of the individual in whom the antibody was first detected. In the revised nomenclature, the term HPA (human platelet antigen) is used to designate the platelet antigen

Table 11-4   Human Platelet Alloantigen (HPA) Systems

Antigen System (Original Name)	Alleles	Glycoprotein Location	Clinical Significane NATP*	PTP**
HPA-1 (PL^A,Zw)	HPA-1a(PL^{A1}) HPA-1b(PL^{A2})	GPIIIa	Yes	Yes
HPA-2 (Ko,Sib)	HPA-2a(Ko^b) HPA-2b(Ko^a)	GPIb		Yes
HPA-3 (Bak,Lek)	HPA-3a(Bak^a) HPA-3b(Bak^b)	GPIIb	Yes	Yes
HPA-4 (Pen,Yuk)	HPA-4a(Pen^a) HPA-4b(Pen^b)	GPIIIa	Yes	
HPA-5 (Br,Hc,Zav)	HPA-5a(Br^b) HPA-5b(Br^a)	GPIa	Yes	

*NATP: Neonatal alloimmune thrombocytopenia
**PTP: Post transfusion purpura

systems. The systems were named chronologically and the alleles are designated alphabetically. HPA-1a corresponds to PL^{A1} in the old nomenclature (although the latter term remains in common use). The first 5 of the 14 identified antigen systems, their alleles, phenotypic frequency, glycoprotein location, and primary clinical significance are summarized in Table 11-4.

GRANULOCYTE ANTIGENS

Granulocytes express three types of surface antigens:

Common Antigens include Class I HLA antigens (HLA-A,-B,-C), and some of the red cell antigens (eg, P, I, and Lewis blood group systems).

Shared Antigens are expressed on granulocytes as well as on mononuclear cells. They include 5a and 5b (HNA-3a), 9a, Mart (HNA-4a), and Ond (HNA-5a). Some of these antigens are associated with alloimmune neonatal neutropenia (ANN) or transfusion-associated lung injury (TRALI); others are of unknown significance.

Granulocyte Specific Antigens initially were defined through the investigation of infants with alloimmune neonatal neutropenia (ANN) and in the study of patients with autoimmune neutropenia (AIN), transfusion associated lung injury (TRALI), and febrile

Table 11-5   Granulocyte Specific Antigen Systems

Antigen	HNA*	Location	Clinical Significance			
			ANN	AIN	TRALI	DIN
NA1	HNA-1a	FcRIIIb	Yes	Yes		
NA2	HNA-1b	FcRIIIb	Yes	Yes	Yes	
NB1	HNA-2a	56-64 kDa Glycoprotein	Yes	Yes	Yes	Yes

* HNA: human neutrophil antigen
ANN: alloimmune neonatal neutropenia
AIN: autoimmune neutropenia
TRALI: transfusion associated lung injury
DIN: drug-induced neutropenia

transfusion reactions. They include the NA antigen system which consists of two antithetical antigens, NA1 (HNA-1a) and NA2 (HNA-1b), and the NB antigens that are inherited independently of the NA system. The NB1 (HNA-2a) antigen is associated with drug-induced neutropenia (Table 11-5).

LABORATORY TESTS

The **direct antiglobulin (direct Coombs) test** (DAT) is used to determine the presence of antibody or complement on the surface of the red cell, i.e. red cell sensitization that has occurred *in vivo*. An antihuman globulin (AHG) reagent, containing both anti-IgG and anti-C3d is added to patient red cells that have been washed to remove unbound immunoglobulins. Agglutination is indicative of the presence of IgG and/or complement fixed to the surface of the red cell. This test is used in the investigation of hemolytic disease of the newborn, autoimmune hemolytic anemia, and transfusion reactions (Figure 11-3).

The **indirect antiglobulin (indirect Coombs) test** (IAT) is used to determine the presence of anti-red cell antibodies in serum. In this test, red cell sensitization is produced *in vitro*: patient serum is incubated with normal control red cells that express clinically significant antigens; the red cells then are washed to remove unbound immunoglobulins, and AHG is added. Agglutination suggests that the patient serum contains IgG antibodies that have fixed to the test red cells. These antibodies are capable of hemolyzing transfused red cells that express the same antigens. This test is used to determine the presence of an antibody in the patient's serum as part of pretransfusion compatibility testing, in routine prenatal testing, and in antibody identification (Figure 11-4).

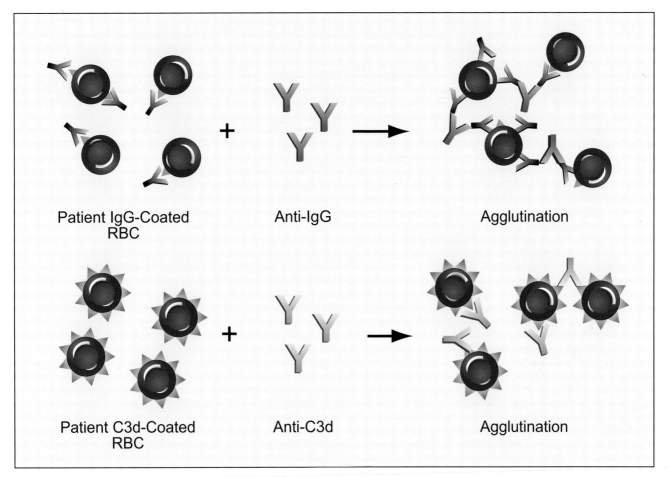

Figure 11-3 Direct Antiglobulin Test (DAT) with Anti-IgG and Anti-C3d

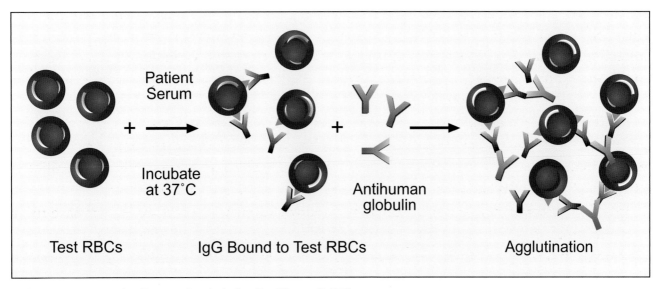

Figure 11-4 Indirect Antiglobulin Test (IAT)

CLINICAL CORRELATES

RED CELL ANTIGENS (Table 11-2)

Hemolytic Disease of the Newborn (HDN) is the result of fetal-maternal blood group incompatibility. There are two primary types: 1) HDN caused by antibodies to antigens such as Rh, Kell, Duffy or Kidd, and 2) HDN due to ABO incompatibility.

Rh Hemolytic Disease is the most common form of HDN. It develops in the fetus of an Rh negative mother sensitized to red cell Rh antigens (usually D) either by transfusion or, most often, by a previous pregnancy. During a subsequent pregnancy in the sensitized mother, there is a secondary immune response with maternal generation of IgG anti-D antibodies that cross the placenta and fix to the Rh positive fetal red cells. As the antibody-coated red cells are destroyed by the fetal reticuloendothelial system, anemia and jaundice result. The fetal DAT is strongly positive. The severity of HDN varies from mild to the development of hydrops fetalis and intrauterine death. Treatment may include intrauterine transfusion, postnatal exchange transfusion, phototherapy and/or red cell transfusions.

Passive immunization of Rh negative mothers with Rh (D) immune globulin can prevent Rh (D) immunization as the anti-D rapidly eliminates the fetal red cells from the maternal circulation, thereby removing antigen stimulation. Rh immune globulin (RhIG) is administered routinely, at 28 weeks gestation and within 96 hours of delivery, to every Rh negative mother delivering an Rh positive baby. It should also be administered after every antenatal bleed or abortion, or at the time of any invasive procedure during pregnancy. The **Kleihauer-Betke test** can be performed to determine the presence and size of the fetal-maternal bleed. This test is based on the differential solubility of Hemoglobin A (HbA) and Hemoglobin F (HF) under acid conditions; the fetal cells containing the less soluble HbF can be identified and quantitated on a maternal blood smear. The calculated approximate volume of feto-maternal hemorrhage is a guide to the amount of RhIG required to prevent alloimmunization.

ABO Hemolytic Disease of the newborn is less severe than HDN associated with other alloantibodies. Maternal anti-A or anti-B is primarily IgM that does not cross the placenta. IgG antibodies are the result of previous immunization (pregnancy or transfusion). Fetal red cells contain fewer A and B antigenic sites and the IgG anti-A and/or anti-B that does cross the placenta encounters many antigenic sites, other than red cells, that soak up the antibody. The cord blood or newborn DAT is negative or weakly positive. Clinical disease is usually mild – only a small percentage of these infants require treatment such as phototherapy or exchange transfusion.

Hemolytic Transfusion Reactions

Acute (immediate) hemolytic transfusion reactions usually are caused by the infusion of ABO incompatible red cells that react with the naturally occurring anti-A and/or anti-B antibodies. These IgM antibodies activate complement, resulting in membrane lysis and the rapid release of free hemoglobin into the circulation. Disseminated intravascular coagulation may be triggered by tissue factor release from red cell membranes. Most cases result from an error in patient or specimen identification.

Delayed hemolytic transfusion reactions are the result of either a primary immunizing event or a secondary response. With primary immunization, there is a slow production of an antibody against the specific antigen that is absent in the recipient – the antigen-antibody reaction may not be obvious clinically because hemolysis is mild. In previously sensitized patients, however, there is a rapid secondary antibody response to the transfusion of the antigen-positive red cells, resulting in major hemolysis accompanied by chills, fever, jaundice and a falling hemoglobin.

Autoimmune hemolytic anemia (AIHA) is associated with the development of autoantibodies (usually IgG). This may occur de novo or be part of a generalized autoimmune disease (eg, disseminated lupus erythematosus). The presence of the antibody on the red cell usually can be demonstrated by the direct Coombs test (DAT).

Disease Association

Malaria – The Duffy gene encodes a membrane glycoprotein that is the receptor for certain malarial parasites, notably *Plasmodium vivax*. Fy(a-b-) individuals (a common phenotype in Blacks) therefore are resistant to *Plasmodium vivax* (but not to *Plasmodium falciparum*).

GI – A number of gastrointestinal diseases are influenced by red cell antigens. Gastric carcinoma is associated more frequently with group A, and duodenal ulcer with group O. One of the receptors for **Helicobacter pylori** is the blood group antigen Le^b which is synthesized and secreted by gastric and intestinal mucosa and secondarily attaches to red cell membranes. *Helicobacter* does not bind to blood group A-Le^b cells, accounting for the higher incidence of *Helicobacter*-induced peptic ulcer in blood group O individuals. Group A$_1$ patients with gastrointestinal malignancies or infections may develop B-like red cell antigens and, as a result, may be typed incorrectly as group B.

The **McLeod phenotype** is a Kell variant with weak expression of Kell antigen. It is associated with a syndrome that may include acanthocytosis, mild congenital hemolytic anemia, neuromuscular abnormalities, or such X-linked disorders as chronic granulomatous disease, retinitis pigmentosa and Duchenne-type muscular dystrophy.

The **Rh deficiency syndrome** is present in individuals with Rh deletions, Rh_{null} and Rh_{mod}. Although no specific membrane function has been identified with the Rh proteins, their absence does result in an abnormal red cell membrane that may manifest as stomatocytosis, increased red cell fragility, and a shortened red cell survival. Patients present with a compensated hemolytic anemia of variable severity. The clinical manifestations usually are corrected by splenectomy.

PLATELET ANTIGENS (Table 11-4)

In **post-transfusion purpura** (PTP), Pl^{A1} negative (Pl^{A1-}) individuals become sensitized to blood products from Pl^{A1+} (HPA-1a) donors. The development of Pl^{A1} antibodies induces severe thrombocytopenia in the recipient. The mechanism is unclear, as the antibody (anti-Pl^{A1}) should not react with recipient Pl^{A1-} platelets. The hypotheses proposed to explain this phenomenon include: 1) formation of anti-Pl^{A1}/Pl^{A1} immune complexes that bind non-specifically to the recipient's platelets and result in platelet destruction, 2) transfused Pl^{A1} soluble antigen from the donor plasma is adsorbed to the Pl^{A1-} platelets which then are destroyed by the alloantibody, or 3) an autoantibody, produced in response to an incompatible platelet specific antigen, reacts with all platelets resulting in their destruction and thrombocytopenia.

In **neonatal alloimmune thrombocytopenia** (NATP), a Pl^{A1-} mother develops anti-Pl^{A1} antibodies after a feto-maternal hemorrhage of Pl^{A1} positive fetal platelets. The maternal antibody crosses the placenta and destroys the Pl^{A1+} fetal platelets. The pathogenic process is similar to that of hemolytic disease of the newborn, however, sensitization may occur during the first pregnancy and the firstborn child may be affected. Although other antigens may be involved, the Pl^{A1} system is the most common.

The anti-platelet antibodies that occur in **autoimmune thrombocytopenia** appear to be directed against any of a variety of antigens associated with platelet membranes, including antigenic sites carried on glycoprotein IIb/IIIa, GPIb/IX, GPIa/IIa and GPIV, but distinct from the HPA antigen systems. Autoantibodies that react with membrane proteins or integrins may induce defects in platelet aggregation and clot retraction.

GRANULOCYTE SPECIFIC ALLOANTIBODIES (Table 11-5)

In **alloimmune neonatal neutropenia** (ANN), the mother is immunized to a granulocyte antigen that the fetus has inherited from the father. The maternal antibody crosses the placenta and destroys fetal granulocytes. The mechanism of granulocyte destruction is the same as for HDN and neonatal alloimmune thrombocytopenia. The granulocytopenia is transient; as the maternal IgG antibody disappears, the granulocyte count gradually returns to normal, usually between the ages of 2 weeks to 6 months.

Febrile transfusion reactions may be associated with granulocyte specific antibodies in the recipient.

Transfusion associated lung injury (TRALI) is a severe reaction with acute respiratory distress and pulmonary edema. This syndrome most commonly is associated with the transfusion of plasma containing either antibodies to HLA or neutrophil-specific antibodies that react with recipient granulocytes.

Granulocyte Autoantibodies

Primary autoimmune neutropenia most commonly is seen in children ages 3 to 30 months. The neutropenia resolves spontaneously. Granulocyte specific antibodies are present in the majority of these patients.

Secondary autoimmune neutropenia usually is associated with an autoimmune disease such as Felty's syndrome or systemic lupus erythematosus, or with a malignancy, eg, lymphoma. Laboratory demonstration of these granulocyte-specific antibodies is difficult.

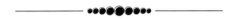

SUGGESTED READING

Bux J. Challenges in the determination of clinically significant granulocyte antibodies and antigens. Trans Med Rev 10:222-232, 1996.

McFarland JG. Platelet immunology and alloimmunization. In: Tossi, SC, Simon TL, Moss GD, Gould SA, editors. Principles of Transfusion Medicine. Baltimore: Williams & Wilkins, pp. 231-244, 1996.

Mollison PL, Engelfriet CP, Contreras, M, editors. Blood Transfusion in Clinical Medicine, 10th edition, Oxford: Blackwell Science, 1997.

Schroeder, ML. Red cell, platelet, and white cell antigens. In: Lee RG, Foerster J, Lukens J, Paraskevas F, Greer, JP and Rodgers GM, editors. Wintrobe's Clinical Hematology, 10th edition. Baltimore: Williams & Wilkins, 1999.

HEME SYNTHESIS AND PORPHYRIN METABOLISM

"Werewolf? ... There wolf!"
[Gene Wilder – Marty Feldman – Young Dr. Frankenstein.]

In plants and animals porphyrins are central to the processes of energy capture, transport, and utilization. Magnesium-porphyrins (chlorophyll) in plants and iron-porphyrins (heme) in animals are the compounds that "make grass green and blood red".

Heme proteins are essential to all mammalian cells. They function to: (1) transport oxygen (hemoglobin and myoglobin), (2) transport electrons (cytochromes), and (3) produce or degrade hydrogen peroxide (peroxidase and catalase). As heme is not transported from cell to cell, the mechanism for heme synthesis is integral to each cell. In man, 80-85% of heme synthesis is devoted to hemoglobin formation during erythropoiesis; the remaining 15-20% is associated largely with the synthesis of cytochromes. The turnover of hemoglobin is slow (3 to 4 months); in contrast, the turnover of the cytochromes is measured in hours or days.

Heme is the iron-complex of protoporphyrin IX. Protoporphyrin IX is composed of four pyrrole rings, a tetrapyrrole, with eight side chains. Of the 15 isomers of protoporphyrin, only protoporphyrin IX is found in nature. (It was the ninth isomer to be identified).

Heme Synthesis

Heme synthesis begins in the mitochondria with the condensation of glycine and succinate (as succinyl CoA), in the presence of the cofactor pyridoxal 5′-phosphate, to form *δ-aminolevulinic acid* (ALA). The enzyme catalyzing this reaction is **ALA synthase (ALAS) (1)** (numbers refer to Figure 12-1). ALAS is rate limiting to the remainder of the cascade. The first enzyme (1) and the last three (6) (7) (8) are intramitochondrial; the intervening steps (2) (3) (4) (5) take place in the cytosol.

ALA moves from the mitochondria into the cytosol where **ALA dehydratase (2)** catalyzes the condensation of two molecules of ALA to form the monopyrrole ring compound *porphobilinogen* (PBG) – the building block for tetrapyrroles. **PBG deaminase (3)** removes the NH_2 side chain; the subsequent condensation of four pyrroles forms the linear tetrapyrrole *hydroxymethylbilane* (HMB). This linear tetrapyrrole then cyclyzes, either enzymatically or spontaneously, to produce *uroporphyrinogen.*

In the presence of **uroporphyrinogen III synthase (4)**, the fourth pyrrole of HMB is reversed to form the porphyrin ring of *uroporphyrinogen III*. When this enzyme is absent or decreased (4-), as in congenital erythropoietic porphyria, HMB cyclyzes non-enzymatically without reversing the fourth pyrrole, and the alternate isomer, *uroporphyrinogen I*, is formed. This

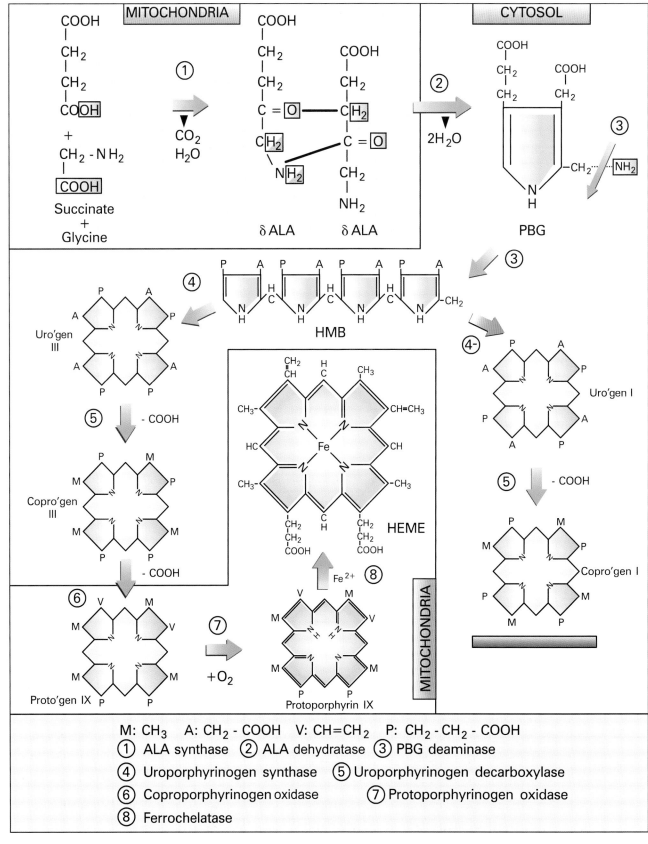

Figure 12-1 Heme Synthesis

latter pathway dead-ends at *coproporphyrinogen I* with accumulation of the two toxic photosensitizing oxidized products *uroporphyrin I* and *coproporphyrin I*.

In the physiological pathway, decarboxylation yields the reduced colourless intermediates, *coproporphyrinogen III* (5) and *protoporphyrinogen IX* (6); the latter is oxidized to *protoporphyrin IX* (7). The final step is the insertion of iron into *protoporphyrin IX* by the enzyme **ferrochelatase** (8) to form *heme*.

The biosynthetic pathway intermediates are in the reduced porphyrinogen state; they are colourless and cannot be photoactivated. The oxidized derivatives, the porphyrins, are purple in colour and absorb intensely near 400 nm in the long ultra-violet portion of the spectrum. On exposure to the exciting wave-length, the porphyrins are photoactivated, fluoresce, and the energy released in the form of singlet oxygen ($^1O_2$) produces tissue damage. The deposition of porphyrins in skin results in photosensitivity.

The early products, *ALA* and *PBG*, are water soluble and are excreted in the urine, as are the highly carboxylated porphyrins (uroporphyrin and the incompletely decarboxylated coproporphyrin). With stepwise decarboxylation, water solubility decreases so that the more fully decarboxylated coproporphyrins and the protoporphyrins are excreted in bile into the stool.

Regulation of Heme Synthesis

As an integral component of the electron transport cytochrome system, heme is a vital constituent of all body cells. Because preformed heme cannot be transported from cell to cell, each cell is dependent on its own synthetic supply. There are two major sites of heme production – 80% of total body heme synthesis takes place in red cell precursors, 10% in hepatocytes. The same precursors and intermediate products are present at all sites and synthesis is regulated by the same rate-limiting enzyme ALAS. There are two isoforms of this enzyme: the ALAS1 gene on chromosome-3 is expressed ubiquitously, ALAS2 (on the X chromosome) is restricted to erythropoietic cells. Different mechanisms regulate these two isoenzymes: in erythropoietic cells, heme synthesis is controlled by the supply of iron; in hepatocytes and other non-erythroid cells, the control depends upon the intracellular content of heme (Figure 12-2).

Heme regulation of ALAS1 depends on three mechanisms: suppression of ALAS1 gene transcription, reduction of the half-life of the ALAS1 mRNA and, at the post-transcriptional level, inhibition of ALAS1 translocation from the cytoplasm into the mitochrondrial matrix. ALAS1 can be downregulated by the infusion of heme. ALAS1 synthesis can be upregulated by drugs and chemicals (eg, barbiturates) that are metabolized via the cytochrome p450 pathway; these agents are inducers of cytochrome p450 – the increase in these heme-containing cytochromes requires upregulation of hepatic ALAS1 synthesis. The role of these controls can be seen in the clinical setting: drugs that induce cytochrome p450 exacerbate the clinical expression of acute intermittent porphyria (AIP) as ALAS1 is increased; the therapeutic use of heme to

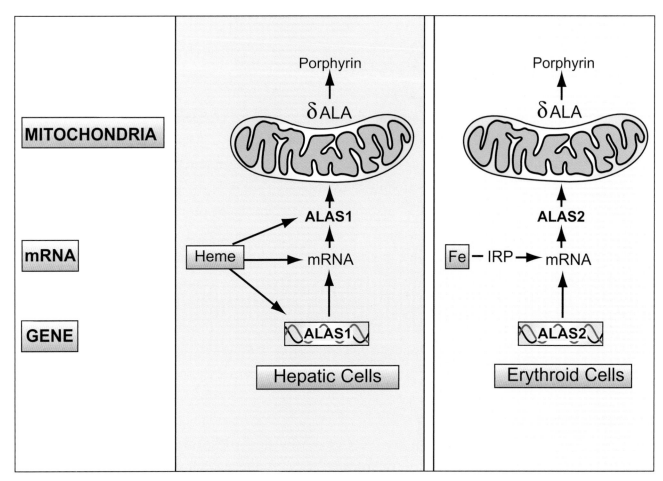

Figure 12-2   Regulation of ALAS1 and ALAS2

downregulate ALAS1 reduces AIP symptoms (see below).

Due to its potential toxicity, it is imperative that during erythropoiesis protophorphyrin production does not exceed the requirements of heme synthesis – and this depends upon the availability of iron. The balance is achieved through iron regulation of ALAS2: when cytosolic iron is available, porphyrin synthesis proceeds expeditiously; when cytosolic iron is low, porphyrin synthesis decreases. There is a unique iron responsive element (IRE) on the 5′ untranslated region of the mRNA for ALAS2 (Figure 12-3). This IRE is recognized by an iron-regulatory protein (IRP) in a manner similar to that which regulates ferritin synthesis (Section 15). In the presence of low cytosolic iron, the iron depleted IRP binds to the mRNA IRE, suppressing the mRNA and ALAS2 synthesis. In the iron replete cell, the IRP is iron-rich and the suppression is lifted, increasing ALAS2 production and porphyrin synthesis. In iron deficiency anemia, although there is some increase in red cell protoporphyrin, this control mechanism ensures that the level remains well below that responsible for the photodynamic effects seen in erythropoietic porphryia.

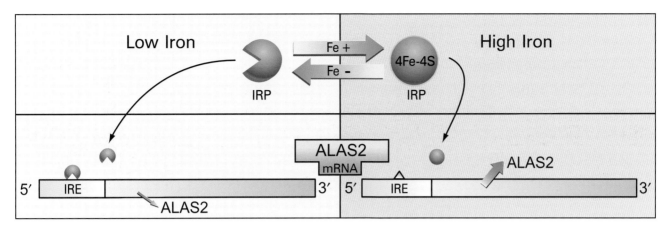

Figure 12-3 Regulation of ALAS2 in Erythropoietic Cells

CLINICAL CORRELATES

THE PORPHYRIAS

These hereditary diseases, characterized by deficiencies in the conversion of the intermediates to end product heme, are due to mutations in the enzymes of the synthetic pathway. Most of these disorders are inherited as autosomal dominants; one exception is the autosomal recessive congenital erythropoietic porphyria. The clinical syndromes result from the accumulation of products behind the metabolic block. The symptoms are those of photosensitivity if the accumulated products are porphyrins, or neurovisceral if the accumulated products are ALA and PBG.

The porphyrias are classified according to whether the major defect in porphyrin metabolism occurs in hepatic cells or in red cell precursors (Table 12-1).

Hepatic Porphyrias

Acute Intermittent Porphyria (AIP). This is an autosomal dominant metabolic disease due to the reduced activity of **PBG deaminase (3)**. Although it is one of the most common of the hereditary porphyrias, many individuals remain clinically asymptomatic unless expression is precipitated by environmental, nutritional or hormonal events. The defect may be amplified, with the induction of the rate-limiting enzyme **ALAS1 (1),** by hormonal stimuli (eg, synthetic estrogens and progesterone) or drugs that induce cytochrome p450. (Induction of heme and cytochrome synthesis in liver is a normal protective mechanism for xenobiotic detoxification and hormonal clearance). The onset or exacerbation of this disease can be precipitated by drugs, such as barbiturates and dilantin, that induce cytochrome p450 – the enhanced demand for heme synthesis upregulates ALAS1 and, as a result, there is increased ALA and PBG synthesis and accumulation behind the metabolic block. As ALA and PBG increase, neurovisceral symptoms appear, including abdominal pain, sensory and motor neuron dysfunction, and psychiatric symptoms. ALA and PBG are excreted in the urine; PBG is a colourless compound that turns brown or black on oxidation to porphobilin. As no excess porphyrin is produced, there is no associated light sensitivity. The acute episode may be terminated by the intravenous infusion of heme (as hematin or heme arginate) which down-regulates ALAS1 with reduction of ALA and PBG synthesis. Similar symptoms have been described in the rare cases of autosomal recessive congenital **ALA dehydratase (2)** deficiency; ALA appears in the urine with little accompanying PBG. The presence of neurotoxic symptoms suggest the importance of ALA as the neurotoxin.

Porphyria Cutanea Tarda (PCT). This disorder is the result of a deficiency of **uroporphyrinogen decarboxylase (5)**; the urinary excretion product is primarily *uroporphyrin III*. The genetic defect, inherited as an autosomal dominant, is present in about 50% of patients – most of these cases are heterozygotes with half the normal amount of uroporphorinogen decarboxylase in all tissues. Expression of this disorder is usually delayed ("tarda") until midlife or later. The major clinical manifestation is photosensitivity. Symptoms are exacerbated by liver disease (hepatitis C), alcohol and iron overload. Sporadic PCT may be associated with hereditary hemochromatosis. As a result of hepatic cell dysfunction due to the iron overload, uroporphyrinogen decarboxylase is decreased, precipitating or exacerbating the clinical disease;

Table 12-1   The Porphyrias

Type	Enzyme Deficiency	Metabolite Excretion Urine	Stool	Photo-sensitivity	Neurovisceral Disease
Hepatic					
AIP - acute intermittent porphyria	PBG deaminase ③	ALA, PBG	–	–	+++
PCT - porphyria cutanea tarda	URO decarboxylase ⑤	URO III	–	+	–
HCP - hereditary coproporphyria	COPRO oxidase ⑥	ALA, PBG, URO III	COPRO III	+	+
VP - variegate porphyria	PROTO oxidase ⑦	ALA, PBG, URO III	COPRO III PROTO	+	+
Erythropoietic					
CEP - congenital erythropoietic porphyria	URO III synthase ④	URO I	COPRO I	++++	–
EPP - erythropoietic protoporphyria	Ferrochelatase ⑧	–	PROTO IX	++	–
Lead Poisoning	ALA dehydratase ② Ferrochelatase ⑧	ALA, URO III, COPRO III	+ –	–	++

⑤
URO I → COPRO I

GLYCINE → ALA → PBG → HMB → URO III → COPRO III → PROTO → PROTO IX → HEME
+   ①   ②   ③   ④   ⑤   ⑥   ⑦   ⑧
SUCCINATE

depletion of hepatic iron stores by phlebotomy can induce clinical and biochemical remission. PCT also can occur in genetically normal individuals upon toxic exposure to inhibitors of uroporphyrinogen decarboxylase such as hexachlorbenzene or dioxin.

Hereditary Coproporphyria (HCP). The deficient enzyme is **coproporphyrinogen-oxidase** (6). The accumulated *coproporphyrin III* is excreted in both urine and stool. During acute exacerbations, *ALA*, *PBG* and *uroporphyrin* also are excreted. Symptoms are those of AIP plus photosensitivity.

Variegate Porphyria (VP). This disease is due to deficient **protoporphyrinogen oxidase** (7). During acute episodes, the accumulated products, *protoporphyrin* and *coproporphyrin,* are excreted in the stool, and *ALA*, *PBG* and *uroporphyrin* in the urine. The manifestations are photosensitivity plus the neurovisceral symptoms of AIP. The incidence is high in a South African population descended from an original Dutch colonist who carried the defective gene. This is presumed to be the disease that affected King George III and contributed to England's loss of its American colonies.

Erythropoietic Porphyrias

Congenital Erythropoietic Porphyria (CEP). The deficiency of **uroporphyrinogen III synthase** (4) diverts the pathway toward *uroporphyrin I* and *coproporphyrin I.* Because this pathway terminates at coproporphyrin I, there is a major accumulation of uroporphyrin I and coproporphyrin I in the normoblasts in the bone marrow (these cells exhibit intense red fluorescence when viewed under U-V light). As these cells break down, the released porphyrins enter the blood and are widely distributed throughout the tissues, including skin where their presence results in severe photosensitivity. Although the level of uro III synthase is low, it is sufficient to maintain heme and hemoglobin synthesis. Large amounts of *uroporphyrin I* and *coproporphyrin I* are excreted in urine and stool. Activation of complement components with release of C3a and C5a leads to increased vascular permeability and edema; formation of the membrane attack complex results in tissue destruction. The extreme photosensitivity, marked by extensive skin necrosis, restricts these patients from venturing outdoors; they can do so safely only after dark. This nocturnal life pattern, associated with tissue necrosis, facial disfigurement and hirsutism, may be the basis of the werewolf myth. Inheritance is autosomal recessive. CEP has been described in cattle. It is interesting that the red squirrel has major deposits of *uroporphyrin I* in various tissues but suffers no ill effects. The grey squirrel does not exhibit this anomaly.

Erythropoietic Protoporphyria (EPP). **Ferrochelatase** (8) activity is reduced resulting in overproduction of *protoporphyrin IX* which accumulates in high concentration in red cells, and is excreted in bile into the stool. Photodermatitis results from light activation of the protoporphyrin in exposed skin.

Lead Poisoning

Lead is an inhibitor of most of the enzymes along the heme biosynthetic pathway, the most sensitive of which are **ALA dehydratase (2)** and **ferrochelatase (8)**. ALA accumulates behind the block of ALA dehydratase and appears in the urine. The inhibition of ferrochelatase results in an increase in red cell protoporphyrin and increased excretion of *uroporphyrin III* and *coproporphyrin III*. Some of the symptoms of lead poisoning, abdominal pain, neuropathy and, in some cases, psychotic behaviour, resemble those of acute intermittent porphyria.

ANEMIAS

Iron Deficiency Anemia

In iron deficiency anemia there is insufficient iron to complete the final step in heme synthesis. As a result, *protoporphyrin IX* accumulates in red cell precursors and increased levels are present in mature red cells. Because iron regulates ALAS2 expression, the amount of porphyrin produced in iron deficiency is insufficient to induce a photodynamic effect.

Sideroblastic Anemias

This heterogenous group of anemias is characterized by the presence of ring sideroblasts in the bone marrow. These are nucleated erythroblasts with a perinuclear distribution of Prussian blue positive iron-laden mitochondria – mitochondrial ferritin is increased. (The structure and control of mitochondrial ferritin differs from that of cytosolic ferritin). The disorder is the result of failure of the final mitochondrial steps in heme synthesis. Although heme synthesis is decreased, iron uptake by the erythroblast is not down-regulated. The erythroid hyperplasia in the bone marrow is a sign of ineffective erythropoiesis and is associated with increased iron absorption.

The most clearly defined entity is the hereditary X-linked sideroblastic anemia due to a mutation of the ALAS2 gene; more than 25 mutations have been identified. The missense mutations result in a reduction in ALA synthesis and reduced porphyrin production. Most mutations are in the region of the ALAS2 molecule that determines the binding of pyridoxal 5-phosphate; the result is decreased affinity for this cofactor. These patients may respond to pyridoxine with an increase in ALAS2 activity. The degree of anemia is variable but, because of the impaired heme synthesis, the red cells are hypochromic and microcytic. Total body iron is increased. Although the mechanism is unclear, the ineffective erythropoiesis leads to increased intestinal absorption of iron. The development of iron overload results in a clinical course indistinguishable from hereditary hemochromatosis (Section 15).

Acquired sideroblastic anemia may be associated with myelodysplastic syndromes and may accompany alcohol or drug myelotoxicity. Both alcohol and isoniazid deplete the ALAS cofactor pyridoxal phosphate; the accompanying anemia may respond to pyridoxine.

PORPHYRIN DERIVATIVES IN THE DETECTION AND TREATMENT OF CANCER

Porphyrins and porphyrin derivatives tend to accumulate in tissues where metabolic activity is high, including some tumors and tumor vasculature. The reason for this is unclear. Synthetic porphyrins (hematoporphyrins and hematoporphyrin derivatives – HPD) have been used for tumor detection and treatment. When a porphyrin molecule absorbs light, it either emits a photon at a longer wavelength or transforms an oxygen molecule to an active state; the fluorescent effect permits localization of tumors, and the oxidizing effect of singlet oxygen has the potential to damage cells.

Following intravenous infusion, the synthetic HPD becomes localized in the tumor and tumor vasculature; superficial lesions fluoresce under UV light (400 nm) because of the photodynamic activation at the Soret band in the near ultraviolet. HPD can be used to identify superficial tumors in bladder, lung, or gastrointestinal tract. Tumor cell kill is minimal, however, because tissue penetration of visible or UV light approximates 1 mm. With the use of light or lasers at long infrared wavelengths, tissue penetration is increased – newer agents that absorb at 760 to 800 nm are activated by deeper penetrating infrared wavelengths. Cell kill results from photodynamic activation of O_2 with formation of the highly reactive singlet oxygen in tumor microvasculature and tumor cell cytoplasm, lysosomes and mitochondria. Tumor cells may die by necrosis or by apoptosis secondary to mitochondrial damage.

SUGGESTED READING

Bottomley SS, Muller-Eberhard U. Pathophysiology of heme synthesis. Semin Hematol 25:282-302, 1988.

Fitzsimons EJ, May A. The molecular basis of the sideroblastic anemias. Curr Opin Hematol 3:167-172, 1996.

Gomer CJ. Photodynamic therapy in the treatment of malignancies. Semin Hematol 26:27-34, 1989.

Kushner JP. Laboratory diagnosis of the porphyrias. N Engl J Med 324:1432-1434, 1991.

May BK, Bawden MJ. Control of heme biosynthesis in animals. Semin Hematol 26:150-156, 1989.

Melfors O, Hentze MW. Iron regulatory factor - the conductor of cellular iron regulation. Blood Rev 7:251-258, 1993.

Moore MR. Biochemistry of porphyria. Int J Biochem 25:1353-1368, 1993.

Mustajoki P, Tenhunen R, Pierach C, Volin L. Heme in the treatment of porphyrias and hematological disorders. Semin Hematol 26:1-9, 1989.

Pass HI. Photodynamic therapy in oncology: mechanisms and clinical use. J Nat Cancer Inst 85:443-456, 1993.

Ponka P. Cell biology of heme. Am J Med Sci 318:241-256, 1999.

Roberts AW, Whatley SD, Morgan RR, Worwood M, Elder GH. Increased frequency of haemochromatosis Cys 282 Tyx mutation in sporadic porphyria cutanea tarda. Lancet 349:321-323, 1997.

Sassa S. Diagnosis and therapy of acute intermittent porphyria. Blood Rev 10:53-58, 1996.

Straka JG, Rank JM, Bloomer JR. Porphyria and porphyrin metabolism. Annu Rev Med 41:457-469, 1990.

THE HEMOGLOBIN MOLECULE

"Haemoglobin or haemoglobulin consists of an albumen and
a colouring matter haematin."
Wagners General Pathology, 1876

This oxygen transport protein constitutes 90% of the dry weight of the red cell. Its intracellular location and intrinsic properties make possible the utilization of some 250 ml of O_2 per minute in the normal adult at rest. The structure of the hemoglobin molecule, dictated by various genes at multiple genetic loci, has a roughly spherical configuration with a molecular weight of 64,500. Hemoglobin consists of two pairs of polypeptide (globin) chains. These polypeptide chains consist of groups of 8 α-helical segments interrupted by linear portions to permit folding. The primary globin chains in the adult are α and β; the assembled hemoglobin tetramer, with its two alpha chains and two beta chains, is designated $\alpha_2\beta_2$. Each chain is non-covalently bound to a single heme group that sits in a hydrophobic pocket. As each heme group can bind a single oxygen molecule, the hemoglobin tetramer can reversibly bind and transport 4 molecules of oxygen. In addition to transporting oxygen to the tissues, hemoglobin delivers CO_2 to the lung and nitric oxide (NO) to the tissues.

Globin Synthesis

The globin polypeptides are synthesized in erythropoietic cells. The paired globin chains are designed by the selective expression of genes on chromosomes 16 and 11 (Figure 13-1). The **alpha gene family**, on chromosome 16, consists of three genes: one zeta (ζ) and two alpha genes (α_2 and α_1); α_2 and α_1 are identical, represent gene duplication, and produce identical α chains. The beta family, on chromosome 11, has five genes: epsilon (ϵ) expressed only in early embryonic life; two gamma (γ) genes that code for γ chains with a single amino acid difference at position 136, (either glycine (Gγ) or alanine (Aγ), a difference that has no functional significance); the delta (δ) gene; and the beta (β) gene. In addition to the exons that dictate the primary structure, promoters 5$'$ to the coding sequence and enhancers in the non-coding regions govern gene transcription, fidelity, and stability of the message. Heme also has a role in the control of globin synthesis: in iron deficiency with reduced heme synthesis there may be selectively reduced globin chain production yielding hypochromic, microcytic red cells – a morphology shared by thalassemia and iron deficiency anemia.

The chronological expression of the globin genes during development in the fetus and newborn roughly follows the gene sequence on the two chromosomes. The defects in globin chain synthesis in the thalassemias are most easily understood by retracing the ontogeny of the molecule. The earliest embryonic hemoglobins synthesized by the erythroblasts in the yolk sac and liver are $\zeta_2\epsilon_2$ (**Gower 1**), $\zeta_2\gamma_2$ (**Portland**), followed by $\alpha_2\epsilon_2$ (**Gower 2**). By week 12 this embryonic form is replaced by $\alpha_2\gamma_2$ (fetal hemoglobin – **Hb F**). The definitive adult β chain comes on line as synthesis moves to erythroblasts in spleen and bone marrow; $\alpha_2\beta_2$ (**Hb A**) increases to replace 25% of $\alpha_2\gamma_2$ (Hb F) at birth, with further increases to 96-97% of circulating hemoglobin by one year of age. Small amounts of $\alpha_2\delta_2$ (**Hb A$_2$**) appear late in gestation.

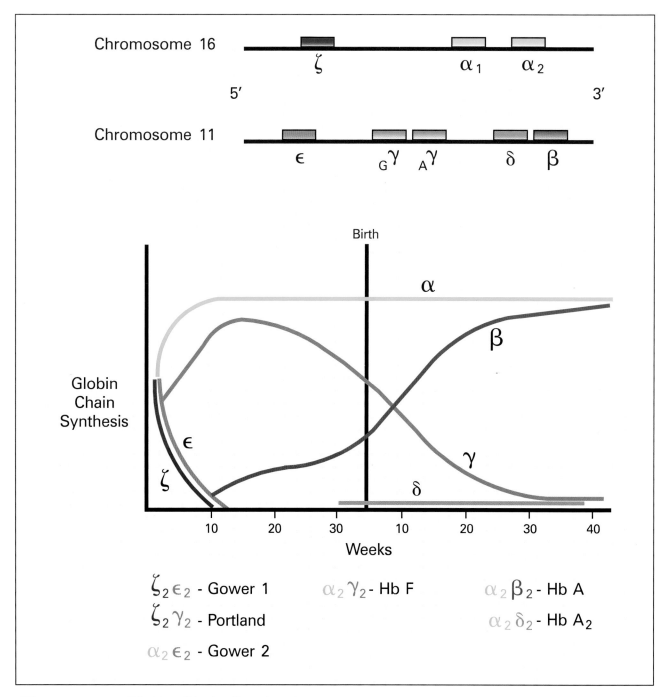

Figure 13-1 Globin Chain Synthesis

Although Hb F and Hb A_2 persist in the normal adult, they account for less than 4% of the total hemoglobin. Throughout normal fetal and adult life there is a balanced expression of the α gene group and the β gene group. The α and β components first combine as $\alpha\beta$ dimers, then spontaneously aggregate to form the hemoglobin tetramer. The tetramer is highly soluble, unpaired globin chains are not; precipitation of residual unpaired chains compromises red cell survival. Small discrepancies in balanced chain production are managed by protease degradation of the excess globin chain. When the discrepancy is major, as in the thalassemias, red cell viability is compromised.

Hemoglobin Structure and Function

Hemoglobin interacts with three diffusable ligands, O_2, CO_2, and NO. Interactions with these molecules result in delivery of oxygen to the tissues, elimination of CO_2 through the lungs, and control of vascular tone by NO.

Hemoglobin and Oxygen. The hemoglobin molecule is designed uniquely for the transport of O_2 from lung to peripheral tissues without oxidation of its heme carrier (i.e. the iron remains in the ferrous state). The two primary units of the molecule, the $\alpha\beta$ dimers, aggregate to form the $\alpha_2\beta_2$ tetramer; the region where the two dimers come into contact is known as the $\alpha_1\beta_2$ region. The dimers have the capacity to rotate on each other along the $\alpha_1\beta_2$ axis to increase and decrease inter-dimer distance, a mechanism that facilitates the uptake and release of O_2. The hemoglobin molecule essentially "breathes in and out" as it takes up and releases O_2. Between the two β chains is the binding site for **2,3 bisphosphoglycerate (2,3 BPG)**, synthesized in the red cell through the Rapoport-Luebering shunt (Section 10). 2,3 BPG is a major regulator of O_2 affinity. As a consequence of 2,3 BPG binding, hemoglobin affinity for oxygen decreases: it moves from an oxygenated to a deoxygenated state as O_2 is released into the tissues.

Hemoglobin exists in two alternating conformations – the **T (taut)** and the **R (relaxed)** states (Figure 13-2). The T (deoxygenated) state has a relatively low O_2 affinity, the R (oxygenated) state has a high O_2 affinity (500 times that of the molecule in its T conformation). As it picks up O_2 in the lung, hemoglobin moves from the T to the R configuration. (The globin units of deoxyhemoglobin are held by electrostatic bonds in a tense conformation.Binding of oxygen induces chemical and mechanical changes that break these electrostatic bonds to produce the relaxed conformation).

In the lung, as "heme one" takes up "O_2 one", it facilitates the uptake of "O_2 two" by "heme two" and so on through hemes "three" and "four" (i.e. once the first oxygen molecule is taken up by hemoglobin, the reaction rate of O_2 with the remaining hemes is accelerated – the transition from low to high affinity). This is reflected in the steeply rising section of the sigmoid

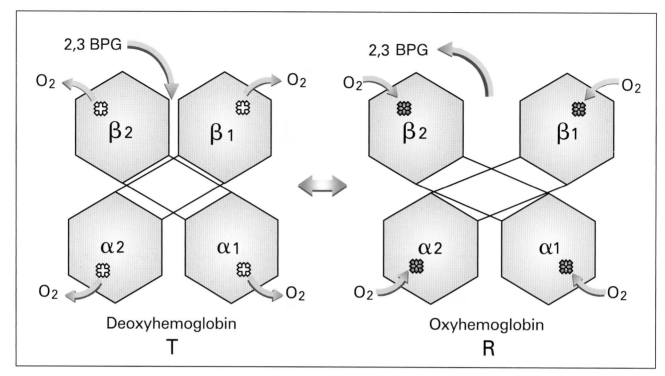

Figure 13-2 Hemoglobin Molecule

O_2 **dissociation curve** (Figure 13-3). With the transition from the T to the R form, the inter-dimer space increases, salt bridges are broken, 2,3 BPG is displaced and O_2 is bound. On reaching the peripheral tissues, in the reverse process, 2,3 BPG re-inserts itself into the pocket between the two β chains, the hemes surrender O_2, the dimers come closer together, the salt bridges reform, and the hemoglobin assumes the T configuration.

Hemoglobin and Carbon Dioxide. In the tissues, CO_2 diffuses freely into the red cell. About 10% binds directly to the amino terminus of the globin chain to form carbaminohemoglobin in a non-enzymatic process. Most of the CO_2 is hydrated by carbonic anhydrase to H_2CO_3, then converted to H^+ and HCO_3^-. The H^+ proton is accepted by hemoglobin, resulting in stabilization of hemoglobin in the T configuration and enhanced O_2 release. CO_2 is carried in the blood primarily as bicarbonate (HCO_3^-). The anion exchange protein (**AE1**), **band 3** in the red cell membrane, is a chloride-bicarbonate exchanger that allows HCO_3^- to cross the membrane in exchange for Cl^-. By making the red cell membrane freely permeable to HCO_3^-, AE1 increases the amount of CO_2 that the blood can deliver to the lungs. (AE1 is a multipass transmembrane protein that traverses the membrane up to 14 times; at approximately one million copies, it is the most abundant membrane protein.) About 80% of CO_2 is transported as bicarbonate (primarily in the plasma as the bicarbonate moves out of the red cell), 10% as carbaminohemoglobin, and 10% in solution. This O_2-CO_2 interaction is a major factor in CO_2 uptake and O_2 release in peripheral tissues. In the lung, the process is reversed: as the hemoglobin is oxygenated, the bound CO_2 is released and converted to HCO_3^-;

CO_2 carried in the plasma as bicarbonate readily diffuses into the alveoli.

Hemoglobin and Nitric Oxide (NO). Hemoglobin is a high-affinity carrier of nitric oxide. NO is synthesized by endothelial cells. Free NO that enters the circulation is scavenged by hemoglobin. In the relatively hypoxic venous blood, Hb is in the T configuration and NO diffusing into the red cell is taken up rapidly by heme. Most of this NO is converted immediately to nitrate. On entering the lung, as Hb takes up oxygen and assumes the R structure, a small fraction of heme-bound NO is shifted intramolecularly to the 93β cysteine residue (a highly reactive site when Hb is in the R configuration). NO binds to a thiol (SH) group on 93β cysteine to form S-nitrosohemoglobin (SNO-Hb). Oxygen release in peripheral tissue begins in the precapillary arterioles, resulting in the allosteric R→T transition of the hemoglobin molecule. This conformational change promotes binding of SNO-Hb to the membrane anion exchange protein AE1, with formation of SNO-AE1. SNO is transferred out of the cell and delivered to the vessel wall, inducing vasodilation and increased blood flow within the precapillary arterioles. Co-ordination of vasodilation with O_2 release ensures optimum tissue oxygenation. (In this capacity, NO also is referred to as endothelial-derived relaxing factor (EDRF), a term originally introduced to describe this activity before it had been identified with NO.)

Oxygen Affinity. The percentage saturation of hemoglobin at different oxygen tensions is described by the oxygen dissociation curve. The heme-heme co-operation sequence results in

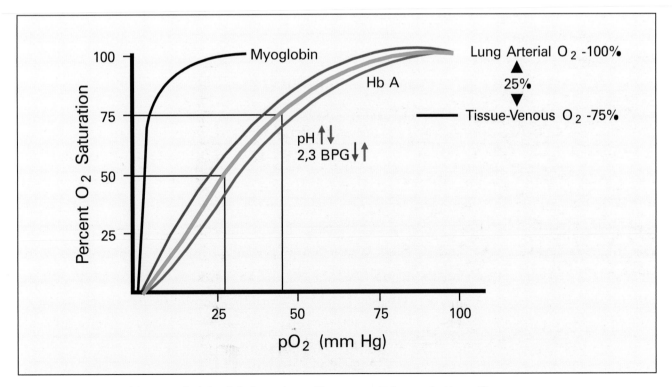

Figure 13-3 Hemoglobin Molecule - Oxygen Dissociation Curve

an O_2 dissociation curve that is sigmoid in shape. The interaction of the heme groups allows 100% saturation in the lungs at an arterial partial pressure of oxygen (pO_2) of 95 mmHg, and desaturation in the peripheral tissues at a pO_2 of 40 mmHg (venous blood) to 75% O_2 saturation – hemoglobin having released 25% of its O_2 load. In the laboratory, O_2 affinity is determined by measuring the partial pressure at which Hb is half-saturated, the p50. For normal HbA the p50 is approximately 28 mmHg (Figure 13-3).

Comparison of the O_2 dissociation curve of hemoglobin with that of **myoglobin** (the oxygen carrying protein of muscle cells) provides a graphic explanation for the different roles of these two heme proteins. Myoglobin is a monomer that has a similar globin and an identical heme unit to that of the monomeric units of hemoglobin but lacks both heme-heme interaction and 2,3 BPG participation. Because of its very low p50 (1-2 mmHg) and high O_2 affinity, it functions efficiently in taking O_2 from hemoglobin and passing it along to the mitochondria in its cell. However, because of its very high avidity for O_2, myoglobin could not function as an intermediate O_2 transporter – the role performed so well by the hemoglobin molecule.

The oxygen affinity of hemoglobin in the red cell is influenced by a number of modifiers. The O_2 dissociation curve is moved to the right (increased O_2 release – i.e. decreased affinity) by the binding of more 2,3 BPG and a drop in pH (acidosis), to the left (decreased O_2 release – i.e. increased affinity) as the pH rises and 2,3 BPG binding falls. HbF binds 2,3 BPG less avidly than does HbA, consequently its oxygen dissociation curve lies to the left of HbA. In placental gas exchange, this increased O_2 affinity of HbF is an advantage in moving O_2 from mother to fetus.

CLINICAL CORRELATES

CONGENITAL ALTERATIONS IN HEMOGLOBIN

Defects In Globin Chain Synthesis

Defective globin chain synthesis, one of the most common genetic disorders, is responsible for a heterogeneous group of inherited anemias termed *thalassemia*. In this syndrome the failure to synthesize normal α or β chains results in decreased hemoglobin synthesis and red cells that are hypochromic and microcytic. Normal hemoglobin tetramers are highly soluble, but unpaired chains are not. With unbalanced chain synthesis, the non-paired globin chains adhere to the cytoskeleton in the erythropoietic cell. The result is either early cell death (ineffective erythropoiesis), or rapid removal of the abnormal red cells from the peripheral circulation (hemolysis) as the impaired deformability of the more rigid red cell membrane results in splenic trapping.

Table 13-1 The Thalassemias

Alpha Thalassemia	α genes	Globin Chains	Hemoglobin	Anemia
Normal	$\alpha\alpha/\alpha\alpha$	$\alpha_2\beta_2$	A	None
Silent Carrier	$\alpha\alpha/\alpha-$	$\alpha_2\beta_2$	A	None
Trait	$\alpha-/\alpha-$ $--/\alpha\alpha$	$\alpha_2\beta_2$	A	Mild
Hb H disease	$--/-\alpha$	$\alpha_2\beta_2, \beta_4$	A, H	Intermediate
Hydrops fetalis	$--/--$	$\gamma_4,$ $\zeta_2\gamma_2$	Barts Portland	Lethal
Beta Thalassemia	**β genes**	**Globin Chains**	**Hemoglobin**	**Anemia**
Normal	β/β	$\alpha_2\beta_2$	A	None
Thalassemia minor	β^+/β β°/β	$\alpha_2\beta_2, \alpha_2\delta_2, \alpha_2\gamma_2$	A, A$_2$, F	Mild
Thalassemia major	β^+/β^+ β°/β°	$\alpha_2\beta_2, \alpha_2\delta_2, \alpha_2\gamma_2$ $\alpha_2\gamma_2, \alpha_2\delta_2$	A, A$_2$, F F, A$_2$	Severe Severe
HPFH *	γ/γ	$\alpha_2\gamma_2$	F	Mild

* — Hereditary persistence of fetal hemoglobin
β° — nonfunctional
β^+ — partial function

The thalassemias are classified according to whether the defect involves the alpha gene or the beta gene family. Some 200 mutations have been described in β thalassemia alone. These molecular anomalies involve both gene exons and introns. The mutations include deletions, point mutations and interruption of the pathways of gene transcription, mRNA processing and translation.

The thalassemias are found along a geographical belt extending from Sardinia and Sicily across the Mediterranean, the Middle East, India and into South East Asia. The β thalassemias predominate in the west, the α thalassemias in the east. That they are commonest in malarial areas suggests thalassemia may provide a survival advantage. In Papua New Guinea, some forms of α-thalassemia appear to provide protection against *Plasmodium falciparum* and, possibly, against *Plasmodium vivax* malaria.

Beta-Thalassemia. The defect in β chain synthesis may result in either complete absence (β°) or partial loss of function (β^+). The possible combinations with the variations in hemoglobin synthesis are shown in Table 13-1. When β chain synthesis fails, there is decreased or absent production of Hb A ($\alpha_2\beta_2$); the β chain is replaced in whole or in part by its counterparts on chromosome 11 with an increase in production of δ chain and γ chain, resulting in increased levels of $\alpha_2\delta_2$ (Hb A$_2$) and $\alpha_2\gamma_2$ (Hg F). In heterozygotes (*thalassemia minor*), the product of one normal β gene is sufficient to maintain Hb A synthesis with little or no accumulation of free α chain; although the red cells are hypochromic and microcytic, these individuals usually are not anemic and the shortened red cell survival clinically insignificant. In patients with minimal β chain synthesis (*thalassemia major*), unpaired α chains accumulate, precipitate to form inclusion bodies which damage red cell membranes and are destructive of immature erythroblasts. Consequently, there is ineffective erythropoiesis and reduced red cell survival as the damaged cells are removed in the spleen, producing hemolysis and severe anemia. The severity of disease is related to the degree of globin chain imbalance. Co-inheritance of α-thalassemia ameliorates the severity of β-thalassemia as the degree of globin-chain imbalance is reduced.

Another variant is the *hereditary persistence of fetal hemoglobin* **(HPFH)** in which β chain synthesis is replaced completely by γ chain ($\alpha_2\gamma_2$). As there is no unpaired α chain accumulation in HPFH, anemia is mild (Table 13-1).

Alpha-Thalassemia is the result of the functional loss of alpha gene expression. As there are two alpha genes on chromosome 16 (α_2 and α_1), there are 4 alpha genes per diploid cell; this is expressed as $\alpha\alpha/\alpha\alpha$. The functional deletion of one gene -$\alpha/\alpha\alpha$ produces a silent carrier with 75% of normal α globin production and normal hematological findings. Loss of two genes --/$\alpha\alpha$ or -α/-α, reduces α globin production to 50% – this is designated α-*thalassemia trait*; there is mild anemia and hypochromic microcytic red cells. Deletion of three genes --/-α, designated **HbH disease**, produces a chronic hemolytic anemia of intermediate severity; there is synthesis of both $\alpha_2\beta_2$ (HbA) and β_4 (Hb H). Deletion of all four α globin genes (--/--) results in complete absence of α chain synthesis with in utero synthesis of γ_4 **(Hb Barts)** and smaller amounts of $\zeta_2\gamma_2$ **(Hb Portland)**; death occurs in utero from hydrops fetalis.

Hemoglobinopathies

The thalassemias are genetic errors that result in *quantitative* defects in globin chain production. The hemoglobinopathies are *qualitative* defects of the globin chains; the mutations give rise to amino acid substitutions, deletions, or elongation of the abnormal globin chain. Abnormalities in chain structure are associated with a number of functional defects.

Abnormal solubility. A single amino acid difference can alter radically the form and function of the hemoglobin molecule and produce major clinical disease. A single amino acid substitution in the β chain, as in *HbC* and *HbS,* results in decreased solubility. In HbC, $\beta6$ glutamine is replaced by lysine; in HbS the $\beta6$ glutamine is replaced by valine.

Homozygous **HbC disease** is characterized by intracellular crystallization of hemoglobin and mild hemolysis. The decreased solubility of deoxygenated HbC with deposition of intracellular crystals accounts for the reduced red cell deformability, splenic sequestration and destruction. Tissue oxygenation is normal despite the mild anemia. There is adequate oxygen delivery to peripheral tissues due to the shift of the oxygen dissociation curve to the right. The shift is the result of a low intracellular pH. (The molecular alteration responsible for the low pH is unexplained.) The red cell morphology includes microcytes, target cells, spherocytes, and cells distorted by the presence of crystalline HbC.

Fully oxygenated HbS is as soluble as HbA. Deoxygenated HbS, however, polymerizes and forms insoluble aggregates that distort red cell shape (sickling). With repeated episodes of polymerization, there is damage to the cell membrane and the sickle shape is no longer reversible. In homozygous **HbS (sickle cell disease)**, splenic trapping of the sickled cell results in hemolysis and severe anemia; microvascular occlusion is responsible for the painful crises associated with this disorder.

Unstable hemoglobins. Historically, this abnormality is known as congenital Heinz body hemolytic anemia. It is the result of amino acid substitutions in the globin chains that compromise the heme-globin linkage with displacement of heme outside its normal globin pocket. Oxidation of the displaced heme leads to globin denaturation and precipitation on the red cell membrane **(Heinz bodies)**. These cells possess a more rigid membrane with decreased deformability; they are trapped in the spleen and "pitted" as the macrophages attempt to remove the Heinz bodies. Further damage to the red cell occurs with the release of free heme into the cell and the generation of reactive oxidants. Splenic removal of these cells results in a shortened red cell life span. Although there are over 100 known globin chain substitutions that result in unstable hemoglobins, many produce little or no clinical hemolysis except when the red cells are exposed to additional oxidant stress (eg, infection or oxidant drugs). During periods of intense hemolysis, heme products (dipyrroles) appear in the urine turning it brown or black. Not all of these hemoglobins have an abnormal electrophoretic pattern, therefore, other procedures are required for their identification. As they are relatively less soluble than normal hemoglobin, a rapid and specific diagnostic test is the demonstration of their insolubility in 17% isopropanol.

Increased oxygen affinity. This is due most frequently to amino acid substitutions in the globin chains at sites that govern heme-O_2 interaction. The abnormality may occur in proximity to the heme pocket or may compromise 2,3 BPG binding. The result is impaired O_2 release in the peripheral tissues; the O_2 dissociation curve is shifted to the left with a lower p50 (Figure 13-3). The tissue hypoxia stimulates erythropoietin synthesis, leading to increased red cell production and polycythemia. Tissue hypoxia and polycythemia also are associated with the rare congenital deficiency of 2,3-BPG mutase; the resulting low level of erythrocyte

2,3-BPG impairs peripheral release of O_2: the O_2 dissociation curve is shifted to the left and the p50 is low (Sections 9 and 10).

Decreased oxygen affinity. This is associated with mutations in the globin chains that result in impaired O_2 binding. In the lung, O_2 binding is usually sufficient to maintain hemoglobin saturation at or near 100%. In peripheral tissues, however, oxygen release is increased – the O_2 dissociation curve is shifted to the right and the p50 is high. As tissue requirements are satisfied at a lower hematocrit, erythropoietin production is reduced and hemoglobin levels are below normal values. (This produces "pseudoanemia": the hematocrit is low, but O_2 delivery is normal). The increased levels of peripheral deoxyhemoglobin may manifest as cyanosis although there is no tissue hypoxia and these individuals otherwise are asymtomatic.

Methemoglobin. Heme iron is maintained in the ferrous state (Fe^{2+}) by methemoglobin reductase. Hemoglobin M is due to globin chain substitutions that destabilize the heme pocket and allow oxidation of heme Fe^{2+} to Fe^{3+}. Although many patients present with cyanosis due to the deep brown colour of methemoglobin, the levels of methemoglobin are usually below those associated with clinical symptoms. Other causes of congenital methemoglobinemia include: methemoglobin reductase (cytochrome b_5 reductase) deficiency, and cytochrome b_5 mutations (Section 10).

ACQUIRED ALTERATIONS IN HEMOGLOBIN

Glycosylation. As the red cell ages, hemoglobin undergoes glycosylation of the amino terminal end of the β chain. There are three glycosylated forms, designated by the order of elution on cation-exchange chromatography. Only HbA1C is of clinical significance. It is formed continuously and cumulatively and, normally, accounts for 3.0 to 3.5% of the total hemoglobin – proportionately more in older than in younger cells. The amount of HbA1C in the cell correlates with blood glucose levels over the previous two to three months (given a normal red cell life span): higher glucose levels result in increased Hb glycosylation. In diabetic patients, the HbA1C level is an index of the degree of hyperglycemia during that period.

Methemoglobinemia. Methemoglobin is produced at a slow rate in normal red cells; because the capacity of the red cell methemoglobin reductase exceeds the rate of heme oxidation, less than 1% of hemoglobin is in the ferric state. Acquired methemoglobinemia develops when the methemoglobin-reducing capacity of the red cell (i.e. the methemoglobin reductase) is exceeded. Various oxidizing agents in food or water (eg, nitrites), drugs (eg, sulfonamides), or chemical agents (eg, aniline dyes) are capable of increasing the rate of heme oxidation up to 1000 fold; infants are particularly vulnerable. These agents also may induce oxidative denaturation of hemoglobin and precipitation of free globin chains (Heinz bodies) which attach to the cell membrane and compromise red cell survival – this mechanism is responsible for the accompanying hemolysis often associated with these toxic agents (Section 10).

Carboxyhemoglobin. Carbon monoxide (CO) binds reversibly to heme with an affinity 200 times that of O_2. Although the binding is reversible, the high affinity can produce a HbCO level of 20% with exposure to an environmental concentration of 0.05% for one hour. The bright red colour of HbCO imparts a cherry red colour to the skin in CO poisoning. Treatment is by ventilation with 100% oxygen or by hyperbaric chamber. Chronically increased levels of HbCO are present in smokers. It is significant that pregnant women who smoke have a carboxyhemoglobin level in the range of 6%. This reduces the fetal O_2 saturation from 75 percent to 58 percent!

———————— •••◐●◐•••• ————————

SUGGESTED READING

Bunn HF, Figure 9-1 in Hematology (ed. 5) Beck WS (ed). MIT Press 174, 1991. With kind permission of the author. (Figure 13-1 in this text).

Bunn HF. Pathogenesis and treatment of sickle cell disease. N Engl J Med 337:762-769, 1997.

Curtin PT, Kan YW. The molecular genetics of hemoglobin. Ann N Y Acad Sci 565:1-12,1989.

Higgs DR, Vickers MA, Wilkie AOM, et al. A review of the molecular genetics of the human α-globin gene cluster. Blood 73:1081-1104, 1989.

Higgs DR. The thalassemia syndromes. Q J Med 86:559-564, 1993.

Hsia CCW. Respiratory function of hemoglobin. N Engl J Med 338:239-247, 1998.

Kazazian HH, Jr. The thalassemia syndromes: molecular basis and prenatal diagnosis in 1990. Semin Hematol 27:209-228, 1990.

Olivieri NF. The β-thalassemias. N Engl J Med 341:99-109, 1999.

Pawloski JR, Hess DT, Stamier JS. Export by red blood cells of nitric oxide bioactivity. Nature 409:622-626, 2001.

Prchal JF, Prchal JT. Molecular basis of polycythemia. Curr Opin Hematol 6:100-109, 1999.

Schrier SL. Thalassemia: pathophysiology of red cell changes. Annu Rev Med 45:211-218, 1994.

Serjeant GR. Sickle-cell disease. Lancet 350:725-730, 1997.

Steinberg MH, Benz EJ. Red Blood Cells. In Hematology: Basic Principles and Practice (ed 3) Hoffman R, Benz EJ, Shattil S, Furie B, et al (eds). Churchill Livingston. pp 356-367 and 485-561, 2000.

Wagner PD. The oxyhemoglobin dissociation curve and pulmonary gas exchange. Semin Hematol 11:405-421, 1974.

Weatherall DJ, Clegg JB. Genetic disorders of hemoglobin. Semin Hematol 36:24-37, 1999.

Weatherall DJ. Phenotype-genotype relationships in monogenic disease: lessons from the thalassemias. Nature Genetics 2:245-255, 2001.

Winterbourn CC. Oxidative denaturation in congenital hemolytic anemias: the unstable hemoglobins. Semin Hematol 27:41-50, 1990.

VITAMIN B_{12} AND FOLATE METABOLISM

"Pernicious Anemia – Arsenic, given in the form of Fowler's solution, or in pill, is the drug upon which the vast majority of physicians still rely."
Richard C. Cabot – In Osler's Modern Medicine – Vol. 4, 1908

In the developing red cell, DNA synthesis is dependent upon both cobalamin (vitamin B_{12}) and folate. In the absence of either, the co-ordinated synthesis of DNA, RNA and protein is disrupted. The result is asynchronous maturation of nucleus and cytoplasm – the nuclei are arrested in S or G_2 phase of the cell cycle while hemoglobinization continues. This gives rise to a series of red cell precursors with a distinct morphological pattern: large nuclei with an open-chromatin structure, although the cytoplasm is that of a more mature cell. These cells are described as megaloblasts; the resulting anemia is termed megaloblastic. The cytological events are not confined to the red cell lineage: analogous defects in cell maturation and replication are present in the myeloid and megakaryocyte series as well as in non-hematopoietic cells (eg, epithelial cells of the buccal mucosa, vagina, and gastrointestinal tract).

COBALAMIN (Cbl)

The cobalamins are a series of compounds consisting of three primary domains: (1) a corrin nucleus which is a tetrapyrolle resembling heme with cobalt replacing iron, (2) a nucleotide, and (3) a β group linked to the cobalt; the β group may be CN *(cyanocobalamin), OH (hydroxycobalamin), CH_3 (methylcobalamin),* or *Ado (adenosylcobalamin)* (Figure 14-1). Cyanocobalamin is the crystalline B_{12} produced during laboratory isolation procedures and is the standard therapeutic form. The primary dietary forms are AdoCbl and CH_3Cbl. These cobalamins have similar nutritional properties. The terms cobalamin and vitamin B_{12} are used interchangeably.

The cobalamins are products of bacterial synthesis and reach humans through fish and animal proteins including dairy products. The standard daily diet contains about 5 µg of cobalamin (Cbl), primarily in the Ado and CH_3 forms. The total body stores in adults average 2 to 5 µg. As the daily requirement is 1-2 µg per day, this storage plus an entero-hepatic recirculation are sufficient to maintain Cbl at functional levels for 3 to 5 years should intake or absorption cease.

Absorption

At the acid pH in the stomach, peptic digestion frees Cbl from its non-specific binding to dietary protein. Cbl then rapidly binds to a pepsin-resistant high-affinity **R protein** (R for

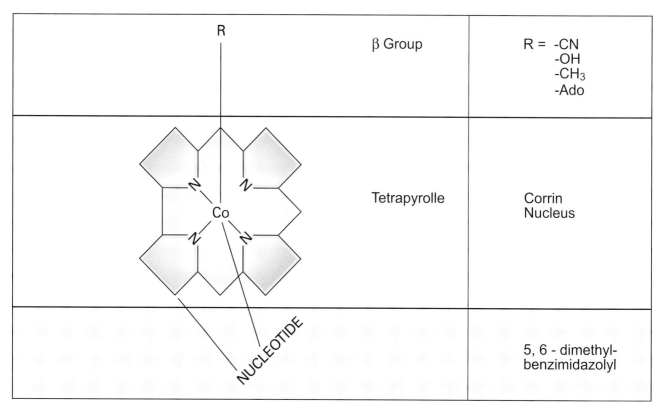

R	β Group	R = -CN -OH -CH$_3$ -Ado
	Tetrapyrrolle	Corrin Nucleus
NUCLEOTIDE		5, 6 - dimethyl- benzimidazolyl

Figure 14-1   Cobalamin Congeners

rapid migration on electrophoresis) present in both saliva and gastric secretions. R protein (**cobalophilin**) has a much higher affinity for Cbl than does *intrinsic factor (IF)*, the specific Cbl-binding glycoprotein produced by gastric parietal cells of the fundus and cardia (Figure 14-2).

In the duodenum, at alkaline pH, the R protein is degraded by pancreatic trypsin. The released Cbl rapidly binds to the C-terminal of the IF that has entered the duodenum along with the Cbl-R complex. IF binds both exogenous Cbl and that re-entering the gut in bile. IF does not bind the inactive Cbl analogues; they are excreted in the stool along with the degraded R proteins. Cbl-IF transits the small bowel; in the terminal ileum, the complex binds to specific Cbl-IF receptors (**cubilin**) on the mucosal cell through the N-terminal binding site of IF. This complex enters the cell by endocytosis where Cbl dissociates from IF; IF is degraded, and Cbl binds to the transport protein **transcobalamin II (TCII)** which carries it into the portal circulation (Fig. 14-2). In the absence of IF, patients will absorb approximately 1% of very large doses (1000 µg) of oral crystalline B$_{12}$. This is of importance in the oral treatment of pernicious anemia and other conditions associated with loss of IF.

Transport

In plasma, there are three Cbl-binding proteins: the transcobalamins – **TC I, TC II** and **TC III**. Approximately 25% of plasma Cbl is bound to TC II, 75% to TC I, and the residual to

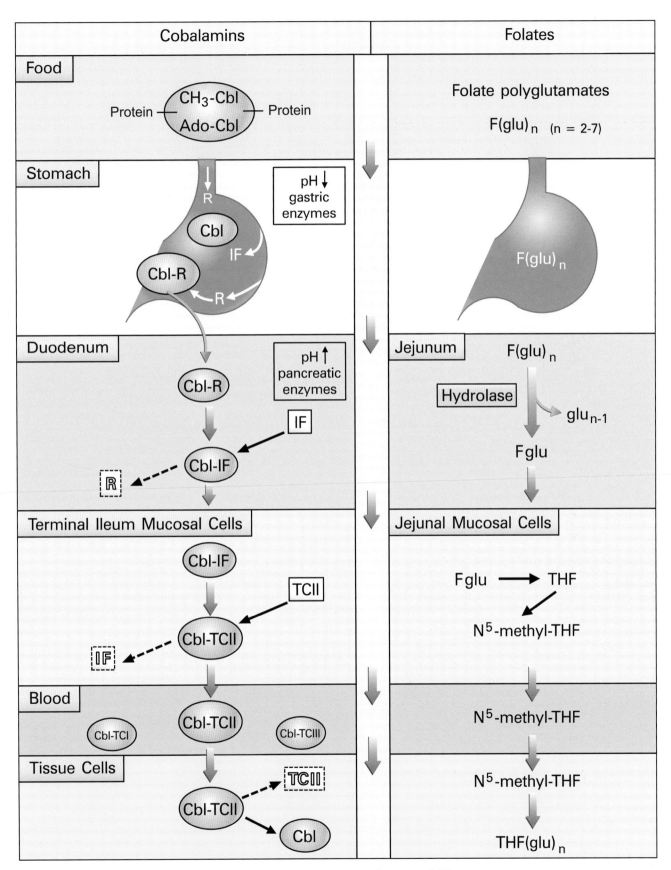

Figure 14-2   Cobalamin and Folate - Absorption and Transport

TC III. TC II, immunologically distinct from the other Cbl-binding proteins, is not an R protein. TC I and TC III are R proteins (cobalophilins) with major homology to the R protein of the saliva and stomach; their function is not clear. TC I-bound Cbl is the major Cbl complex in plasma but the long $t_{1/2}$ of 6-9 days suggests that it does not have a major transport function. TC I probably is derived from the secondary specific granules of mature granulocytes, TC III from earlier granulocyte precursors. Both are increased in patients with high granulocyte counts, accounting for the high serum B_{12} levels in myeloproliferative disorders. TC I and TC III may function as a mechanism for binding and clearance of non-functional cobalamins – these TC I and TC III complexes are cleared by the liver into the bile. In the intestine, functional Cbl is bound by IF and reabsorbed, non-functional analogues are excreted in the stool.

TC II, a 38 kD protein, binds Cbl in a 1:1 molar ratio; it is the specific transport protein for Cbl delivery to systemic cells. Most of the B_{12} in plasma is methyl cobalamin. The cobalt atom in plasma Cbls is in the stable +3 oxidation state (cob(III)alamin). Plasma clearance is rapid ($t_{1/2}$ of 6-9 minutes). For Cbl delivery into cells, TC II-Cbl binds to high-affinity membrane receptors; the complex invaginates the cell membrane and is internalized as an endosome. Within the cell, Cbl is released and TC II is degraded. Intracellular reductases reduce the cobalt atom to the labile +2 or +1 state (cob(II)alamin or cob(I)alamin) before Cbl becomes active as a coenzyme. Most of the Cbl binds to two intracellular enzymes: **methylmalonyl-CoA mutase** and **methionine synthase** – Cbl functions as a coenzyme in these two independent metabolic pathways.

FOLATE

Folic acid *(pteroylmonoglutamate)* consists of three basic segments: (1) a *pteridine* component, (2) a *para-aminobenzoic acid (PABA)* component, and (3) an *L-glutamic acid* residue (Fig. 14-3). It is present in leafy vegetables and animal proteins, and is synthesized by most microorganisms. Although the pharmaceutical product (folic acid) is the monoglutamate *Fglu*, the natural sources primarily are polyglutamates *F(glu)$_n$* with additional glutamic acid residues (n = 2 to 7). The nutritional requirement for adults is approximately 100 µg/day, and up to 500 µg/day during pregnancy. Hepatic folate stores range from 8 to 20 mg. With dietary deprivation, serum levels begin to decline in 3 to 4 weeks and megaloblastic anemia appears in four to six months.

Absorption and Transport

Dietary folates are ingested as polyglutamates but are absorbed as the monoglutamate Fglu. A hydrolase, present in the brush border of jejunal and ileal epithelial cells, deconjugates the polyglutamate $F(glu)_n$ to the monoglutamate Fglu form. The monoglutamate then enters the cell either by simple diffusion or is transported by folate-binding proteins. In the mucosal cell, Fglu is reduced to *tetrahydrofolate (THF)*, then methylated to N^5-*methyl-THF* before release into the portal circulation. Although there is a high-affinity protein binder in plasma, most folate circulates loosely bound to albumin. Normal serum folate levels range from 7 to 25 nmol/L and red cell folate from 430-1200 nmol/L of packed cells. Folate plays no known role in the metabolism of the mature red cell and the level remains relatively unchanged during the life-span of the cell — it probably represents the folate that initially entered the cell during erythropoiesis.

N^5-methyl-THF binds to specific folate receptors on cell membranes; the folate receptors belong to the group of surface molecules attached through the GPI anchor (Section 17). The complex invaginates the membrane to form an endocytotic vesicle. Inside the cell, the N^5-methyl-THF is released into the cytoplasm and the receptor is re-cycled to the membrane. The N^5-methyl group is transferred by a methyl transferase to Cbl and the THF molecule is polyglutamated by a polyglutamate synthase to THF(glu)$_n$. Intracellular retention of folate is dependent upon the formation of *polyglutamates (glu)*$_n$ within the cell. In the absence of polyglutamation, the cell rapidly becomes folate deficient.

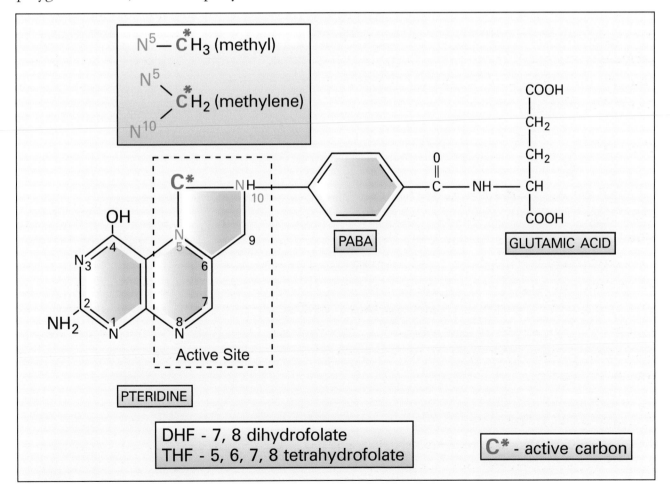

Figure 14-3   Folic Acid

COBALAMIN AND FOLATE IN CELL METABOLISM

The primary role of this system in cell metabolism is the sequential transfer of the single carbon units carried into the cell on the N^5, N^{10} active site of the folate molecule. These carbon units may be carried as methyl (-CH$_3$), methylene (=CH$_2$), formyl (-CHO) or foramino (-CH=NH) groups (Figure 14-3).

Figure 14-4 traces the primary metabolic routes of Cbl and folate in the synthesis of methionine and DNA. Following the entry of N^5-methyl-THF into the cell, the methyl group (*CH$_3$) is transferred to Cbl by a **methyl transferase (methionine synthase)** to form *methyl-Cbl;* with transfer of the methyl group from *N^5-methyl-THF, THF* is formed. The enzyme **polyglutamate synthase** converts THF to its polyglutamated form. THF picks up a methylene group (=*CH$_2$) from *serine*, via **serine methyl transferase,** to form *N^5N^{10}-methylene-THF.* This

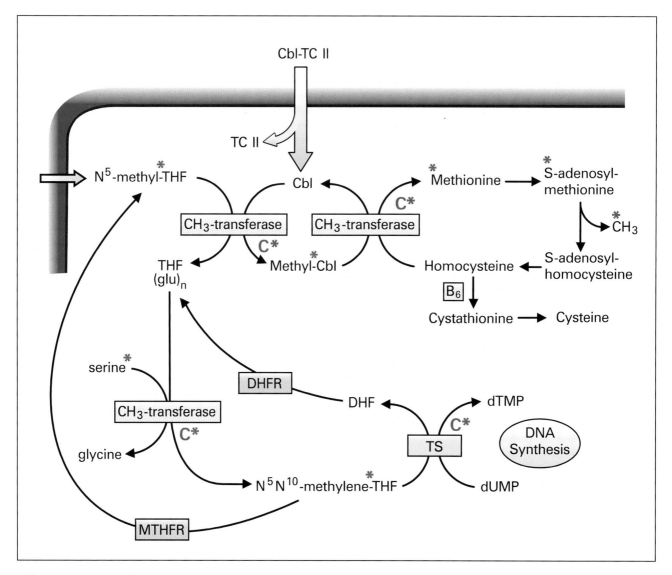

Figure 14-4 Cobalamin-Folate Metabolism

molecule follows two important paths in folate metabolism: (1) N^{5}N^{10}-methylene-THF provides the *CH$_3$ group for the conversion of *deoxyuridine monophosphate (dUMP)* to *deoxythymidine monophosphate (dTMP)* by **thymidylate synthase (TS),** an essential step in DNA synthesis; the demethylated molecule, *dihydrofolate (DHF),* is reduced and recycled to THF by the enzyme **dihydrofolate reductase (DHFR).** (2) N^{5}N^{10}-*methylene-THF* is recycled to N^5-methyl-THF by the enzyme **N^{5}N^{10}-methylene-THF reductase (MTHFR).** This second route supports and amplifies homocysteine metabolism as N^5-methyl-THF is the methyl donor in the homocysteine-methionine cycle.

On entering the cell, Cbl picks up a methyl group from N^5-methyl-THF through the catalytic action of methionine transferase (a methyl transferase) to form methyl Cbl. Methionine transferase then transfers the *CH$_3$ group from methyl cobalamin to homocysteine to form methionine. Methionine is activated by ATP to form S-adenosyl methionine (SAM) – a universal methyl donor (the methyl group is donated to a variety of receptors including nucleic acids). Demethylated SAM is S-adenosyl homocysteine (SAH) – the cycle is complete when SAH is hydrolyzed to homocysteine. (Note: Methionine (methyl-homocysteine) is an essential amino acid derived from dietary sources. There is no exogenous source of homocysteine – it is solely a derivative of methionine metabolism).

Homocysteine may be remethylated to methionine or may undergo transulfuration to cysteine (an irreversible process). In the latter process, homocysteine condenses with serine to form cystathionine in a reaction catalyzed by the vitamin B$_6$-dependent enzyme **cystathionine β synthase**; subsequent hydrolysis converts cystathionine to cysteine. Excess homocysteine is catabolized through this second pathway. Plasma homocysteine levels are increased in both vitamin B$_{12}$ and folate deficiency due to the lack of methyl donors required for the conversion

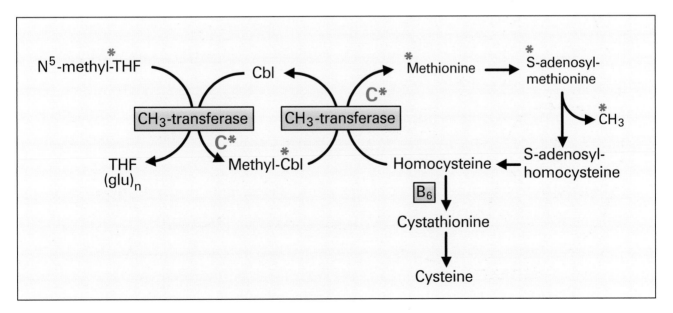

Figure 14-5 Homocysteine Metabolism

of homocysteine to methionine. Hyperhomocysteinemia is a risk factor for vascular thrombotic disease (Section 25).

The absence of Cbl has major consequences: N^5-methyl-THF is not demethylated to THF and, therefore, because polyglutamation cannot occur, N^5-methyl-THF is rapidly lost to the cell; in the absence of THF, there is failure in the transfer of one carbon units with resultant impairment of DNA synthesis. Folate analogues such as *methotrexate (MTX- 4-amino-N^{10}-methyl pteroylglutamic acid)* block DHFR activity thus rapidly depleting the cell of THF; the affinity of MTX for DHFR is some 10,000 times that of DHF. This is the basis of the antiproliferative antitumour effects of the folate antagonist MTX (Section 23).

In mitochondria, the cobalt atom is reduced to the +1 state (cob(I)alamin) and converted to adenosylcobalamin. In the mitochondrial metabolic pathway of propionate metabolism, AdoCbl functions as an essential cofactor for **methylmalonyl CoA mutase**-catalyzed conversion of methylmalonyl CoA to succinyl CoA. In this reaction, Cbl functions as a free radical reservoir, not as a methyl donor (Figure 14-6). In the absence of Cbl, methylmalonate (MMA) levels increase in plasma and urine. Folate does not participate in this reaction – high levels of methylmalonic acid (MMA) in serum and urine are present in Cbl deficiency but not in folate deficiency. In contrast, serum homocysteine levels are increased in both folate and Cbl deficiency. This dichotomy can be used to distinguish B$_{12}$ from folate deficiency.

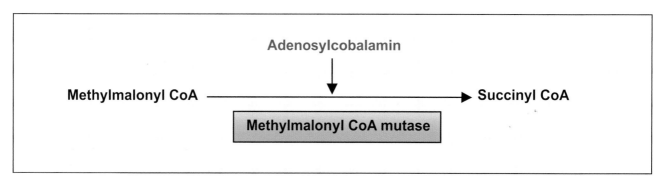

Figure 14-6 Methylmalonic Acid Metabolism

CLINICAL CORRELATES

Because the cobalamin-folate metabolic pathway is essential to purine, pyrimidine, and DNA synthesis, any interruption will impair cell division. This is reflected clinically in the **megaloblastic anemias** characterized by pancytopenia and macrocytic red cells. In addition, there is major ineffective erythropoiesis due to intramedullary cell death; the increased hemoglobin release accounts for the increase in bilirubin formation and the associated hyperbilirubinemia. The macrocytosis is due to impaired cell division with early extrusion of nuclei and relatively uninterrupted hemoglobin synthesis. Abnormal myelopoiesis is reflected in the giant metamyelocytes and hypersegmented neutrophils. Abnormalities in cell production are not confined to hematopoiesis – also present are giant buccal and vaginal mucosal cells.

COBALAMIN DEFICIENCY

Dietary deficiency of cobalamins is rare; it is associated with strict vegetarian diets that exclude all animal-derived foods. The deficiency is more commonly the result of impaired absorption associated with atrophic gastritis, or the absence of gastric IF in pernicious anemia and in postgastrectomy patients. In the presence of pancreatic disease, failure of protease degradation of R protein results in reduced Cbl binding to IF and Cbl malabsorption.

Elderly patients may present with cobalamin deficiency on the basis of hypochlorhydric or achlorhydric atrophic gastritis, although secretion of IF is adequate. The deficiency is due to the inability to release B$_{12}$ from its dietary protein carriers as pepsin requires a low pH for optimum activity. This mechanism is responsible for about one-third of the cases of low serum B$_{12}$ in the elderly. Drug-induced achlorhydria (eg, ranitidine, omeprazole), similarly, results in reduced pepsin release of protein-bound Cbl. Because IF is present, absorption of free crystalline B$_{12}$ is unimpaired – and the Schilling test, which measures the absorption of crystalline B$_{12}$, may be normal.

Other causes of Cbl deficiency include: intestinal malabsorption of the Cbl-IF complex due to intrinsic intestinal disease, resection of the absorptive site in the terminal ileum, competition for Cbl by fish tapeworm, or bacterial overgrowth in blind loops. The rare congenital absence of TC II (but not TC I or TC III) also results in Cbl deficiency. Nitrous oxide (N$_2$O) inactivates intracellular cobalamins by oxidizing the cobalt to the inactive +3 state. Prolonged or repeated exposure to N$_2$O can produce megaloblastic anemia and neuropathy (historically, anaesthesiologists have been at risk).

Pernicious anemia, so called because it was usually fatal before the therapeutic value of liver was demonstrated by Minot and Murphy in 1926, remains the classical megaloblastic anemia. It begins as a chronic atrophic gastritis with achlorhydria and loss of IF production. The submucosa is infiltrated with lymphocytes and plasma cells. Over 50% of these patients have serum antibodies to gastric parietal cells and to IF, often in association with antibodies to thyroid acinar cells (and other autoimmune endocrinopathies). In addition, there may be demyelination of the posterior and lateral columns of the spinal cord and a variety of symptoms due to cerebral demyelination. Although not well-understood, the demyelination may be associated with the inability to synthesize *S-adenosylmethionine;* there is impairment of myelin methylation with subsequent demyelination and clinical neuropathy.

Laboratory Studies

Normal serum B$_{12}$ levels range from 160 to 900 pmol/L. Levels are increased in chronic myelocytic leukemia (due to the high levels of TCI and TCIII derived from granulocytes and their precursors) and are low in Cbl deficiency. It is important to note that neurological symptoms and memory loss that respond to vitamin B_{12} therapy may occur in the presence of normal or borderline low serum levels and in the absence of a megaloblastic bone marrow and associated peripheral blood changes. Population studies have demonstrated a low serum Cbl in about 5% of healthy elderly subjects while approximately 25% had elevated MMA levels.

Serum B_{12} levels may not reflect accurately the requirements of the metabolic processes in which Cbl is an essential cofactor: patients with normal serum levels may have a metabolic Cbl deficiency. It is estimated that many elderly subjects with low normal serum Cbl levels are in fact Cbl deficient. Cbl deficiency is determined more accurately by assays of **serum methylmalonic acid (MMA)** and **homocysteine**. Both are elevated in Cbl deficiency and return to normal with Cbl supplementation. Although homocysteine levels are elevated in both folate and Cbl deficiency, elevated MMA levels are present only in the latter. The combined measurements of MMA and homocysteine are used to distinguish between Cbl and folate deficiencies.

The **deoxyuridine (dU) suppressor test** is a sensitive measure of both vitamin B_{12} and folate deficiency but, because of its complexity, is used infrequently. *In vitro* bone marrow cultures are used to measure the incorporation of ^3H thymidine into DNA in the presence of added dU. In cultures of normal bone marrow, there is sufficient N^5N^{10}-methylene-THF to facilitate dU conversion to dUMP and dTMP, and its incorporation into DNA; therefore, little of the ^3H thymidine tracer is incorporated into DNA. In either B_{12} or folate deficiency, because the level of the methyl donor N^5N^{10}-methylene THF is decreased, dU cannot be converted to thymidine – as a result, there is increased incorporation of the added ^3H thymidine into DNA.

The lack of IF or the inability to absorb the IF-Cbl complex may be established by the **Schilling urinary excretion test**. This test depends upon the ability to absorb oral crystalline $^{57}CoCbl$; a "flushing" dose of non-radioactive cyanocobalamin is injected intramuscularly 1-2 hours after the oral labelled Cbl. Radioactivity is assayed in a urine specimen collected for 24-72 hours. The criterion of normal absorption is the excretion in the urine of 7 percent or more of the labelled Cbl. If excretion does not exceed 7 percent, the test may be repeated by including IF with a second test dose of labelled Cbl. Normalization in the presence of administered IF, establishes IF deficiency as the cause of the failure to absorb Cbl. The test measures only the absorption of crystalline B_{12} (i.e. not bound to dietary proteins) and, therefore, may not mirror the clinical situation that depends on the utilization of dietary B_{12}. This is pertinent in the presence of atrophic gastritis or following gastric surgery – although the Schilling test is often normal in these patients, there may be deficient absorption of dietary B_{12}.

FOLATE DEFICIENCY

The normal serum folate is 7-25 nmol/L. Folate deficiency will develop within 4 to 6 weeks on a folate-free diet. Deficiency results from a dietary lack of folate or a diet in which the folate is destroyed by excessive heat during cooking. Malabsorption in celiac disease or sprue also will produce low serum folate levels. Alcoholics frequently are folate deficient due to poor diet, poor absorption and, possibly, the effect of alcohol on folate metabolism. Oral contraceptives and long term dilantin therapy occasionally result in folate-deficient megaloblastic anemia. There are increased folate requirements in pregnancy and in chronic hemolytic anemias. The most common cause of megaloblastic anemia worldwide is pregnancy associated with a folate-deficient diet.

In pernicious anemia, the megaloblastic changes in the bone marrow can be reversed by folic acid alone without Cbl, but the neurological symptoms are exacerbated. The neurological damage probably is associated with the deficit in S-adenosylmethionine synthesis – the level of Cbl is insufficient to sustain methyl transferase activity in the methionine metabolic pathway.

The incidence of neural tube defects, including spina bifida and anencephaly, can be reduced by folic acid supplementation during pregnancy. Women at risk often have normal serum folate but increased levels of homocysteine. The metabolic abnormality in these women may be due to a defect in the gene coding for methylene tetrahydrofolate reductase (MTHFR); this enzyme recycles N^5N^{10}-methylene-THF to N^5-methyl-THF, a source of the single carbon units required for the conversion of homocysteine to methionine and S-adenosylmethionine (Section 25).

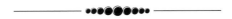

SUGGESTED READING

Antony AC. The biological chemistry of folate receptors. Blood 79: 2807-2820, 1992.

Antony AC. Megaloblastic anemias. In Hematology, Basic Principles and Practice. (Ed 3) Hoffman R, Benz EJ, Shattil SJ, Furie B, et al. (eds) Churchill Livingstone 446-485, 1999.

Carmel R. Megaloblastic anemias. Curr Opin Hematol 1:107-112, 1994.

Carmel R. Subtle cobalamin deficiency. Ann Intern Med 124:338-340, 1996.

Chanarin I, Deacon R, Lumb M, Perry J. Cobalamin and folate: recent developments. J Clin Pathol 45:277-283, 1992.

Epstein FH. Pernicious Anemia. N Engl J Med 337:1441-1448, 1997.

Snow CF. Laboratory diagnosis of vitamin B$_{12}$ and folate deficiency. Arch Intern Med 159:1289-1298, 1999.

Tefferi A, Pruthi RK. The biochemical basis of cobalamin deficiency. Mayo Clin Proc 69:181-186, 1994.

Toh BH, van Driel IR, Gleeson PA. Pernicious anemia. N Engl J Med 337:1441-1448, 1997.

Whitehead AS, Gallagher P, Mills JL, Kirke PN, et al. Genetic defect in 5, 10 methylene-tetrahydrofolate reductase in neural tube defects. Q J Med 88:763-766, 1995.

Wickramasinghe SN. The wide spectrum and unresolved issues of megaloblastic anemia. Semin Hematol 36:3-18, 1999.

Zittoun J, Zittoun R. Modern clinical testing strategies in cobalamin and folate deficiency. Semin Hematol 36:35-46, 1999.

IRON METABOLISM

"Virchow's hypothesis that the disease chlorosis is due to a congenital hypoplasia of the heart and blood vessels seems incompatible with the fact that the disease can be promptly cured by the administration of iron."
Richard C. Cabot – In Osler's Modern Medicine, 1908

Iron is the essential element of the heme complex, central to the function of hemoglobin, myoglobin, and the cytochromes, but also found in iron-dependent non-heme proteins. As a component of these systems, it participates in oxygen and electron transport and is an integral catalyst of oxidation-reduction systems, functions that depend on its ability to cycle readily between the reduced ferrous (Fe^{2+}) and oxidized ferric (Fe^{3+}) forms. Unbound iron generates free radicals with peroxidation of membrane lipids and tissue damage. Because free elemental iron is cytotoxic, the iron absorbed from the bowel is transported in combination with a carrier protein, then passed to protein-associated functional or storage forms. Iron deficiency results in decreased levels of iron-dependent compounds; iron overload results in cell and organ damage. Total body iron, absorption, transport and storage are adjusted continuously on the basis of physiological requirements. As iron excretion is limited, body iron is regulated almost exclusively by absorption from the upper small bowel.

The total body content of elemental iron ranges from 2 to 5 Gm consistent with body size – approximately 40 mg/kg in adult females and 50 mg/kg in adult males. Two-thirds of the iron is present in hemoglobin and one-third in tissue and transport forms. Storage iron, in the form of ferritin and hemosiderin, approximates 6 to 12 mg/kg; transport iron in transferrin is less than 0.1 mg/kg; the heme and non-heme iron-containing enzymes average 2 mg/kg.

Iron Intake and Absorption

The primary regulator of iron homeostasis is intestinal iron absorption. As stores decline absorption increases and, as stores are replenished, absorption decreases. Iron loss normally is small, averaging 1 mg per day in males and 2 mg per day in menstruating females. (Hemoglobin contains 3.46 mg of iron per gram of hemoglobin – each milliliter of blood loss (Hb 150 g/L) is equivalent to the loss of 0.5 mg of iron). In the iron-replete adult, maintenance of iron stores within this highly conserved system requires 1 - 2 mg of absorbed iron per day; this rises to 4 - 6 mg during pregnancy and lactation. An adequate diet contains about 15 mg/day of iron; 10 percent of this is absorbed – sufficient to maintain iron balance in men and most non-pregnant non-lactating women. Approximately 20-30% of dietary iron present in heme is absorbed from the gut, only about 5% of dietary non-heme iron is absorbed. In areas where meat is available, about one-third of dietary iron may be provided by heme; the incidence of iron-deficiency anemia increases in areas where consumption of meat is low.

Absorption increases in the presence of: (1) low total body iron stores, and (2) increased erythropoiesis. The relationship of these two regulatory elements is unclear. Absorption decreases as iron stores rise. Regulation of iron absorption is related to the ferritin content of the enterocytes present at the bottom of the intestinal crypt before they move up to assume an absorptive role. The mediation by erythropoiesis, however, appears to be independent of iron stores – in some chronic hemolytic anemias (eg, thalassemia), iron absorption continues despite the presence of iron overload, in others (eg, spherocytosis) iron overload is not significant (Figure 15-1).

Iron absorption takes place primarily in the duodenum by the enterocytes at the tip of the intestinal villi; the iron must pass through the apical and then the basolateral membranes of these cells to reach the circulation. The apical membrane transports both heme and ferrous iron into the cell. Heme is absorbed directly into the mucosal cell where it is degraded by heme oxygenase and Fe^{2+} is released – this pathway of heme-iron uptake is very efficient but the molecular mechanisms are unknown. Dietary inorganic iron is primarily in the ferric form; it is reduced enzymatically to the more efficiently absorbed ferrous form by a brush border **ferric reductase** (denoted as FeRed in Figure 15-2), facilitated by the low gastric pH and the presence of reducing agents such as ascorbic acid. The ferrous iron is transported across the apical membrane into the enterocyte by the **divalent metal transporter DMT1** (a twelve transmembrane domain protein). DMT1 is up-regulated in iron deficiency and down-regulated

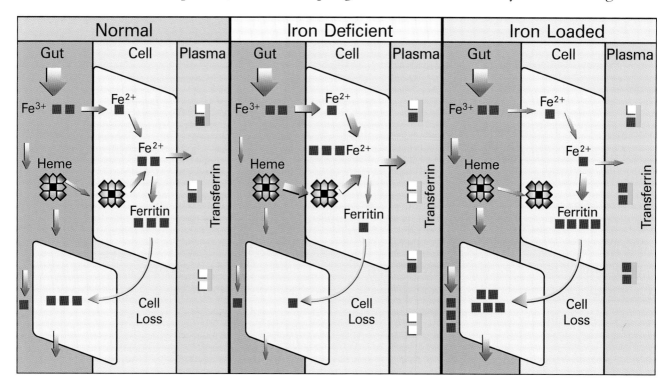

Figure 15-1 Iron Absorption

as body iron stores increase. The iron from all dietary sources either transits the cell and moves into the circulation as a complex with transferrin or is sequestered in the enterocyte as ferritin (Fe^{3+}). This ferritin is lost into the lumen of the gut as the enterocytes are sloughed in the process of normal mucosal cell turnover (Figure 15-1).

The uptake of iron by the enterocytes is determined by their iron content, and this depends upon the amount of transferrin-bound iron that was deposited as ferritin in the basal crypt cells prior to migrating upwards to their absorptive location. The iron content of the crypt cells reflects total body iron stores and is linked closely to body need. **Transferrin receptors,** in association with the MHC class 1-like protein **HFE,** determine the iron content of these cells. In the presence of a low plasma iron, the level of iron in the crypt cells is low; as these iron-deprived enterocytes migrate to the top of the villus to become the absorptive cell there is upregulation of DMT1, resulting in greater iron influx. In the iron replete state, the iron content of the villus cell is high and DMT1 is downregulated – iron uptake is decreased (Figure 15-2).

HFE

A gene closely linked to the HLA site on chromosome 6 encodes a novel MHC class 1-like protein designated HFE; like other MHC class I molecules, HFE associates with β_2-microglobulin (β_2m). HFE is expressed in varying degrees on all cells but is expressed most strongly by the deep crypt cells of the duodenum. The association with β_2-microglobulin is essential for HFE localization on the cell surface. HFE also binds with high affinity to the transferrin receptor (TfR); this trimolecular complex (HFE, β_2m, TfR) assembles on the cell membrane. Binding of HFE to TfR is pH dependent and is optimum at the cell surface pH of 7.4; it fails to bind at the endosomal pH of 6.2 (Figure 15-2).

HFE, as an integral part of this trimolecular complex, modulates the uptake of transferrin-bound iron into the duodenal crypts cells. In the normal iron replete state, the high level of plasma iron results in increased TfR-HFE-β_2m-mediated transfer of iron into the crypt cells and, ultimately, in reduced iron absorption. When HFE is mutated (in hereditary hemochromatosis), the uptake of transferrin iron is reduced, resulting in low iron levels in the crypt cells and falsely signaling that body stores are low; the result is an inappropriate increase in iron absorption.

Iron Transport – Intestine to Plasma

In the intestinal lumen, ferric iron is reduced to ferrous iron by ferric reductase; ferrous iron is transported across the apical surface of the enterocyte via the divalent metal transporter DMT1. Inside the cell, iron can be oxidized to Fe^{3+} for storage as ferritin or transported across the basolateral membrane of the enterocyte by a transmembrane ferrous iron transporter

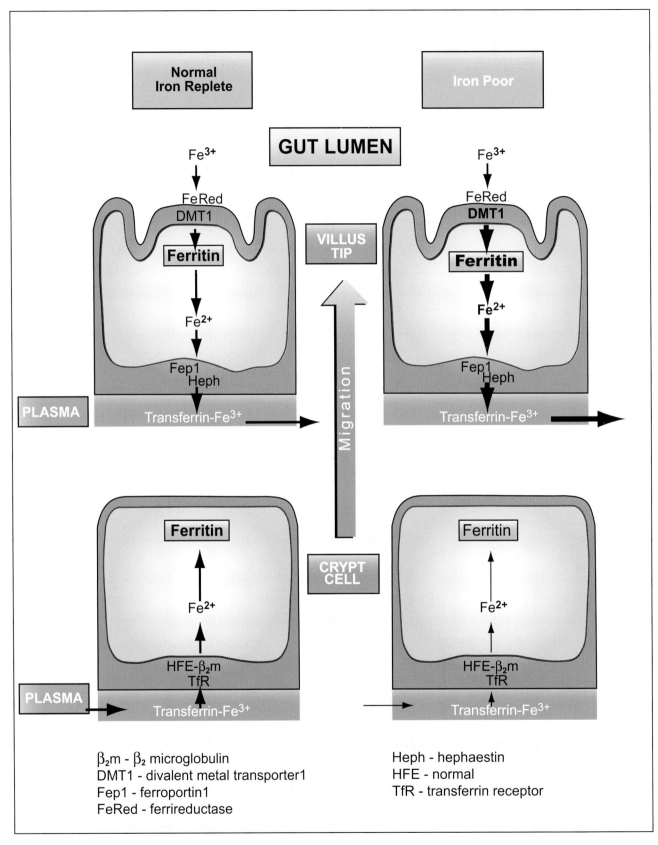

Figure 15-2   Regulation of Iron Absorption

ferroportin 1(Fep1). An associated ceruloplasmin homologue, the transmembrane multicopper ferroxidase **hephaestin (HEPH)**, facilitates iron export and oxidation to the ferric state. (Hephaestin: the Greek god of metal working, a.k.a. Vulcan). It is unclear whether HEPH functions independently or in association with ferroportin 1.

Iron Transport in Plasma

In plasma, the ferric iron circulates tightly bound to **transferrin**, an 80,000 kD glycoprotein synthesized in the liver that is distributed equally between the vascular and extra-vascular space. Chelation of iron by transferrin-binding maintains iron in a soluble form. Transferrin is a bi-lobed molecule; a pocket in each lobe is available for binding one molecule of Fe^{3+}. Binding to either pocket is random – circulating transferrin is present in diferric, monoferric and apoferric (iron-free) forms. At the plasma pH of 7.35, transferrin binds iron tightly. The amount of transferrin in plasma is capable of binding about 300 µg/dl (60 µmol/L) of iron – referred to as the *total iron binding capacity (TIBC)*. Transferrin normally is one-third saturated, carrying 100 µg/dl (20 µmol/L) of iron (referred to as *serum iron*). In the presence of iron deficiency, as the plasma iron falls there is increased hepatic synthesis of transferrin with an increase in the TIBC.

Iron Uptake (Figure 15-3)

Transferrin-bound iron is moved into tissue cells through the **transferrin receptor (TfR)**, a transmembrane glycoprotein dimer with a large extracellular domain, a transmembrane

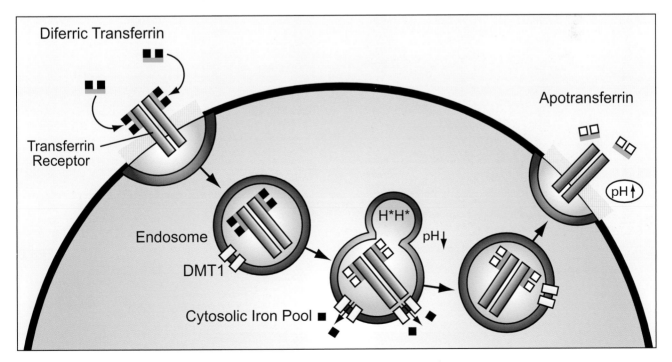

Figure 15-3 Iron Uptake

region and a short cytoplasmic component. HFE is an important modulator of this interaction. TfR is capable of binding two molecules of transferrin, each carrying one or two molecules of iron. At physiological pH, affinity of the receptor is greatest for diferric transferrin, less for monoferric and least for apotransferrin. Because of the universal cellular requirement for iron, transferrin receptors are present on most cells, their number reflecting cell need and function; the largest numbers are found on erythrocyte precursors, hepatocytes, placental trophoblasts, and replicating cells. In the red cell synthetic line, the number of receptors peak at approximately 800,000 per cell in intermediate (polychromatophilic) normoblasts, decrease to about 100,000 on reticulocytes and are absent from mature red cells. The transferrin receptor may undergo proteolytic cleavage at the cell surface and appear in soluble form in the plasma – plasma TfR is increased in iron deficiency.

The diferric or monoferric transferrin bound to the transferrin receptor is internalized within an endocytotic vesicle. An ATP-dependent proton pump in the membrane of the endosome maintains the internal pH at about 5.5; at this acidic pH, the iron dissociates from the transferrin which remains bound to the receptor. The released ferric iron is reduced to its more soluble ferrous form as it enters the cytoplasmic pool via the endosomal iron transporter DMT1 (the same iron transporter that is present in the enterocytes of the intestinal villi). The receptor-apotransferrin complex returns to the cell surface where the receptor is re-incorporated into the cell membrane; with exposure to the ambient pH of 7.35 at the cell surface, the iron depleted apotransferrin is released into the plasma; both receptor and transferrin now are available to repeat the cycle. On entry into the cytoplasm the iron may associate with: (1) *heme-proteins*, (2) *non-heme iron-containing proteins*, (3) *ferritin*, or (4) the *iron-regulatory protein (IRP)*.

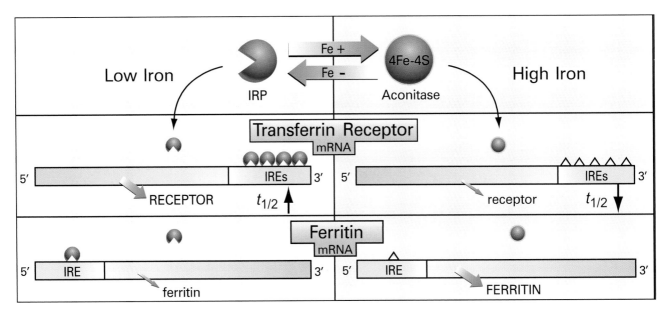

Figure 15-4 Iron - Intracellular Regulation

The iron content of the cell is regulated by control of the iron uptake and storage capacity in a reciprocal fashion. When cellular iron falls, the levels of ferritin decrease and transferrin receptors increase; as cellular iron increases, ferritin levels rise and transferrin receptors fall. This mechanism is regulated by the **IRP** (iron-regulatory protein), a delicate biosensor of iron load; IRP itself is regulated by the level of iron in the cell. IRP is an iron-sulphur protein with two different functions that depend on the iron content of its central *4Fe-4S cluster*. In the presence of a low cytoplasmic iron pool, the iron content of this cluster falls and the conformation of the protein changes: a deep cleft opens to produce the active configuration of the IRP (Figure 15-4).

Iron responsive elements (**IREs**) are present on the specific mRNAs for the transferrin receptor and ferritin. The mRNA for the transferrin receptor has 5 IREs at its untranslated 3′ end. Binding of IRP to these sites protects the mRNA from endonuclease cleavage, stabilizing the mRNA and prolonging its half-life. As a result, there is increased synthesis of transferrin receptors followed by increased iron uptake into the cell. The mRNA for apoferritin has one IRE at its untranslated 5′ end. When IRP binds to this IRE, the translation of apoferritin mRNA is repressed – consequently, ferritin synthesis and iron storage are reduced. Thus, low cytosolic iron increases iron uptake and decreases iron storage; by limiting storage, the iron in the cell is made available for critical metabolic processes. Note: binding of IRP to the mRNAs of these two proteins, the transferrin receptor and apoferritin, upregulates the first and downregulates the second.

When the cell is iron replete, the iron content in the 4Fe-4S cluster of the IRP is restored, the cleft closes and binding to the IREs ceases. This results in a shortened $t_{1/2}$ for transferrin receptor mRNA with a drop in receptor synthesis; at the same time the suppression of apoferritin mRNA is lifted and ferritin levels increase. The overall result is decreased iron uptake and increased storage. Note: (1) the regulatory IRP protein in its 4Fe-4S mode functions as the mitochondrial enzyme *aconitase* that mediates the conversion of citrate to isocitrate in the

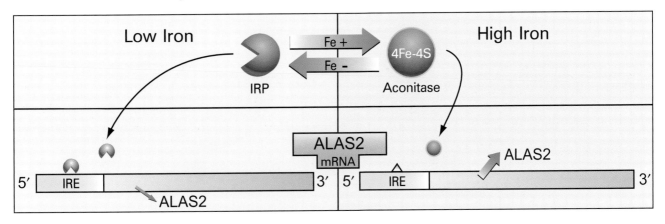

Figure 15-5 Regulation of ALAS2 in Erythropoietic Cells

Krebs cycle; (2) DMT1 mRNA, governing the endosomal transport of iron, also has an IRE site which is upregulated by IRP binding – as a result, endosomal transport is facilitated in parallel with increased expression of the transferrin receptor when the cell is iron depleted.

In red cell precursors, iron utilization is coupled to heme synthesis and is regulated by an IRP-dependent mechanism (Figure 15-5). In these cells, an IRE site is present on the 5' untranslated region of the mRNA for δ-aminolevulinic acid synthase (**ALAS2**), the rate limiting enzyme for red cell porphyrin synthesis. The iron-depleted IRP binds to the ALAS2 IRE site in the mRNA and inhibits ALAS2 synthesis. Decreased ALAS2 synthesis in iron-deficient red cell precursors down-regulates porphyrin synthesis (Section 12). Thus, when there is insufficient iron to complete heme synthesis, the accumulation of potentially toxic porphyrin is reduced. This control mechanism, however, is not absolute – some excess protoporphyrin does accumulate in the red cells in iron deficiency anemia.

Iron Storage

Iron taken up by the cell in excess of that required for heme synthesis is stored in two forms, *ferritin* and *hemosiderin*. The major iron stores are in the form of ferritin. The ferritin molecule is a hollow protein shell, *apoferritin*, composed of 24 subunits (polypeptide chains of two types, the H and L subunits) with intervening hydrophobic channels that allow passage of iron into the internal core. The ferroxidase activity of the H subunit converts Fe^{2+} to Fe^{3+} for storage. The storage capacity is about 4300 iron atoms per unit, but normally averages half that number. Ferritin is water soluble – this storage iron is returned readily to the metabolic pool.

As iron continues to accumulate in the cell, a second storage form, hemosiderin, appears. Hemosiderin has a higher iron to protein ratio and is not water soluble; it can be visualized in tissue sections as Prussian blue positive granules and aggregates. (Ferritin is seen only on

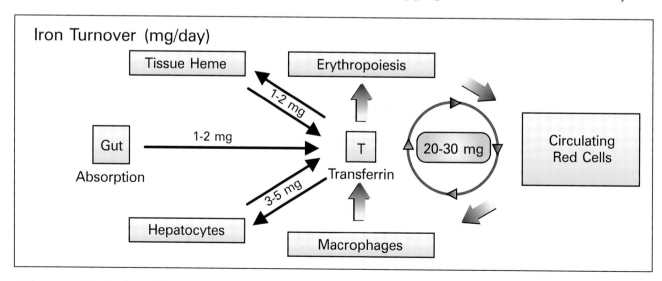

Figure 15-6   Iron Turnover

electron microscopy). Hemosiderin, although less easily mobilized for metabolic need than ferritin, does become available in iron deficiency; when stores are mobilized, this stainable iron disappears as it moves into the metabolic pool.

Internal Exchange (Figure 15-6)

The major pathway for internal iron exchange cycles through the erythroid precursors in the marrow and specialized macrophages (the reticuloendothelial system) in the spleen, bone marrow, and liver. This circuit accounts for 80% of iron exchange, i.e. 20-30 mg/day. Time-expired or damaged red cells are taken up by macrophages; iron is removed from the hemoglobin by heme oxygenase and either stored as ferritin or released to plasma transferrin. The mechanism of iron release from the macrophage is not clear: it has been suggested that the exit of iron from the macrophage may be dependent on ferroportin 1, and that the re-oxidation of iron (Fe^{2+} to Fe^{3+}) for incorporation into transferrin may depend on the ferroxidase **ceruloplasmin**. HFE also may be involved in modulating the iron content of these cells – in the presence of the mutated *HFE* gene, little iron is stored in reticuloendothelial cells despite the increase in total body stores. Transferrin transports the iron to erythropoietic sites for re-synthesis of heme. The macrophage, in response to the degree of erythropoiesis, maintains an equilibrium between the amount of iron stored and the amount released. Note: (1) The macrophage receives little iron from transferrin; (2) A recently described receptor (CD163) on tissue macrophages/monocytes may be involved in the clearance of hemoglobin-haptoglobin complexes from the circulation (Section 16).

The liver takes up iron bound to transferrin via surface transferrin receptors. Another source of hepatic iron is the hemoglobin iron that appears in plasma as a result of intravascular hemolysis, ineffective erythropoiesis, and the hemoglobin that accompanies the nuclear extrusion of maturing normoblasts. The hemoglobin binds to plasma haptoglobin or hemopexin for transport to the hepatocyte (Section 16). Hepatocytes have a storage pool equivalent to about 20% of that in macrophages. The storage pool (primarily in macrophages and hepatocytes) provides a supply of mobilizable iron in the event of blood loss or other causes of iron depletion. In the normal iron replete state when erythropoiesis declines, iron accumulates in the storage pool as ferritin or hemosiderin, to be mobilized again when erythropoiesis increases.

CLINICAL CORRELATES

Laboratory Evaluation of Iron Status

Serum Iron is a measure of transferrin-bound iron (60 - 150 µg/dl; 10 - 27 µmol/L). **Total Iron Binding Capacity** (TIBC) is the total amount of iron that can be bound by the transferrin in serum (250 - 435 µg/dl; 45 - 78 µmol/L). The binding capacity normally is

Table 15-1　　　　　　　　　　Clinical Laboratory Data

Clinical State	Serum			Bone Marrow		Red Cell	
	Iron µg/dl *(µmol/L)	TIBC µg/dl *(µmol/L)	Ferritin ng/ml *(µg/L)	Stainable Iron	Sideroblasts	Morphology	Protoporphyrin µg/dl
Normal	60 – 150 *(10 – 27)	250 – 435 *(45 – 78)	15 – 250 *(15 – 250)	+ + +	+ + +	N	40±20
Iron Depleted	↓	N or ↑	↓	+	+	N	N or ↑
Iron Deficiency Anemia	↓	↑	↓	–	–	Hypochromic Microcytic	↑
Iron Overload	↑	N or ↓	↑	+ + + +	+ + +	N	N
Anemia of Chronic Disease	↓	↓	↑	+ + +	+	N (Hypochromic)	N
* SI Units							

one-third saturated. Circulating **ferritin** is an indirect measure of the storage pool – note the wide normal range (15 - 250 ng/ml; 15 - 250 µg/L). When low, plasma ferritin is a good index of iron depletion. It is high in iron overload and in liver disease. Because ferritin is an acute phase reactant, it is increased in inflammatory states unrelated to body iron stores.

Bone Marrow - The identification of hemosiderin by Prussian blue staining is a direct measure of iron stores. Hemosiderin is graded from 1+ to 3+ in normal bone marrow; it is absent in iron deficiency when stores are depleted, and increased (4+ to 5+) in iron overload. Stainable iron granules in normoblasts (sideroblasts) represent iron replete red cell precursors. In sideroblastic anemias there is failure in heme synthesis, the iron accumulates in the mitochondria of the erythroblasts – the iron-laden mitochondria surround the nucleus; the cells are referred to as ring sideroblasts (Section 12).

Iron Deficiency

Iron deficiency may be the result of: (1) increased iron requirements in pregnancy and lactation and during rapid growth in infants, (2) an iron deficient diet, (3) impaired intestinal absorption, or (4) external blood loss. As iron deficiency develops, the depletion of iron stores is followed by falling serum iron and rising transferrin (TIBC) levels; eventually, there is a decrease in the number of red cells and a reduction in their hemoglobin content with the appearance of hypochromic microcytic red cells. Because some protoporphyrin continues to be synthesized even when iron is unavailable to complete heme synthesis, red cell protoporphyrin levels increase.

In copper deficiency (a rare clinical entity), there may be an associated iron-deficiency anemia despite adequate levels of iron in the diet; iron enters the intestinal mucosal cell normally in these patients but cannot exit into the circulation. The discovery of hephaestin has provided the link between copper and iron metabolism. Egress of iron from enterocytes into the circulation is facilitated by the multicopper ferroxidase hephaestin. In the absence of copper, iron release from enterocytes fails due to the absence of hephaestin activity: the anemia responds to copper administration, not to iron. Ceruloplasmin and hephaestin are homologous proteins – both are multicopper ferroxidases that regulate tissue iron efflux although their sites of action are distinct. Ceruloplasmin has a primary role in the mobilization of iron from liver and other tissue sites. **Aceruloplasminemia**, an autosomal recessive disease, is characterized by iron overload in parenchymal cells resulting in diabetes and neurodegeneration of the retina and basal ganglia. Because hephaestin activity is normal, iron does not accumulate in intestinal endocytes and anemia, if present, is mild.

Iron Overload

As iron stores are regulated primarily by uptake into a closed system, inappropriately increased absorption will produce iron overload. Iron overload occurs in a number of hereditary disorders, including atransferrinemia, aceruloplasminemia, X-linked hereditary sideroblastic anemia, thalassemia major, and hemochromatosis. The progressive accumulation of iron in body parenchymal cells eventually results in cellular damage.

Hereditary hemochromatosis (Figure 15-7) is an autosomal recessive disease with an incidence in Caucasians of 3 to 5 per 100,000. The gene mutation is present in 5% of northern Europeans. Two missense mutations in the HFE gene are associated with hemochromatosis. Sixty to ninety percent of patients are homozygous for the C282Y mutation (substitution of tyrosine for cysteine). This mutation is in the HFE binding site for β_2-microglobulin – because HFE is not displayed on the cell surface, the interaction with the transferrin receptor is lost. The H63D mutation (substitution of aspartate for histidine) does not interfere with β_2-microglobulin binding and iron overload is less severe. Clinical disease is manifest in C282Y homozygotes and in C282Y / H63D double heterozygotes. There is a wide variation in the clinical presentation and severity.

As a result of the HFE mutation, uptake of transferrin-bound iron by duodenal villi crypt cells is decreased and ferritin levels in the crypt cells are low. This conveys a message of iron depletion in spite of large iron stores – intestinal absorption in these patients is 2-3 times normal. There are marked deposits of iron in parenchymal cells; less in macrophages which indeed may be empty. Serum iron is high and the TIBC at or near saturation; serum ferritin levels usually are increased. Diagnosis is confirmed by liver biopsy with demonstration of increased iron in hepatic parenchymal cells. Deposition of iron in the parenchymal cells of liver,

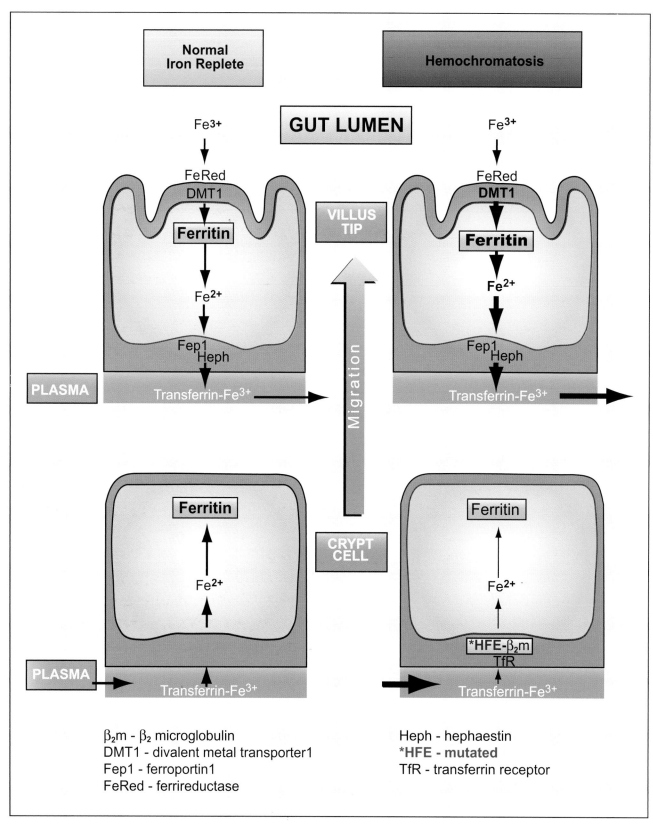

Figure 15-7 Hemochromatosis

heart, pancreas, and endocrine organs evolves to eventual organ failure. Skin pigmentation, cirrhosis, diabetes, arthropathy and testicular atrophy, all due to iron deposition, are hallmarks of the untreated disease. As iron accumulation is slow, the disease usually manifests after age 40. The persistence and prevalence of the gene suggests that it may provide a genetic advantage, perhaps by maintaining iron stores in women during their reproductive years. Therapy is based on iron removal by phlebotomy.

Other Forms of Iron Overload

African iron-overload is more common in sub-Saharan Africa than hereditary hemochromatosis in Europe. The disorder has a genetic basis although the pattern of inheritance has not been established; it is not due to mutations in the *HFE* gene. **Juvenile hemochromatosis** becomes manifest clinically during the second or third decade, at an earlier age than hereditary hemochromatosis. Although not linked to the *HFE* gene, the pathophysiology of the disease suggests that the defect resides in the same iron-regulatory pathway. A locus for juvenile hemochromatosis maps to chromosome-1.

Iron overload also occurs in some chronic hemolytic anemias (eg, thalassemia) where the stimulus of increased erythropoiesis mediates increased iron absorption. In all types of refractory anemias requiring repeated transfusion, patients may sequester up to 10 Gm of iron per year (each unit of blood introduces 200 - 250 mg of iron into a closed system). There is initial macrophage loading followed by involvement of parenchymal cells and organ failure. Repeated transfusion in patients with hemolytic anemia may result in body burdens of 40-50 Gm of iron. Iron mobilization is achieved by chelation therapy.

Anemia of Chronic Disease

One of the most common anemias is associated with infectious, inflammatory or neoplastic disease. The anemia is due to defective iron reutilization – macrophages appear unable to release storage iron (obtained by red cell phagocytosis) to the circulating pool. The increased ferritin storage may result from increased intracellular apoferritin synthesis in response to the cytokines IL-1 and TNFα induced in macrophages as an expression of the primary disease. These cytokines and TGFβ (transforming growth factor β) also may interfere with EPO production. The anemia usually is normocytic and normochromic, only occasionally is it hypochromic and, rarely, microcytic. It is characterized by low serum iron, normal or decreased transferrin (TIBC) and, frequently, increased serum ferritin; the marrow macrophages contain increased amounts of iron, but the number of sideroblasts is decreased. Erythropoietin (EPO) levels frequently are inappropriately low for the degree of anemia; some patients do respond to EPO. These patients also may have a shortened red cell life span and decreased erythropoiesis due to increased levels of circulating Fas ligand; binding of the ligand to the Fas membrane receptor of the normoblast induces apoptosis by activation of the caspase system (Section 4).

Some of these patients may be iron deficient. In the anemia of chronic disease, the plasma transferrin receptor concentration is normal or low. In contrast, the plasma transferrin receptor concentration is high in iron deficiency. (Soluble transferrin receptor is derived from normoblasts). A sensitive means of differentiating these two anemias is by determination of the plasma transferrin receptor/ferritin index: it is low in the anemia of chronic disease, and high in iron-deficiency anemia.

––––––––––– •••◗◖••• –––––––––––

SUGGESTED READING

Andrews NC. Disorders of iron metabolism. N Engl J Med 341:1986-1995, 1999.

Andrews NC, Levy JE. Iron is hot: an update on the pathophysiology of hemochromatosis. Blood 92:1845-1851, 1998.

Andrews NC, Fleming MD, Levy JE. Molecular insights into mechanisms of iron transport. Curr Opin Hematol 6:61-64, 1999.

Bacon BR, Powell LW, Adams PC, Kresina TF, Hoofnagle JH. Molecular medicine and hemochromatosis: at the crossroads. Gastroenterology 116:193-207, 1999.

Cazzola M, Bergamaschi G, Dezza L, Arosio P. Manipulations of cellular iron metabolism for modulating normal and malignant cell proliferation: achievements and prospects. Blood 75:1903-1919, 1990.

Conrad ME, Umbreit JN. Iron absorption and transport – an update. Am J Hematol 64:287-298, 2000.

Cook JD, Skikne BS, Baynes RD. Serum transferrin receptor. Annu Rev Med 44:63-74, 1993.

Drakesmith H, Townsend A. The structure and function of HFE. BioEssays 22:595-598, 2000.

Finch CA. Regulators of iron balance in humans. Blood 84:1697-1702, 1994.

Harris ZL, Durley AP, Man TK, Gitlin JD. Targeted gene disruption reveals an essential role for ceruloplasmin in cellular iron efflux. Proc Natl Acad Sci 96:10812-10817, 1999.

Harrison PM, Arosio P. The ferritins: Molecular properties, iron storage function and cellular regulation. Biochim Biophys Acta 1275: 161-203, 1996.

Henderson BR. Iron regulatory proteins 1 and 2. BioEssays 18:739-746, 1996.

Hershko C, Link G, Pinson A. Principles of iron chelating therapy. Semin Hematol 27:91-94, 1990.

Klausner RD, Rouault TA, Harford JB. Regulating the fate of mRNA: the control of cellular iron metabolism. Cell 72:19-28, 1993.

McKie AT, Marciani P, Rolfs A, et al. A novel duodenal iron-regulated transporter, IREG1, implicated in the basolateral transfer of iron to the circulation. Molec Cell 4:299-309, 2000.

Montosi G, Paglia P, Garuti C, et al. Wild type HFE protein normalizes transferrin iron accumulation in macrophages from subjects with hereditary hemochromatosis. Blood 96: 1125-1129, 2000.

Vulpe CD, Kuo YM, Murphy TL, Cowley L, et al. Hephaestin, a ceruloplasmin homologue implicated in intestinal iron transport, is defective in the sla mouse. Nat Genet 21:195-199, 1999.

RED CELL LIFE SPAN & BILIRUBIN METABOLISM

"What grief hath set the jaundice on your cheeks?"

Troilus & Cressida, Act I Scene III

Normal red cell life span averages 120 days. Determination of the sequential biochemical changes that define the aging cell is hampered by the difficulties with *in vitro* separation of cells on the basis of age. However, good evidence does exist for an age-dependent reduction in red cell glycolytic enzymes manifest by decreased glycolysis, ATP production, and generation of NADH and NADPH. As a result, cellular function is impaired: (1) cation exchange, ionic equilibrium, and membrane maintenance (ATP), (2) the hexose monophosphate shunt and its capacity to respond to oxidative injury (NADPH and GSH), and (3) the reduction of methemoglobin (NADH) (Section 10). Finally, the cells fail to pass inspection within the spleen and are culled from the circulation. Under physiological conditions and in low-grade chronic hemolytic anemias, red cell destruction takes place primarily within the macrophages outside the vascular stream – termed **extravascular hemolysis**. In acute hemolytic states (eg, transfusion reactions, malaria), major red cell lysis occurs within the circulation – **intravascular hemolysis**. These two forms of red cell lysis give rise to different products and different clinical events.

MEASUREMENT OF RED CELL SURVIVAL (Figure 16-1)

Red cell survival may be measured either by: (1) labelling a single cohort of cells of comparable age, or (2) labelling a mixed population of cells of all ages.

In vivo cohort labelling is accomplished by the intravenous injection of 2-^{14}C glycine – this label is incorporated into globin during a brief period of hemoglobin synthesis. Labelling takes place in the bone marrow during the period when hemoglobin synthesis coincides with the presence of the isotope (2 to 5 days); the labelled cells emerge into the circulation, plateau in number and then decline. Normally, the median time to plateau and decline is about 80 days. The disadvantages of this technique include: (1) differences in rates of red cell production under abnormal conditions, (2) the long interval required to determine outcome, (3) the difficulty in interpreting the curve when red cells are destroyed at random rather than on the basis of age, and (4) the reutilization of the label.

The first determination of normal red cell survival was performed by Ashby who infused a population of donor cells that could be identified by antigenic blood group difference from the cells of the recipient. The linear disappearance of these normal cells (with a random distribution of cells of all ages and identified by differential agglutination), took place over a period of 100 - 120 days.

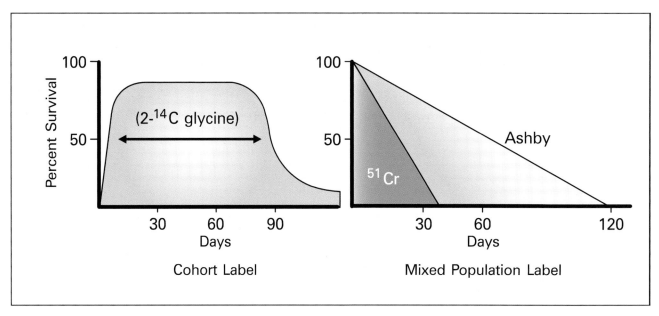

Figure 16-1 Red Cell Survival

As Ashby's technique is laborious and requires compatible but identifiable donor cells, it has been replaced by a shorter simpler method that uses the patient's own cells. The patient's blood is labelled ex-vivo by incubation with ^{51}Cr which diffuses into the cell and binds to hemoglobin. This technique labels cells of all ages; in the normal state tagged cells represent a linear spectrum from 1 to 120 days of age. Because this label is not reutilized, if all the tag remained in the cells, 1/120 of the tagged population would disappear each day – the last tagged cells disappearing on day 120. However, ^{51}Cr is eluted from the red cells at a constant rate of about 1% per day and this must be taken into account in the interpretation of results. The disappearance of ^{51}Cr is curvilinear but assumes linearity on a semilogarithmic plot. In normal individuals, the ^{51}Cr tag has a $t_{1/2}$ that falls between 25 and 30 days (equivalent to a red cell survival of 120 days). This is presently the standard clinical method of determining red cell survival.

THE ROLE OF THE SPLEEN (Figure 16-2)

The primary site of red cell destruction is the spleen; the liver normally subserves a minor role. The spleen is the more discerning organ in selecting out old, effete or damaged cells. However in the presence of gross red cell damage, the liver has a more significant role because of its relatively greater blood flow. The life span of red blood cells in splenectomized patients is unaltered as macrophages in other organs assume this function.

The spleen fulfils the dual role of both a red cell and an immunological filter; these functions are served by the filtration beds in the white pulp, the marginal zone and the red pulp.

On entering the parenchyma of the spleen, the arterial vessels divide into central arterioles that are surrounded by aggregates of lymphoid tissue referred to as the white pulp. It consists of two elements: (1) a periarterial sheath of T-lymphocytes where circulating T cells may selectivel-home, and (2) lymphoid follicles that are collections of B lymphocytes – these are recovery areas available to circulating B cells. In the marginal zone, arterioles terminate in an anastomosing

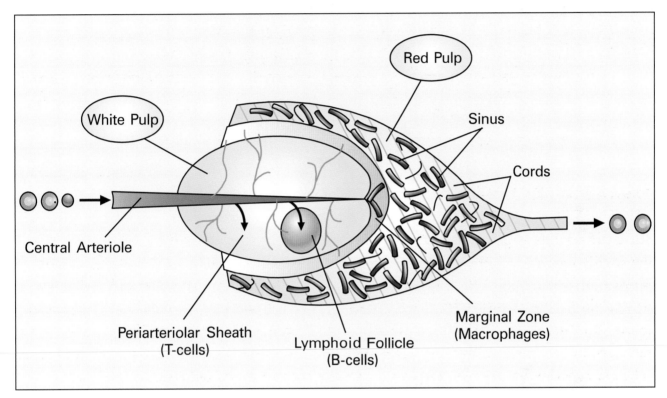

Figure 16-2 The Splenic Filter

complex of discontinuous vessels. This allows close contact of the blood with the cells of the zone, primarily with the large number of macrophages that remove damaged leukocytes, bacteria, platelets and red cells.

The red pulp derives its name from the macroscopic appearance due to the large number of erythrocytes contained within its cords and sinuses. The sinuses are composed of a discontinuous endothelial lining and a fenestrated basement membrane. The red cells are able to leave the containment of the vascular channels and percolate through the cords which consist of a network of macrophages, fibroblasts and collagen. It is here that granulocytes and platelets are stored and monocytes are detained as they differentiate into macrophages. How red cells are selected for destruction is uncertain, but several mechanisms have been proposed: (1) Red cells sequestered in this maze for extended periods may be in a relatively hypoxic state and deprived of glucose as the plasma drains away and the hematocrit rises. To survive, the red cells must maintain osmotic and membrane integrity – red cells that are unable to meet this metabolic challenge because of age or defect are ingested and destroyed by macrophages. (2) As red cells age, they may expose surface markers that lead to their recognition and destruction by macrophages.

As the red cells pass through the interstices of the cords that are smaller than the circumference of the cell, their biconcave shape and deformability allow a slow but safe passage. Cells may be retained for longer periods if: (1) their shape is less adaptable (spherocytes), (2) the membrane less pliable (older cells), or (3) there are inclusions or particles stuck to the membrane. These particles, such as Heinz bodies (denatured hemoglobin), siderotic granules (ferritin), or Howell-Jolly bodies (nuclear remnants), are removed or bitten-off ("pitted") by the macrophages; the red cell then reseals itself, somewhat smaller and, because of loss of membrane, more spherical than before. In splenectomized patients or in patients who have lost splenic function (eg, splenic infarction), this role is not performed. The hallmark of this loss of splenic function is the presence of Howell-Jolly bodies in circulating red cells as well as varying numbers of spherocytes – both identifiable in the peripheral blood smear.

Not all red cells are subjected to examination on each splenic pass. Only 10% are detained and inspected at any one time – the remaining 90% flow through a functionally closed sinusoidal system to rapidly exit into the collecting venous channels. At a flow rate of 300 ml per minute in an adult with a blood volume of 5,000 ml, it would be possible to screen all circulating red cells every three hours. However, the random nature of the screen makes the spleen a less than high performance filter, but adequate under normal conditions.

EXTRAVASCULAR HEMOLYSIS (Figure 16-3)

Following red cell ingestion by the macrophage, the hemoglobin is split into its heme and globin components. The globin is degraded into its constituent amino acids for re-cycling. **Heme oxygenase**, a microsomal enzyme, splits the porphyrin ring of heme at the α-methene bridge (between the two vinyl bearing pyrroles); the bridging carbon is converted to CO (the only CO generated in the body), and the iron molecule is removed. This first product is *biliverdin*. It is reduced by the enzyme **biliverdin reductase**, in the presence of NADPH, to form *bilirubin*. Bilirubin exits the macrophage and complexes with plasma albumin in a 2:1 ratio for transport to the liver. This bilirubin is referred to as *unconjugated bilirubin*. It is lipid soluble and readily crosses cell membranes; excess accumulation may be toxic to some cells (eg, development of kernicterus in the newborn with hyperbilirubinemia).

There are two distinct forms of heme oxygenase, HO-1 and HO-2, transcribed by separate genes. HO-1 is the principal form in spleen, HO-2 in liver and brain. HO-1 is induced by heme and also by hormones, organic compounds, various oxidants, and stress. Degradation of heme by HO-1 releases three biologically active molecules: iron, CO and biliverdin. Iron is a

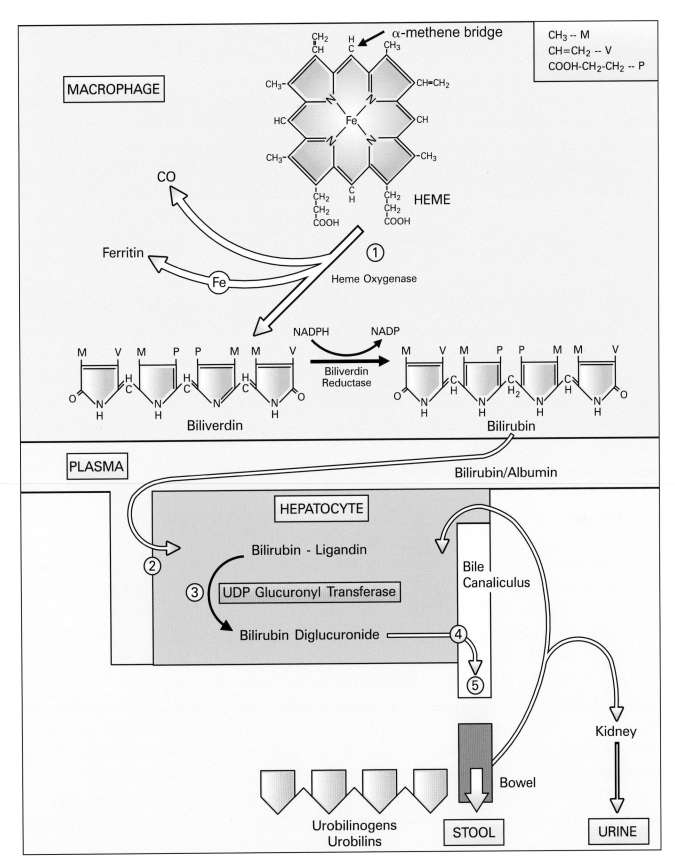

Figure 16-3 Bilirubin Synthesis and Metabolism

strong oxidizing agent; it is bound rapidly by apoferritin to form the less reactive ferritin and recycled into the iron pool. CO is a vasodilator of both small and medium sized vessels. Bilirubin and its precursor biliverdin are strong antioxidants. The antioxidant activity of bilirubin is of major significance; it may be a negative risk factor in coronary artery disease as it prevents oxidation of low density lipoproteins (LDLs). HO-1 deficiency is associated with oxidative endothelial cell injury: major endothelial damage was observed in a two-year-old child with a congenital HO-1 deficiency. (Similar lesions are known to occur in HO-1 deficient mice). It is postulated that the normal hyperbilirubinemia of newborns may be protective before they have access to dietary antioxidants, although abnormally high levels of unconjugated bilirubin are toxic (kernicterus).

Approximately 15-20% of plasma bilirubin arises from sources other than the destruction of mature red cells. This bilirubin comes from: (1) the more rapidly turning over cytochromes and other heme proteins in liver, and (2) the hemoglobin derived from ineffective erythropoiesis due to intramedullary destruction of defective red cells and hemoglobin lost at the time of nuclear extrusion. This is termed the *"early labelled bilirubin"* because it can be identified in plasma shortly (within 2-3 days) after the administration of the heme label 2-^{14}C glycine – in contrast to the labelled bilirubin that appears between 80 and 100 days concurrent with the destruction of the cohort of labelled red cells as they reach senescence. The early-labelled bilirubin becomes a major component when ineffective erythropoiesis is significant (eg, in pernicious anemia or thalassemia).

The bilirubin/albumin complex dissociates on reaching the hepatic cell where bilirubin crosses the hepatocyte membrane. Bilirubin uptake is carrier-mediated, ATP-dependent, saturable and bi-directional – approximately 40% of this unconjugated bilirubin is returned to the plasma along with some bilirubin originating from the hepatic heme pool (heme carried to the liver by haptoglobin, hemopexin, and that derived from hepatic cytochromes). That bilirubin remaining within the hepatocyte binds to a cytosolic receptor *ligandin,* a glutathione-S-transferase (GST). This GST isoform probably acts only as a receptor-transport protein, not as an enzyme. The microsomal enzyme **uridine diphosphate-glucuronyl transferase (UDP-GT)** catalyzes the transfer of glucuronic acid from *uridine diphosphate glucuronic acid* to bilirubin, first producing *bilirubin monoglucuronide* and then *bilirubin diglucuronide*. These forms, referred to as *conjugated bilirubin,* are water soluble and transit the hepatic cell for excretion into the bile canaliculus. (Because of their reaction in the *in vitro* assay for bilirubin, unconjugated bilirubin is often referred to as indirect (reacting) bilirubin and conjugated bilirubin as direct bilirubin).

The canalicular membrane houses an ATP-dependent **MRP2** unidirectional transport system that drives biliary products, including bilirubin diglucuronide, from the hepatocyte into the canaliculus for excretion. MRP2 (multidrug resistance-associated protein 2) is an isoform of the MRP2 protein transport system that removes glucuronide-conjugated xenobiotics and drugs from hepatic cells and some tumor cells (Section 23). Excretion into the canaliculus is the rate limiting step in hepatic bilirubin transport. A small amount of conjugated bilirubin is retained in the hepatocyte and leaks back into the plasma.

When conjugated bilirubin reaches the terminal ileum and colon, bacteria remove the glucuronic acid and reduce the bilirubin to a series of *urobilinogens*. Most of this colourless product is excreted in the stool as fecal urobilinogen; it is readily dehydrogenated to form orange-yellow *urobilins* that contribute to the color of the stool; some 10-20% of urobilinogen is re-absorbed into the plasma. Most of the re-absorbed urobilinogen is excreted back into the gut by the liver (entero-hepatic circulation), a minor component reaches the kidney to be excreted in the urine.

INTRAVASCULAR HEMOLYSIS (Figure 16-4)

Hemoglobin (Hb) that directly enters the plasma is cleared: (1) via the liver as a hemoglobin/haptoglobin complex, or as heme complexed to hemopexin or albumin; or (2) through the kidney.

Hepatic Clearance

Haptoglobin (Hp) is a specific hemoglobin-binding α_2- glycoprotein synthesized in the parenchymal cells of the liver. The haptoglobins are tetramers with two alpha chains and two beta chains linked by disulfide bonds. When not bound to hemoglobin, the $t_{1/2}$ of plasma Hp is 3.5 to 5 days. As Hp is an acute phase reactant, plasma levels are increased in infections or inflammatory disease. It is absent in the newborn; detectable levels are present at three months of age.

In plasma the hemoglobin tetramer dissociates into $\alpha\beta$ dimers; the dimer quickly binds to Hp, in a 1:1 ratio, to form an irreversible noncovalent complex. The hemoglobin-binding capacity of plasma ranges from 0.5 to 2.0 G of Hb/L. The Hb/Hp complex is cleared from the plasma, with a $t_{1/2}$ of 10-30 minutes, by a specific hepatocyte receptor and internalized. The heme moiety is detached from the complex; globin and Hp are degraded. The heme is catabolized to bilirubin and the iron is stored as ferritin. Approximately 15% of red cell hemoglobin normally follows this pathway: this includes the free Hb in bone marrow derived from that accompanying the nuclei of normoblasts as they are extruded, and from red cell fragments not ingested by macrophages. Hp mops up Hb that has spilled into the plasma during intravascular hemolysis; when hemolysis is massive and acute there is rapid saturation of Hp and clearance of the Hb/Hp complex; Hp is replaced slowly over a period of days. The absence or low level of plasma Hp is an indicator of recent or ongoing intravascular hemolysis.

Hemopexin and Methemalbumin – Hemopexin is a β_1 glycoprotein with a high affinity for heme. When the Hp system is overloaded, the circulating free Hb is rapidly oxidized

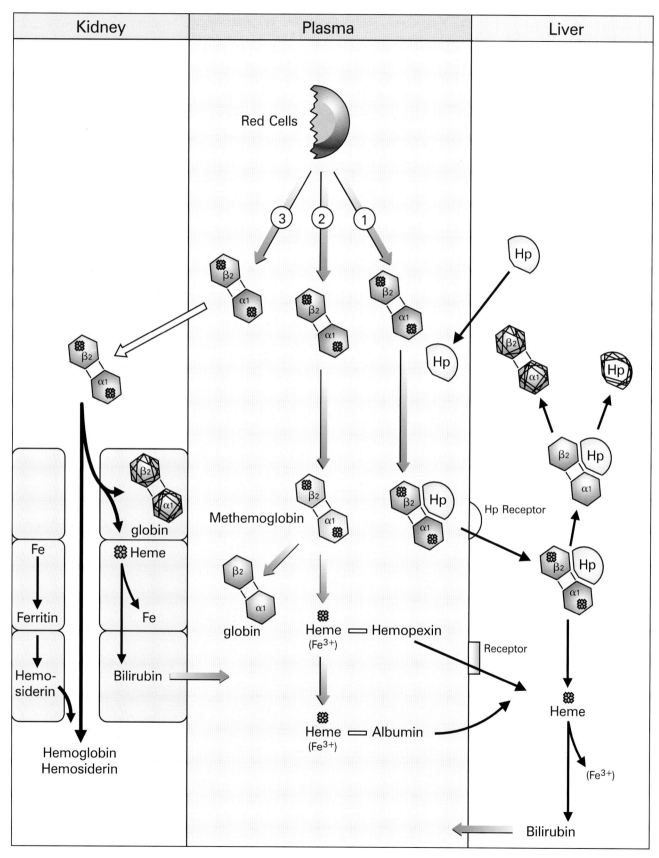

Figure 16-4 Intravascular Hemolysis

to *methemoglobin*. Methemoglobin dissociates non-enzymatically into globin and heme – the free oxidized heme (Fe^{3+}) binds rapidly (in a 1:1 molar ratio) to *hemopexin* and is removed from the plasma with a $t_{1/2}$ of 8 hours. The complex is taken up by specific hepatic receptors and internalized; the heme is converted to bilirubin and the hemopexin is returned to the plasma. In addition, free heme can bind to albumin as *methemalbumin*, which either carries the heme to the liver directly, or acts as an intermediate carrier in the transfer of heme to hemopexin.

Renal Clearance

Free Hb (64kD) is too large to pass the glomerular filter but dissociation of the tetramer into $\alpha\beta$ dimers (32kD) allows their entry into the tubular system. A large proportion of this Hb is reabsorbed into the cells of the proximal tubules – the globin is degraded and the residual heme is catabolized to iron and bilirubin by the heme oxygenase in these cells. In acute intravascular hemolysis, as the Hp and other plasma binding proteins are saturated and the capacity of tubular reabsorption is exceeded, Hb appears in the urine. When Hb is present in large amounts, it may precipitate in the tubules causing tubular cell necrosis and acute renal failure. In low grade continuous intravascular hemolysis, ferritin and hemosiderin accumulate in the tubular cells; subsequent loss of these cells into the urine can be demonstrated by Prussian blue staining for hemosiderin in the desquamated cells.

CLINICAL CORRELATES

Hyperbilirubinemia

Prehepatic. This hyperbilirubinemia may result from either shortened red cell survival or an increase in the production of early-appearing bilirubin due to increased abortive erythropoiesis; both mechanisms play a role in pernicious anemia. Unconjugated bilirubin accumulates in plasma at a rate greater than can be accommodated by hepatic uptake and conjugation. The increase in bilirubin production and hepatic throughput into the bile produces a secondary increase in fecal and urine urobilinogen (①-Figure 16-3).

Shortened red cell survival, with increased bile pigment production, may be due to *intrinsic* red cell defects or to factors *extrinsic* to the cell. Intrinsic defects include: (1) structural membrane defects (congenital spherocytosis and elliptocytosis), (2) red cell enzyme defects (G6PD and PK deficiency), and (3) hemoglobinopathies. Extrinsic causes include: (1) immune hemolytic anemia, (2) sepsis, (3) parasitic diseases (malaria), or (4) exposure to toxic drugs and chemicals (Sections 10 and 13).

Hepatic. *Gilbert's disease* is a common cause of hyperbilirubinemia, present in 2-5% of the population. This may result from a decreased rate of bilirubin transport into the hepatic cell (②-Figure 16-3), but is usually associated with a deficiency of **UDP-glucuronyl transferase** (③-Figure 16-3) – the genetic abnormality has been identified in the promoter region of this gene. Although the serum level of unconjugated bilirubin is increased, it rarely rises above 100 μmol/L (5-6 mg/dL); urobilinogen levels in stool and urine are usually normal. The serum bilirubin increases on fasting. It decreases in patients given a short course of phenobarbital, an inducer of hepatic UDP-glucuronyl transferase.

A major congenital deficiency of UDP-glucuronyl transferase is present in the autosomal recessive *Crigler-Najjar Syndrome (CNS)*. In Type I CNS, complete or almost complete absence of glycuronyl transferase results in severe neonatal unconjugated hyperbilirubinemia with kernicterus. In Type II CNS, the enzyme is reduced but present, therefore, the jaundice is less severe; unconjugated bilirubin levels range from 170 - 250 μmol/L (10-15 mg/dL).

A defect at site ④-Figure 16-3 with a reduced capacity of the hepatic parenchymal cell to move conjugated bilirubin into the bile canaliculus is a manifestation of the congenital autosomal recessive *Dubin-Johnson Syndrome.* This disorder is due to a mutation of the multidrug-resistance protein gene (*mrp2*) that results in the absence of a functional MRP2 in the canalicular membrane. MRP2 is an ATP-dependent export pump for both endogenous and exogenous lipophilic compounds conjugated with glucuronate, sulfate or glutathione. Several mutations of the gene have been identified that compromise the transport and canalicular excretion of xenobiotics and endogenous conjugates. As a result of this defect, bilirubin glucuronide excretion is reduced and increased levels of conjugated bilirubin are present in plasma. As bilirubin glucuronide is water soluble, it is excreted by the kidney and bilirubin appears in the urine; urobilinogen production and excretion are decreased and stools are pale.

Posthepatic. Biliary obstruction at level ⑤-Figure 16-3 results in obstructive jaundice with increased levels of conjugated bilirubin in the plasma; the conjugated water-soluble bilirubin is excreted by the kidney producing bilirubinuria. Little or no bilirubin reaches the bowel, therefore, urobilinogen production and excretion are decreased and stools are pale.

——————— •••●●●••• ———————

SUGGESTED READING

Aono S et al. Analysis of genes for bilirubin UDP glucuronosyl-transferase in Gilbert's syndrome. Lancet 345:958-959, 1995.

Bunn HF. Erythrocyte destruction and hemoglobin catabolism. Semin Hematol 9:3-17, 1972.

Chapman WC, Newman M. Disorders of the spleen. Wintrobe's Clinical Hematology (Ed. 10). Lee GR, Foerster J, Lukens JN, Paraskevas F, Greer JP, Rodgers GM (eds), Lea and Febiger pp 1969-1989, 1999.

Deiss A. Destruction of erythrocytes. Wintrobe's Clinical Hemtology (Ed. 10). Lee GR, Foerster J, Lukens JN, Paraskevas F, Greer JP, Rodgers GM (eds), Lea and Febiger pp 267-299, 1999.

Galbraith R. Heme oxygenase: who needs it? PSEBM 222:299-305, 1999.

Keppler D, Arias IM. Transport across the hepatocyte canalicular membrane. FASEB J 11:15-18, 1997.

Keppler D, König J. Expression and localization of the conjugate export pump encoded by the MRP2 (cMRP/cMOAT) gene in liver. FASEB 11:509-516, 1997.

Keppler D, König J. Hepatic secretion of conjugated drugs and endogenous substances. Semin Liver Dis 20:265-272, 2000.

Platt JL, Nath KA. Heme oxygenase: protective gene or Trojan horse. Nature Med 4:1364-1365, 1998.

Powell LW. Clinical aspects of unconjugated hyperbilirubinemia. Semin Hematol 9:91-105, 1972.

Tenhunen R. The enzymatic degradation of heme. Semin Hematol 9:19-29, 1972.

THE IMMUNOGLOBULIN MOLECULE

Frixos Paraskevas

Bricolage (Fr.) –
A structure assembled from available bits and pieces.

Humoral immunity is the functional responsibility of circulating antibodies synthesized by plasma cells and their B cell precursors. Antigen-specific antibodies function to neutralize toxic substances (as antitoxins), agglutinate particles (as agglutinins), destroy microorganisms (as lysins), and facilitate phagocytosis (as opsonins). Antibodies belong to the immunoglobin (Ig) family.

GENERAL STRUCTURE OF THE Ig MOLECULE

The Polypeptide Chains

The Ig molecule consists of four polypeptide chains: two identical long or **heavy (H) chains** (about 50,000 MW), and two identical short or **light (L) chains** (about 25,000 MW). Each L chain is bound to one H chain through a disulfide bond, and two or more disulfide bonds join the two H chains, forming a symmetrical molecule that is usually diagrammed in the shape of a "Y". There are two types of L chains, designated kappa (κ) and lambda (λ); these light chains are functionally identical. The five types of heavy chains have been assigned lower case Greek letters, μ, γ, α, ϵ, and δ. The heavy chains dictate the five functional **classes** or **isotypes** of the Igs: IgM, IgG, IgA, IgE, and IgD. Their structural and functional properties are listed in Table 17-1.

Each antigen-binding site of the Ig molecule is formed by the combination of the N-terminal regions of one H chain and one L chain (Figure 17-1). Although presented with a myriad of antigens, the two binding sites of an Ig molecule interact with only one particular antigen of a specific structure. The structural diversity of the N-terminals of both H and L chains provides the unique conformation that determines antigen recognition; these areas are referred to as the variable (V) regions or domains. The remainder of the H and L chains are invariant or constant (C) domains. V_L/C_L designates the L chain, and V_H/C_H the H chain.

The Ig chains fold into compact three-dimensional units of about 110 amino acids, referred to as **domains**. The domain folding is maintained by an intrachain disulfide bond. The L chain consists of two domains corresponding to the V_L and C_L regions; the H chain consists of one V_H and three C_H domains (C_H1, C_H2, and C_H3), with the exception of IgM and IgE classes that have four C_H domains. The isotype and the functional activity of the antibody are determined by the C domains of the H chain.

Table 17-1 The Immunoglobulins

	IgG	IgA	IgM	IgD	IgE
Molecular Weight	150 000	160 000	900 000	180 000	190 000
Heavy Chain	γ	α	μ	δ	ε
Light Chain	κ/λ	κ/λ	κ/λ	κ/λ	κ/λ
Half-life (days)	21	6	5	3	2
Concentration (g/L)	7.2-16.9	0.7-3.8	0.6-2.8	0-0.14	<0.005
Complement Binding	+	+	+++	-	-
Phagocyte Binding	+++	-	+/-	-	-
Placenta Crossing	+	-	-	-	-

The Fab and Fc Fragments

The structure of the Ig molecule originally was determined by proteolytic splitting of the molecule with specific enzymes (Figure 17-1). Limited digestion of the Ig molecule with the proteolytic enzyme **papain** generates three fragments: two identical fragments each containing one antigen-binding site referred to as **Fab** (Fragment antigen-binding), and a third named the **Fc fragment** because it crystallizes upon isolation (Fragment crystallizable). **Pepsin** digestion generates one large piece consisting of both Fab fragments – it is bivalent (consisting of both antigen-binding sites) and is known as the **F(ab′)$_2$ fragment**; the Fc fragment is degraded.

Although these constituent pieces are identified by *in vitro* enzymatic digestion, the terms are used clinically to describe the fragments (Fab) that interact with antigen, and the part of the molecule (Fc) that interacts with the Fc receptor on cell membranes. Each Fab proteolytic fragment consists of one L chain associated through a disulfide bond to an H chain; the disulfide bond links the C_L to the C_H1 domain. The Fc fragment consists of the C_H2 and C_H3 domains of both H chains. The Fab fragments are joined to the Fc fragment in the intact Ig molecule by a region of the H chains known as the **hinge**, which allows the two arms of the molecule a degree of flexibility during antigen binding. The hinge region is located between the C_H1 and C_H2 domains; because of the large number of proline residues, the hinge region is susceptible to proteolytic cleavage. The IgM and IgE classes lack a hinge region but this function is performed by the C_H2 domain in each of these molecules.

Structural Organization of the Ig Molecule

The polypeptide chains of the Ig molecule, like other proteins, are folded into a three

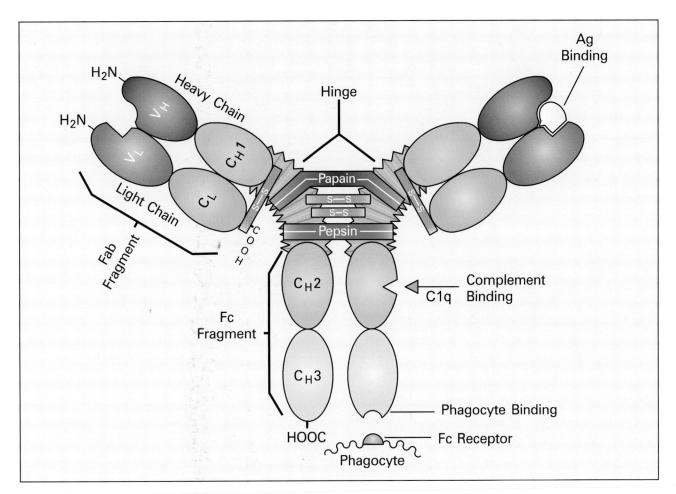

Figure 17-1 The Immunoglobulin Molecule

dimensional configuration. **The primary structure** refers to the linear amino acid sequence. The **secondary structure**, known as the **immunoglobulin fold**, is the most characteristic configuration of the Ig molecule: the amino acid sequences are arranged in β strands that run in opposite directions, i.e. anti-parallel, to form a β-pleated sheet (Figure 17-2). (Proteins are folded primarily into one of two forms: an **α-helix** that can be visualized as a staircase, or a **β-sheet** formed by two side-by-side pleated chains, i.e. folded like an accordion). If both chains run in the same direction (indicated by the correspondence of the N-terminal and C-terminal of one chain relative to the second), the sheet is called **parallel,** and **anti-parallel** if the chains run in opposite directions.

The **tertiary structure** is realized when two β-pleated sheets are fully folded into globular forms or **barrels,** the structural basis of each **Ig domain**. Central to the domain structure are two cysteine residues that form the intradomain disulfide bond joining the β-pleated sheets. In addition, the two β-sheets are linked by hydrophobic bonds in the interior of the barrel. The structure can be visualized as a sandwich: the two slices of bread represent the β-pleated sheets and the butter the hydrophobic bonds. (This Ig domain structure has been identified in over 100

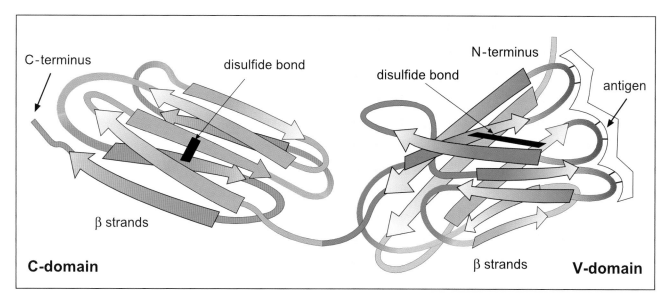

Figure 17-2 Secondary Structure of the Light Chain

proteins other than antibodies – they constitute the **Ig superfamily;** most are adhesive proteins involved in cell-cell interaction. Members of the Ig superfamily occur in disparate species, suggesting that the primordial Ig domain structure may antedate eukaryotic evolution).

The quarternary structure of the polymeric Igs. Two of the Ig classes, IgM and IgA, form multimeric complexes. The increased number of potential antigen-binding sites enhances the avidity of binding to pathogenic targets. Polymerization of IgA and IgM is dependent on the small **J (joining) chain** synthesized in plasma cells (Figure 17-5 and 17-6).

Ig FUNCTIONS

The Ig molecules perform diverse functions that are designed and coordinated to neutralize and efficiently dispose of invading microorganisms and their products. These functions are best understood in the context of the basic structural unit, the **domain.**

Antigen binding: variable (V) domains (Figure 17-1)

The V_L and V_H domains contribute to the formation of a pocket that binds antigen. The variability of each V domain is concentrated within three specific areas known as **hyper-variable regions (HVR)**; the remainder of the domain exhibits far less variability and is known as the **framework region (FR)**. The HVRs, that form the antigen-binding pocket, also are known as **complementarity determining regions** or **CDRs**. There are three CDRs in each V domain (CDR_1, CDR_2, and CDR_3) that correspond to the loops of amino acids joining the β strands (Figure 17-2). The FRs correspond to the β strands. CDRs vary not only in amino acid composition but also in length, attributes that contribute to the variation in size and shape of the antigen-binding pocket.

Effector functions : constant (C) domains

Complement fixation and opsonization are two important effector functions of the Ig molecule. Complement fixation is mediated through the constant domains: the second constant ($C\gamma2$) domain of IgG and the third constant ($C\mu3$) domain for IgM. These domains contain sites for C1q binding (Section 20). The IgM antibody, which consists of five subunits, is more efficient than IgG in activating complement as it possesses multiple binding sites for the C1q component of complement: a single IgM molecule is capable of activating the complement cascade, while a minimum of two precisely spaced IgG molecules are required.

The IgG antibody bound to bacteria acts as an opsonin, i.e., it enhances phagocytosis by granulocytes and macrophages. **Phagocytosis** is mediated through interaction of the Fc segment of the bound IgG with Fc receptors on phagocytes (Figure 17-1). The Fc domain also mediates IgG crossing of the placenta (Section 11).

GENERATION OF DIVERSITY

Two fundamental properties of the antibody response are **specificity** and **diversity**. **Specificity** defines the binding of an antibody only to the antigen that triggered its production. **Diversity** refers to the ability of the immune system to produce specific antibodies to almost an unlimited number of antigens.

Originally, two hypotheses (now discarded) were considered to explain the diversity of the immune response: (a) **germline theory** – one gene, one antibody, and (b) **somatic mutations** of a limited number of genes. In fact, antibody diversity is based on the formation of specific antibodies by somatic **gene rearrangements** of a relatively small number of DNA segments. These rearrangements generate new V genes, but do not affect the genes which encode the constant region – it is the constant region that determines the isotype or class of the Ig molecule.

The H chains in all isotypes are encoded by four DNA segments: three of the coding segments, **V (variable)**, **D (diversity)**, and **J (joining)**, come together to form a complete **new V gene** that encodes the V domain of the H chain involved in antigen binding. All constant regions of the H chain are encoded by one C_H gene. For the L chains, the variable (V) region is encoded by V and J segments (no D segments), and the constant (C) regions by one C_L gene.

Immunoglobulin production depends on the somatic sequential recombination of the germline genes for both H and L chains. Rearrangement begins in the pre-B cell. The heavy chain genes destined to produce IgM are the earliest Ig class to be synthesized (Section 18).

The Heavy Chain (Figure 17-3)

The heavy chain genes are located on chromosome 14. Each of the V, D, and J genes are present in multiple copies arranged in families based on structural similarities; the C_H gene exists as a single copy. There are about 100 V_H genes (only 50 of them are functional), 30 D_H

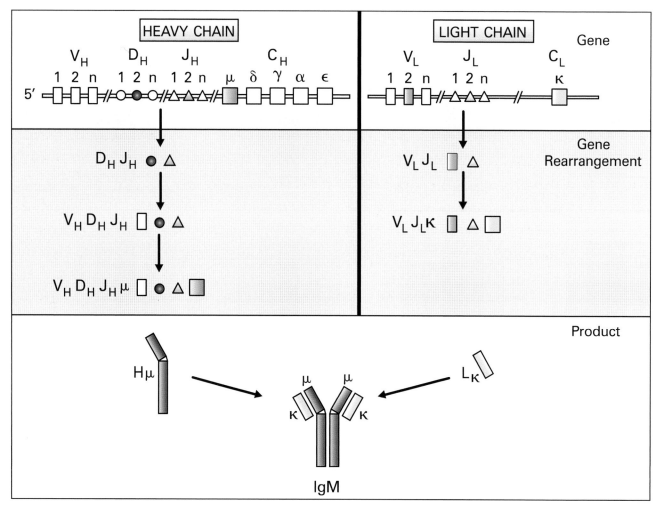

Figure 17-3 Ig Gene Rearrangements

genes and 6 J_H genes. Generation of a complete H chain requires two rearrangements for the formation of the complete V gene. First a D_H segment joins a J_H segment, then the $D_H J_H$ complex is joined by a V_H segment. By a process of recombination, the DNA segments are brought together to form the complete V gene. This is achieved by two enzymes (recombinases), encoded by genes known as **recombination activating genes, RAG-1** and **RAG-2**; both are required for recombination. The new complete V gene then is transcribed with the $C\mu$ gene as well as the entire intervening DNA sequence. The J_H segments between the complete V gene and the C_μ gene, that are superfluous to the recombination, must be removed; this is accomplished during RNA processing, resulting in formation of the mature mRNA which is translated to produce the complete IgM heavy or μ chain. The IgD heavy chain (or δ) is transcribed at the same time as the IgM heavy (μ) chain; this is accomplished by the association of the same V gene with the $C\delta$ gene. Thus, the variable region of the IgD heavy chain is identical to the variable region of the IgM heavy chain, but the constant region is distinct.

The Light Chain (Figure 17-3)

Upon completion of the H chain rearrangements, the signal is given for the initiation of the light chain rearrangements, first to the κ gene cluster and, if unsuccessful, then to the λ genes. Each light chain gene has two opportunities to establish a successful rearrangement (since there are two alleles). There are approximately 27 $V_κ$ and 5 $J_κ$ genes; in the $V_λ$ cluster, there are about 30 $V_λ$ and 4 $J_λ$ segments. If all the attempts at rearrangement are unsuccessful, the B cell dies. Less than 20% of the rearrangements are successful, indicating that the vast majority of young B cells do not advance to the mature stage.

Antibody Diversity (Figure 17-4)

Considering all the available functional segments, it is possible to produce 3.2×10^7 different antibody specificities. This is known as **combinatorial diversity**. The actual number of possible specificities is greater because of imprecisions in the joining of the DNA segments – a feature known as **junctional diversity**.

Tracing the steps required for joining the heavy chain D and J segments demonstrates the complexity of the process. The recombinases (RAG-1 and RAG-2) initiate recombination by recognizing nucleotide sequences known as **recognition signal sequences (RSS)** (Figure 17-4). The RSS consists of two conserved sequences with **seven (heptamer)** or **nine (nonamer)** base pairs, separated by 12 or 23 non-conserved base pair sequences known as **spacers**. The heptamers are positioned at the ends of the DNA segments that are to be joined. The process of recombination is described in the following steps: (1) The RAG-1:RAG-2 enzymes cut one strand of the DNA precisely at the heptamer end next to the D and J segments (Panel 1). (2) Each cut single strand interacts with the other strand and breaks it – severing the double strand completely (Panel 2). (3) The two heptamers (one next to each segment) join head to head to form the **signal joint,** which consists of: the two heptamers, the two spacers, and the two nonamers (Panel 3). The joining of the two heptamers forms a circular structure which includes not only the signal joint but also the areas that lie between the joined D and J segments. This circular piece of DNA is discarded. The 12/23 spacer arrangement is critical in terms of ensuring the recombination of proper segments and in the appropriate order, i.e. the spacers prevent inappropriate joining.

The D and J segments now join to form the **coding joint**, which will be modified by two types of nucleotides, known as **P-** and **N-nucleotides**. The P-nucleotides, originally present in the germline DNA sequence, are translocated to a new position. The N-nucleotides are random new additions, i.e. they were not present in the germ line. (4) The new single strands of the cut ends of the two segments (D and J) to be joined, form a hairpin, known as a **palindrome** (Panel 4). (5) These hairpins are cleaved by an endonuclease (Panel 5). (6) As a result, a single stranded overhang is formed containing the **palindromic (P) nucleotides** (Panel 6). (7)The coding joint is modified further by the addition of random nucleotides (**N-nucleotides**) through the action of the **terminal deoxynucleotidyl transferase (TdT)**, which is expressed early in B cell development (Panel 7). (8) An exonuclease removes improperly paired nucleotides (Panel 8). (9) The coding joint is completed by the addition of complementary nucleotides as needed by a DNA polymerase and the two segments finally are joined by a DNA ligase (Panel 9). The N- and P- nucleotides constitute unique markers of the B cell clone.

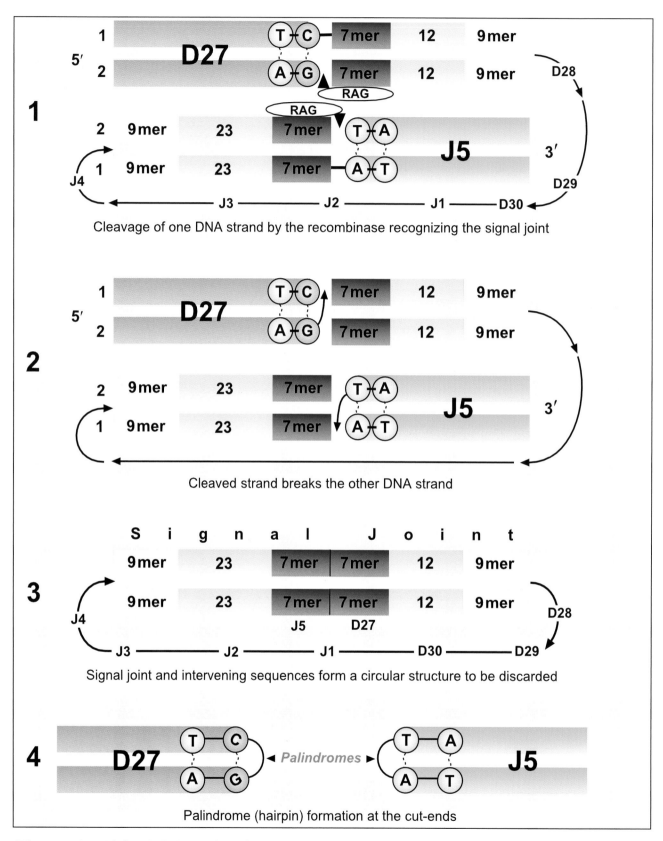

Figure 17-4(a)   Joining of H Chain D and J Segments

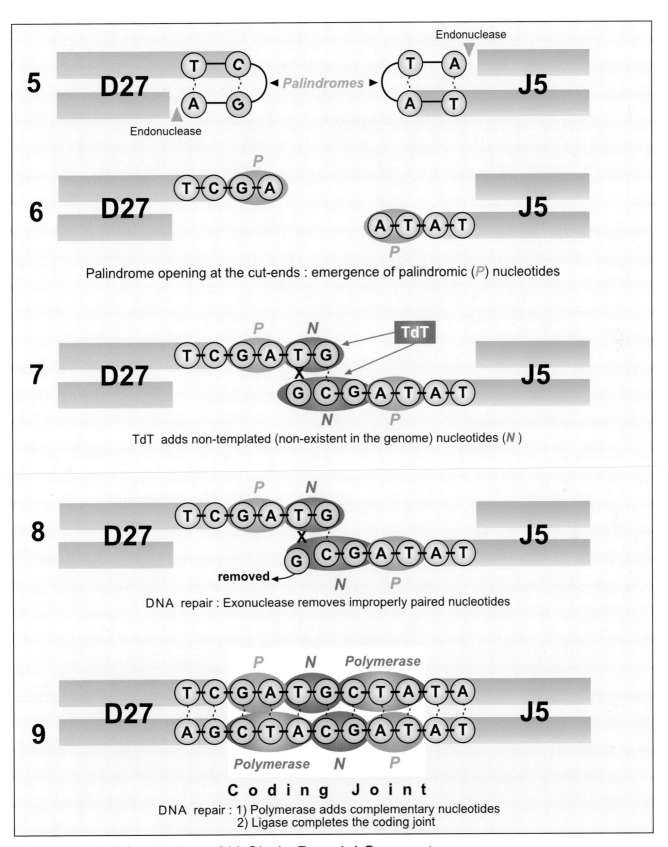

Figure 17-4(b) Joining of H Chain D and J Segments

Class Switch

During an immune response, the production of antibody switches from IgM to the production of the other Ig classes. The formation of a new antibody class (IgG, IgA, IgE), known as **class switch,** takes place in the germinal centres. In this process, the V_H gene (that was produced during IgM synthesis) is translocated next to a different C_H gene, resulting in the synthesis of a second Ig class. Because the same V_H gene combines with a new isotype C_H gene, the antibody specificity of the initial IgM antibody is retained but its effector function is altered.

Class switch is accomplished through a DNA segment located 5′ to each H chain gene known as the **switch region**. The IgD gene, however, lacks its own switch region and therefore is transcribed in the same primary transcript with the IgM gene; subsequent differential splicing generates the two separate transcripts, i.e. IgM and IgD. Class switch is regulated by T cells and involves the participation of specific cytokines.

The Isotypes

The function of each isotype is determined by the structure of the heavy chain constant domains. The isotype can determine the location of the antibodies by limiting their distribution across membranes, and can enhance their interaction with transporter proteins and with the Fc receptors on cell membranes.

IgG is a monomeric immunoglobulin that is distributed equally between the intravascular and extravascular space. Over 75% of plasma immunoglobulin is IgG: it readily crosses the placenta. IgG functions primarily as an antitoxin and an opsonin. The Fc domain of IgG binds to Fc receptors on phagocytic cells, while the two Fab arms interact with the antigen. Complement activation by IgG is relatively weak as this function requires the co-operative participation of at least two IgG molecules associated in a precise spatial relationship, a configuration necessary for binding and activation of the C1q component of complement. IgG is comprised of four subclasses, IgG1, IgG2, IgG3, and IgG4. The most abundant is IgG1; IgG3 is present at the lowest concentration. The involvement of the individual IgG subclasses in immune responses depends on the nature of the antigens: responses against polysaccharides trigger predominantly IgG2 antibodies; antiprotein and antiviral antibodies are mainly IgG3 and IgG4; and the IgG1 subclass responds to both types of immunogens. The efficiency with which IgG activates complement varies with the subclass in the following order: G3>G1>G2>G4.

IgA can be divided into two systems: (1) The IgA (IgA1) in serum and internal secretions (eg, synovial, pleural and peritoneal fluids) is synthesized by plasma cells in bone marrow, lymph nodes and spleen. It is primarily monomeric, about 20% is polymeric. (2) The IgA (IgA2) in external secretions (eg, in saliva, milk, tracheobronchial, genitourinary and gastrointestinal secretions) is present as a dimer; it is produced by plasma cells in submucosal tissues (eg, intestine and respiratory tracts). The formation of the **secretory IgA** dimer depends

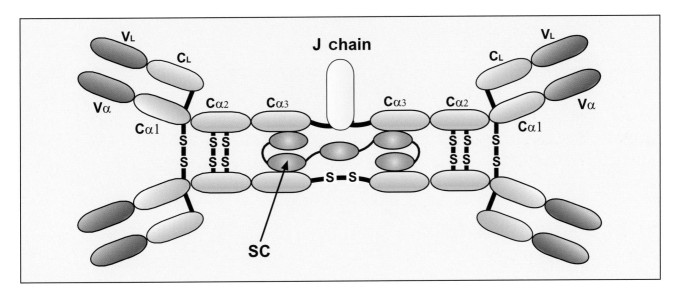

Figure 17-5   The IgA Dimer

upon interaction with the J chain, a 15kD protein that is involved in the formation of the disulfide bond between the two monomers (Figure 17 -5).

The IgA dimer is captured by a receptor for polymeric Ig on the basal membrane of epithelial cells in the respiratory, gastrointestinal and genitourinary tracts. The IgA interacts with the extracellular domain of this receptor, is endocytosed and transported to the cell's apical surface (transcytosis) where the IgA dimer is released still attached to the extracellular portion of the receptor – the **secretory component** (SC). The SC protects the IgA dimer from intraluminal degradation by proteolytic enzymes. Additional protection is provided by deletion of most of the hinge region in the secretory IgA, rendering it resistant to an IgA-specific bacterial protease. The protection afforded by these two mechanisms allows the IgA dimer to survive exposure to bacteria on mucosal surfaces. Secretory IgA has a key role in blocking the attachment of bacteria, such as N. gonorrhoeae and V. cholerae, to mucosal surfaces as well as preventing the absorption of antigenic molecules.

IgM is a pentamer consisting of five subunits or monomers, joined by disulfide bonds between $C\mu 3$ and $C\mu 4$ of the monomers (Figure 17-6). In a process similar to IgA, the small J chain is involved in the formation of a disulfide bond between two of the subunits; this configuration allows IgM to be transported as secretory IgM to mucosal surfaces. Because IgM contains 10 antigen binding sites, it is very efficient in binding large antigens such as bacteria or red blood cells – its potency as an **agglutinin** is up to a thousand-fold greater than IgG. IgM also is an effective **lysin** as it activates the complement system by a stoichiometric (1:1) interaction with C1q. IgM macromolecules remain primarily within the vascular system and do not cross the placenta. IgM monomers function as antigen receptors on the surface of B lymphocytes (Section 18). IgM was the first Ig to appear during evolution, it is the first Ig expressed on the

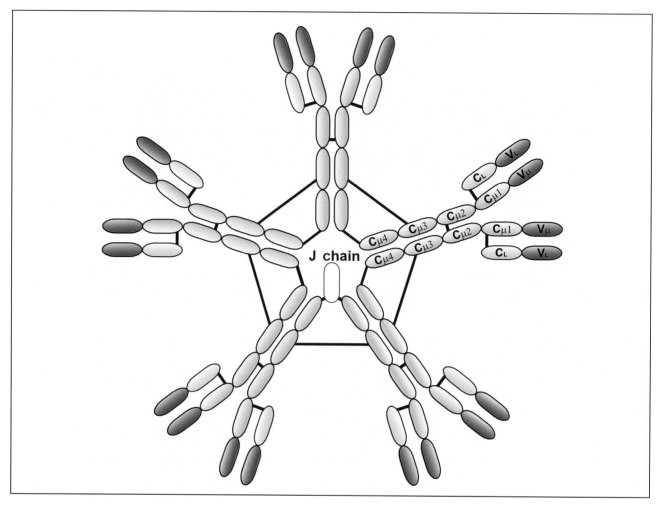

Figure 17-6 The IgM Pentamer

surface of B cells, and the first antibody to be produced during an immune response.

IgD is expressed on the membrane of B cells. Its concentration in serum is low. The function of IgD is unknown.

IgE is present in the serum in low concentration; most is bound to specific Fc receptors on mast cells and basophils. Cross-linking of cell-bound IgE by multivalent antigen triggers mast cell and basophil degranulation with release of histamine and other mediators of the allergic response (Section 8).

CLINICAL CORRELATES

Immunodeficiency

Congenital immunodeficiency diseases arise from genetic defects in one or more components of the immune system. Antibody deficiency may result from abnormal B cell development or from defects that affect development of both B and T cells. These are discussed in Section 19. **Acquired hypogammaglobulinemia** frequently is present in the lymphomas and chronic lymphocytic leukemia.

Hypergammaglobulinemia.

High levels of serum Ig can be separated into two groups: monoclonal gammopathies that involve one specific Ig, and polyclonal gammopathies that produce a spectrum of Ig molecules. The former usually are associated with malignancies of the Ig producing B cells, the latter with autoimmune disease or chronic infection.

Monoclonal Igs are demonstrated as narrow bands on electrophoresis, reflecting a homogeneous population of molecules with identical mobility; these are referred to as paraproteins. Paraproteins are present in a variety of disorders but occasionally are found in otherwise normal individuals. High levels of IgG or IgA paraproteins usually are indicative of **multiple myeloma;** high levels of IgM paraproteins are associated with **macroglobulinemia.** Lower levels of paraproteins may occur in lymphoproliferative disorders, in other malignancies, and in some autoimmune diseases. The term "monoclonal gammopathy of undetermined significance" **(MGUS)** is used to denote relatively low levels of monoclonal Ig in the absence of recognizable disease. This is a chance observation in up to 3% of the population over the age of seventy. Up to 30 % of cases of MGUS eventually evolve into overt myeloma.

In about 20% of patients with myeloma, the paraproteins consist exclusively of L chains **(light chain disease);** they are excreted in the urine as *Bence Jones protein (BJP)*. Some myeloma patients may develop amyloidosis; the amyloid in these patients consists of either intact monoclonal light chains (BJP) or fragments of these chains, most frequently the V region. Approximately 15 to 20% of BJPs are amyloidogenic.

The coupling of the two halves of the Ig molecule, to form the complete molecule, is dependent upon the presence of a normal C_H1 domain. Rarely, patients with a lymphocytic malignancy produce and secrete free H chains **(heavy chain disease)**, a consequence of major deletions in the C_H1 domain.

Monoclonal Antibodies

Injection of an antigen (or immunogen) into an animal yields an antiserum which consists of a variety of antibody molecules, each one specific for a single epitope or antigenic determinant. For example, injection of an antigen that consists of four epitopes, A, B, C, and D, may induce antibodies specific for A, B, C and D (Figure 17-7). Since each of these antibodies is produced by a different B cell clone, the antiserum is **polyclonal.**

When spleen cells from an immunized mouse are mixed with mouse myeloma cells that do not produce Ig, the fusion of a myeloma cell with **one** B cell (of the spleen cell suspension) generates a hybrid – the **hybridoma.** The hybridoma cell retains the properties of the malignant

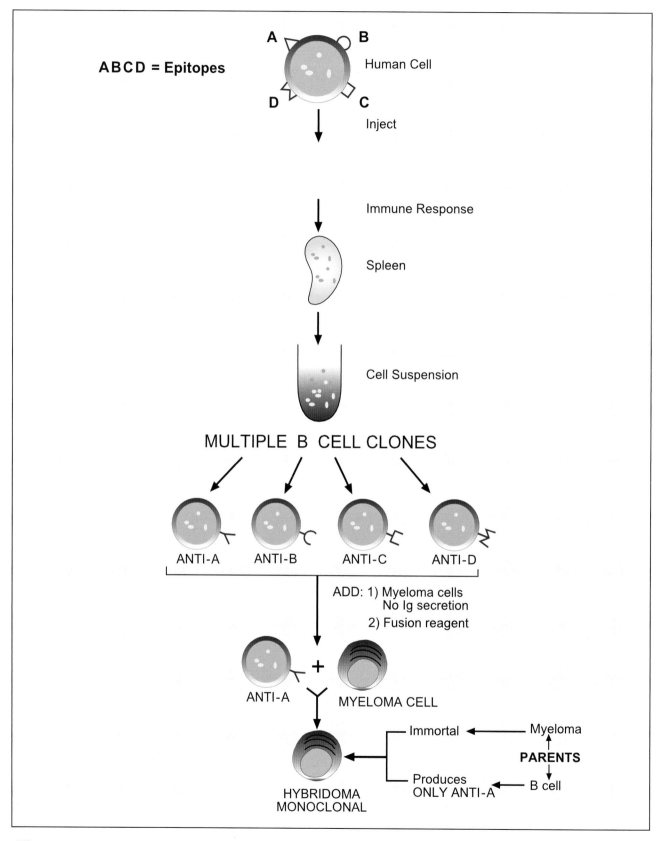

Figure 17-7 Monoclonal Antibody Production

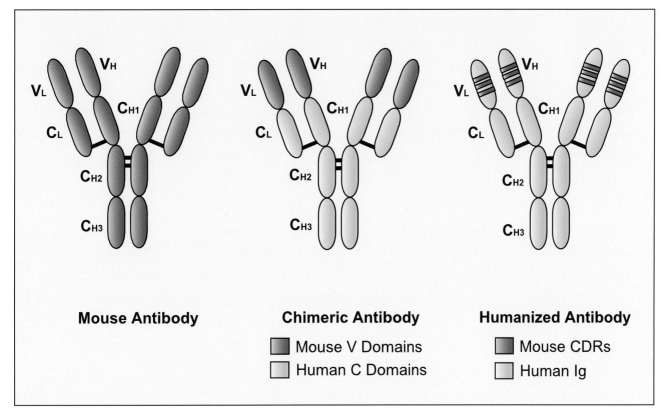

Mouse Antibody   **Chimeric Antibody**   **Humanized Antibody**

Mouse V Domains   Mouse CDRs

Human C Domains   Human Ig

Figure 17-8 Humanization of Monoclonal Antibodies

myeloma cell parent (i.e. it is immortal), but it also inherits the ability to produce the same antibody as the non-malignant parent spleen B cell. Since the proliferating hybridoma cells produce an antibody derived from **one** B cell, it is **monoclonal**.

Monoclonal antibodies have broad applications as diagnostic tools and as therapeutic agents in clinical medicine. They are used to identify differentiation antigens on hematopoietic cells, facilitating precise classification of various hematopoietic malignancies. The development of rapid and simple monoclonal antibody-based laboratory assays has facilitated the identification of enzymes, clotting factors, specific proteins and microbial organisms.

More recently, monoclonal antibodies have been used in the treatment of certain lymphocytic malignancies. Their immunogenicity, however, presents a major problem. Because the monoclonal antibodies are of mouse (or other animal) origin, they induce a humoral immune response when administered to humans. These antibodies are specific for either the Fc (constant) domain (anti-isotypic) or the antigen-binding variable domain (anti-idiotypic) of the mouse immunoglobulin. As a result, these antibodies neutralize the monoclonal antibodies, forming Ag/Ab complexes that are removed from the circulation; in a severe response, they may induce anaphylaxis.

The immunogenicity of the monoclonal antibodies may be reduced by genetic engineering procedures that involve DNA recombinant technology. In one process, the "foreign" (mouse) immunogenic sequences within the constant region are replaced by human sequences: this process is known as **chimerization** (Figure 17-8). In a modified technique, the complementarity determining regions (CDRs) of the rodent monoclonal antibody (which are involved in antigen binding) are "grafted" onto human framework (FR) and constant (C) regions; this process is called **humanization**. Such "reshaping" of the antibodies results in molecules that are less immunogenic than the original rodent monoclonal antibody or the chimeric antibodies; some of these are in clinical use. The humanized antibodies may become immunogenic in some patients following repeated administration.

Monoclonal antibodies also have been conjugated with protein toxins, such as ricin or diphtheria toxins, to produce **immunotoxins,** and also with radionuclides or chemotherapeutic drugs. These conjugated monoclonal antibodies, targeted to specific tumor cell antigens, kill the primary target via the active passenger. Monoclonal antibodies also are used as immunosuppressive agents in certain autoimmune diseases, in organ transplantation, and as inhibitors of platelet function (Section 30).

••••◉••••

SUGGESTED READING

Dreyer WJ, Bennett JC. The molecular basis of antibody formation: a paradox. Proc Natl Acad Sci 54:864-869, 1965.

Frazer JK, Capra JD. Immunoglobulins: structure and function. In Fundamental Immunology, 4th Edition, Paul WE (ed). Ch 3:37, 1999.

Janeway CA, Travers P. Immunobiology. Garland, 1999.

Paraskevas F. Cell interactions in the immune response. In Wintrobe's Clinical Hematology (Ed 10) Lee R, Foerster J, Lukens J, Paraskevas F, Greer JP, Rodgers GM (eds). Williams and Wilkins Vol 1:544-614, 1999.

B LYMPHOCYTES

Frixos Paraskevas

*"The hour of departure has arrived, and we go our separate ways –
I to die, and you to live. Which is better, the gods only know."*
Socrates in: Plato's Apologia

The role of B lymphocytes is to produce antibodies in response to environmental antigens. B cell development from the stem cell to the differentiated plasma cell is under the control of signals generated on its surface following interactions with other cells and stimulation by growth factors and foreign antigens. This is accomplished in two stages. During the first stage in the bone marrow, the immunocompetent B cells are derived from undifferentiated stem cells. Under the guidance of stromal cells, but in the absence of antigenic stimulation, they acquire the potential (the repertoire) for antibody production. The cells that emerge from the bone marrow are referred to as **naïve B cells** because they have not yet been in contact with antigen. During the second stage, which evolves in the secondary lymphoid organs, antigenic stimulation drives the differentiation of naïve B cells into antibody-producing **plasma cells**.

The interaction of the B cell with its environment involves appropriate "receptors" that develop on the cell surface. They serve as markers that define the precise stage of the developing B cell during the process of differentiation. These markers are known as CDs, "clusters of differentiation".

Transcriptional Regulation of B Lineage Development

All hematopoietic lineages derive from pluripotent hematopoietic stem cells (HSC) (Section 5). These primitive HSCs are lineage negative, i.e. they do not express the markers detected on cells committed to a specific lineage. Signals generated on the cell surface of HSCs induce transcription factors (TF) – regulatory proteins that bind to specific DNA sequences and activate appropriate genes in a hierarchical manner. Some TFs, such as TAL-1 and GATA-2, act at a very early stage; experimental blocking of their expression stops development of all hematopoietic lineages. The commitment of cells to lymphocytic differentiation is controlled by the **Ikaros gene** which encodes specific TFs; these TFs target genes that are essential for lymphocyte development, such as the recombination activation genes (**RAGs**) and the terminal deoxynucleotidyl transferase (**TdT**) gene, both involved in immunoglobulin (Ig) (Section 17) and T cell receptor (TCR) gene rearrangements (Section 19).

Progression to B lineage is regulated by another set of genes (E2A, EBF, SOX-4, and PAX-5), encoding TFs that act in the early stages of B cell development. With disruption of the **E2A gene**, which affects only B cell development, transcripts of RAG-1 and CD19 are absent. The product of the **PAX-5 gene**, the TF known as BSAP (B Cell Specific Activator Protein),

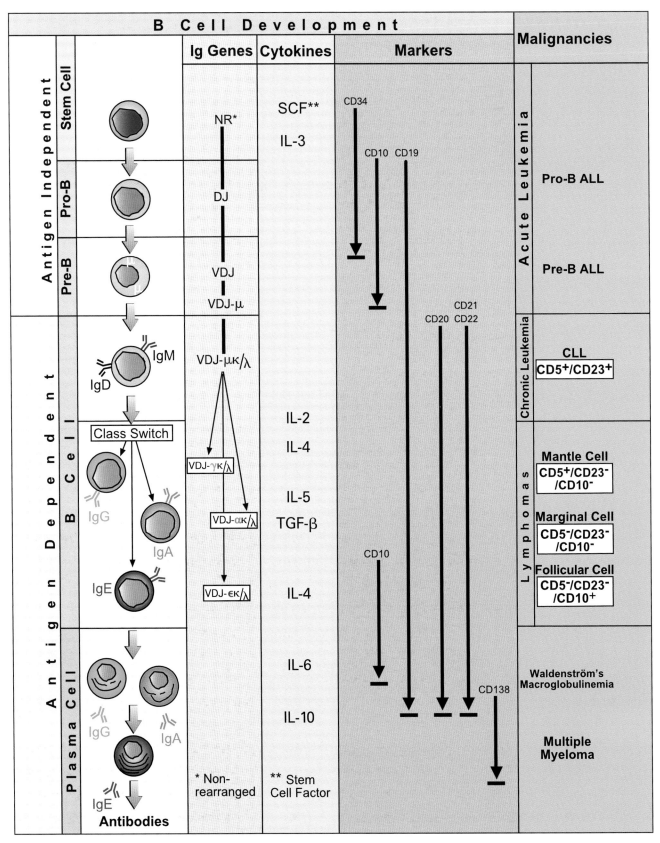

Figure 18-1 Normal B Cell Differentiation and B Cell Malignancies

binds to the promoter regions of CD19, λ5, and Vpre-B genes; the products of the last two genes are proteins that form the pre-B cell receptor, crucial in the initial stages of B cell differentiation.

Antigen-Independent Differentiation in The Bone Marrow (Figure 18-1)

The sites of B lymphocyte generation vary with the different developmental stages. During embryonic development, the first B cell precursors are detected in the omentum and the liver. After birth, the bone marrow takes over as the major site of B cell development, which begins near the endosteum and moves toward the centre of the marrow cavity as the cell differentiates. The hallmark of this stage of B cell differentiation is rearrangement and expression of the immunoglobulin genes; in addition, there are changes in expression of cell surface and intracellular proteins.

Development of mature B cells from HSCs depends on contact with stromal cells; different stromal cells are involved at various stages of differentiation. Stroma (Greek: mattress) is a generic term that includes a variety of cells such as fibroblasts, endothelial cells, macrophages, and adipocytes. Stromal cells regulate B cell development in a number of ways: (1) by direct interaction, (2) by formation of the extracellular matrix (collagen, proteoglycans) which regulates cell migration and binds growth factors, and (3) by release of cytokines.

B Cell Precursors (Figure 18-1)

The earliest stage in B cell development, known as the **pro-B cell**, is characterized by the CD34, CD10, CD19 phenotype, and the intracellular enzymes TdT and RAG. Ig gene rearrangements in these cells involve only D_H/J_H segments; therefore, pro-B cells do not express surface Ig, but a protein complex known as **pro-B cell receptor** that consists of a **surrogate light chain (SL)** in association with a complex of glycoproteins. (The SL consists of two non-covalently linked proteins known as **Vpre-B** and **Vλ**). The next stage, known as the **pre-B cell**, is characterized by a productive $V_H/D_H/J_H$ rearrangement, which results in the formation of a complete μ heavy chain. Because the L chain genes are still in the germ line configuration, the μ heavy chain is present in the cytoplasm and also in association with the SL on the cell surface forming the **pre-B cell receptor (pre-BCR).** The function of the pre-BCR is related to **allelic exclusion**, i.e. the prevention of expression of immunoglobulin H chains from the second (alternate) allele after the successful rearrangement of the first (Section 17). The pre-BCR also gives a proliferative burst to pre-B cells which at this stage are large, cycling cells with a longer life span due to the expression of the *bcl-x* gene, a member of the bcl-2 family that blocks apoptosis (Section 4).

In the subsequent stage, the cells are small, non-cycling, and lose the pre-BCR. Their phenotype changes to CD34⁻/CD10⁻, while new markers (CD20/CD21/CD22) appear. At this stage, light chain rearrangements proceed. With the completion of a successful light chain gene rearrangement, the complete IgM molecule appears on the cell surface as the receptor for antigen, the **B cell receptor (BCR)**. At this stage, the B cell is only IgM$^+$ and is immunologically **immature**. Interaction of the BCR with antigen may "paralyze" the cell (i.e. induce tolerance). Subsequent expression of IgD on the surface endows the cell with immunological competence (**mature B cell**) and signifies the end of the first, antigen-independent, stage of differentiation.

Homing

B cells leave the bone marrow and **home** to the secondary lymphoid organs. Lymphocyte homing is regulated at the molecular level by interaction of lymphocytic **homing receptors** with appropriate ligands on the endothelial cells which function as **addressins**. As lymphocytes pass through the capillary bed in the lymph node (LN), they encounter a unique vascular structure which is anatomically part of the venular system but differs from venules because of the tall cuboidal endothelium – these are known as **high endothelial venules (HEVs)**. As the lymphocytes come in contact with the surface of these cells, they interact with adhesion molecules on the endothelial cell surface; the lymphocytes slow, roll, adhere to the endothelium, and migrate through the HEV wall into the tissues. The **initial interaction** involves the **L-selectin** on lymphocytes and its ligand on the HEV cell, known as **peripheral node addressin (Pnad)**. Arrest and tight adhesion of the lymphocyte to the endothelium is mediated by the lymphocyte β_2 **integrin**, CD11a/CD18 ($\alpha_L\beta_2$). Following chemokine activation, CD11a/CD18 interacts with its counter receptor on the HEV surface, **ICAM-1** (intercellular cell adhesion molecule-1). Tight adhesion is followed by transmigration between the endothelial cells into the tissues (Section 7). Integrin-mediated transmigration is regulated by a CC chemokine known as **SLC (secondary lymphoid tissue chemokine)** produced by the HEV cells. SLC is strongly chemotactic for naïve T cells and, to a lesser extent, for B cells. These cells bind to the HEVs by the SLC receptor, CCR-7, expressed on the surface of lymphocytes. Some B cells may exit venules directly into the follicles. Most B cells traverse a unique vascular labyrinthine network of corridors and conduits within the T cell zone, finally arriving at the **follicle**. The movement of the B cells to the follicles, after exiting the paracortical HEV, is triggered by a CXC type of chemokine secreted by the follicular dendritic cells, **BCA-1 (B cell-attracting chemokine 1)**, also known as **BLC (B lymphocyte chemoattractant)**. BCA-1 specifically attracts B cells which express the BCA-1 receptor CXCR5. If the follicle has not been the site of a previous immune response, it is referred to as a **primary follicle**; it consists of a loose collection of naïve small B cells within a loose network of **follicular dendritic cells (FDC)**. A follicle that has been the site of a previous immune response is known as a **secondary follicle**; it consists of a dense collar of small compact lymphocytes, **the mantle**, which surrounds large blast-like cells that form the **germinal centre**.

Homing to Peyer's patches depends on the lymphocyte **mucosal homing receptor**, the

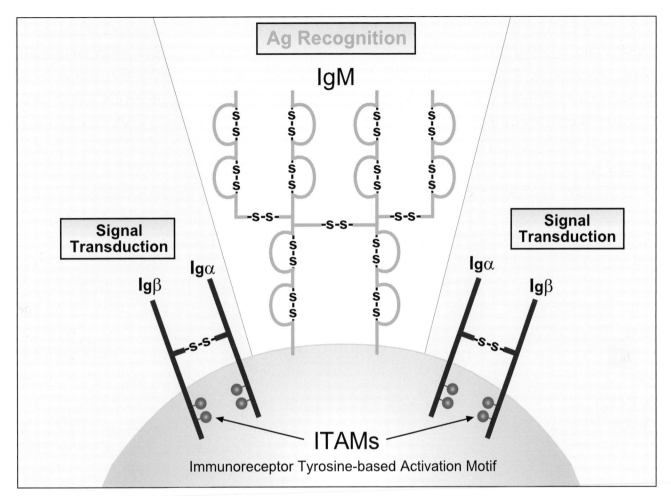

Figure 18-2 B Cell Receptor Complex

integrin $\alpha_4\beta_7$, which interacts with a mucosal addressin, **MAdCAM-1** (Mucosal Addressin Cell Adhesion Molecule-1), on the endothelial cell. In Peyer's patches, segregation of T and B cells involves distinct HEVs. The HEVs near follicles support B cell accumulation, while T cells gather around interfollicular HEVs. As in the peripheral LN, T and B lymphocytes are guided by specific chemokines produced by different HEVs.

The B Cell Receptor (BCR) and Coreceptors

(a) BCR Complex (Figure 18-2)

The antigen receptor of the B cell consists of the membrane IgM and two heterodimers, one on each side. The heterodimers consist of two polypeptide chains, **Igα** and **Igβ**, linked by a disulfide bond. **Recognition of antigen** is mediated by IgM, and **signal transduction** is mediated by the Igα and Igβ polypeptides. Initially, IgM is the only membrane immunoglobulin (**mIg**), joined later by IgD. (IgG, IgA, and the other immunoglobulins are expressed on memory B cells).

The surface IgM is monomeric, i.e. it consists of only one of the five subunits that make up the pentameric serum IgM (Section 17). The mIg consists of three domains: **extracellular** (similar to the monomer of serum IgM molecules), **transmembrane** (20-25 amino acids), and **intracellular** (3 amino acids). Because the intracellular domain of mIg is only three amino acids long, it is unable to initiate signal transduction. This function is carried out by its associated Igα/Igβ polypeptides – their long cytoplasmic tails facilitate interactions with protein tyrosine kinases of the signaling cascade. These interactions are mediated by a unique amino acid sequence present in the Igα amd Igβ cytoplasmic tails, known as the **Immunoreceptor**

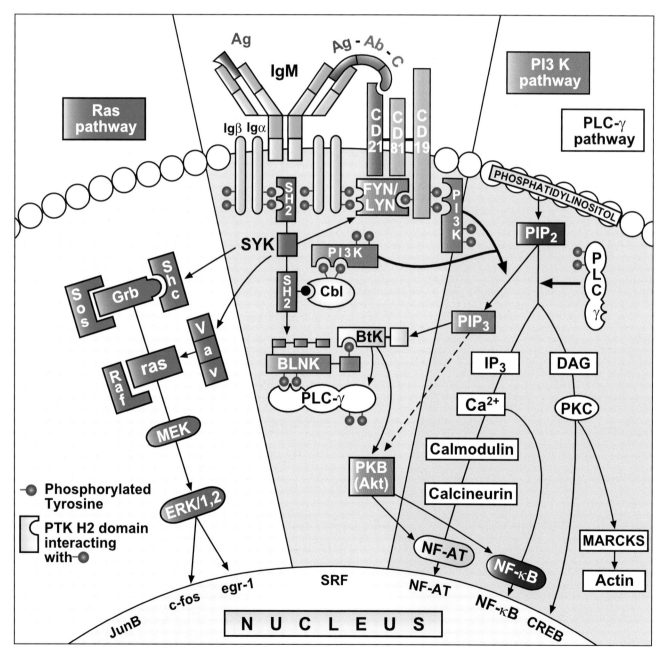

Figure 18-3 B Cell Activation Pathways

Tyrosine-based Activation Motif or **ITAM.** It contains two YxxL sequences (Y = tyrosine; L = leucine; x = any amino acid) separated by 6-8 non-conserved amino acids.

(b) Coreceptors (Figure 18-3)

BCR signaling is influenced by two coreceptors, one a promoter and the other an inhibitor of B cell activation. The **activation-promoting coreceptor** is a complex of three proteins: CD19, CD21 (complement receptor 2), and CD81 (or TAPA-1, Target of Anti-Proliferative Antibody). Antigen-antibody-complement complexes induce aggregation of the coreceptor with the BCR through binding of the complement component to CD21 and the antigen component to the IgM of the BCR. These complexes are bound to follicular dendritic cells in the germinal centres and is the form by which antigen is presented to B cells (Section 21).

The **inhibitory coreceptor** is the receptor for the Fc domain of IgG; **the FcγIIB isoform (CD32)** is the most important inhibitory coreceptor. The cytoplasmic domain of the FcγIIB receptor has a sequence known as **ITIM, immunoreceptor tyrosine-based inhibitory motif,** which contains a single tyrosine. ITIM that has been phosphorylated by tyrosine kinases recruits and interacts with inhibitory tyrosine phosphatases, thereby interfering with signal transduction.

B Cell Activation (Figure 18-3)

(a) BCR in B Cell Activation

The production of protective levels of antibody depends upon the **clonal expansion** (increase in numbers) of B cells and their **differentiation** into plasma cells that are capable of synthesizing antibody at a high rate.

Proliferation and differentiation of B cells are triggered by signals received by the BCR that activate intracellular signaling pathways. (For a general discussion of signaling, see Section 1). The initial event, subsequent to engagement of the BCR by antigen, is the phosphorylation of tyrosine in the Igα and Igβ ITAMs, followed by **phosphorylation of protein tyrosine kinases (PTKs).** The PTKs that are activated within seconds after BCR engagement are: (a) the Src group, (b) **Syk,** and (c) **Btk.**

The Src (Fyn, Lyn) and Syk PTKs, via their SH2 domains, dock on the phosphorylated ITAMs of the BCR complex. The Syk kinase plays a central role in initiating multiple downstream signaling cascades, involving three pathways: (a) phospholipase C-γ (PLC-γ), (b) phosphatidylinositol-3 kinase (PI3-K), and (c) Ras. Syk activates Bruton's tyrosine kinase (Btk) through the adaptor protein BLNK. (A mutation of Btk is the cause of X-linked agammaglobulinemia). PI3-K and PLC-γ act on plasma phospholipids, generating second messengers that regulate the activity of downstream signaling proteins (Section 1). PI3-K is activated by Syk through the intermediate linker Cbl. PI3-K converts PIP_2 to PIP_3 which binds to PTKs with a **pleckstrin** homology domain, such as Btk and protein kinase B (PKB or Akt). Akt has prosurvival functions as it regulates activation of transcription factors such as NF-kB and NF-AT.

PLC-γ is activated by Syk and Btk. Hydrolysis of membrane phospholipids by PLC-γ generates diacylglycerol (DAG) and inositol-1,4,5-triphosphate (IP_3). DAG activates protein kinase C (PKC), while IP_3 increases intracellular Ca^{2+} by release from intracellular sources. Ca^{2+} activates transcription factors NF-AT and NF-κB. PKC, through the MARCKS proteins, mediates actin cross-linking and association with the cell membrane. The Ras pathway leads to activation of other transcription factors (eg, egr-1 and c-fos). Signals originating from the BCR and other receptors follow diverse pathways to the nucleus and regulate B cell survival, differentiation, and proliferation, depending on the nature of the ligands and their receptors.

(b) Coreceptors in B Cell Activation

The CD19/CD21/CD81 activating coreceptor reduces, by 1000-fold, the threshold of antigen required for activation. Two of the tyrosines in the cytoplasmic domain of CD19 are phosphorylated upon activation and serve as binding sites for PI3-kinase. The inhibitory coreceptor (Fc-receptor) has a single tyrosine in its ITIM. When this tyrosine is phosphorylated, the ITIM binds and activates an **inositol phosphatase** known as **SHIP**. How SHIP inhibits BCR-mediated activation is not clear, however it does inhibit CD19 phosphorylation and also degrades PIP_3.

Antigen-Dependent Differentiation in Secondary Lymphoid Organs (Figure 18-1)

The B cells that leave the bone marrow have antigen receptors (IgM) that are of low affinity. Furthermore, antigen-specific B cells are rare. Therefore, these cells are ill-equipped to provide protection from an infectious threat. Pathogens that enter the body may be carried through the lymphatic system to the peripheral lymphoid organs; naïve B cells that encounter these foreign antigens are stimulated to become antibody-producing cells.

The objectives of the antigen-driven second stage of B cell differentiation are well defined: (a) increase the number of antigen-specific cells (**clonal expansion**), (b) increase antibody affinity (**affinity maturation**), (c) selection of cells capable of making high affinity antibodies (**clonal selection**), (d) generation of cells with rapid rates of antibody production (**plasma cell differentiation**) capable of producing antibodies of all classes (**class switch**) for immediate protection, and (e) generation of large numbers of cells that are prepared to respond when they again encounter the same antigen (**memory B cells**) for future protection.

Antibody responses to foreign antigens are designated as: (1) **primary** – occurring within the first 3-4 days following encounter with an antigen and consisting of the IgM class; or (2) secondary – occurring within 7-15 days, or later, following antigen stimulus and consisting predominantly of IgG and IgA.

Germinal Centre Reaction (Figure 18-4)

The first encounter with an antigen by a naïve B cell entering the lymph node is believed to take place in the paracortical or T cell zone near the follicle. Activation of the B cell in this location generates a B-blast which, subsequently, follows one of two possible pathways: (1) rapid differentiation to short-lived plasma cells secreting IgM can be detected in the first 3-4 days after exposure to antigens – this is the primary IgM antibody response; (2) migration into the follicle where rapid proliferation initiates the **germinal centre (gc) reaction**.

The blasts that migrate to the follicle are known as **centroblasts**; they are surface Ig negative or very weakly positive. As they multiply, they form the **dark zone** of the gc (located next to the T cell zone). **Follicular dendritic cells (FDCs)** with fine dendritic processes, $CD23^-$, penetrate the dark zone. (Phenotypically the centroblasts are $CD19^+$, $CD10^+$, $CD20^+$, and $CD38^+$).

At this stage, the B cells undergo a second round of **antigen receptor diversification**. The first diversification took place in early maturing B cells, within the bone marrow, during the antigen-independent phase, and involved rearrangement of the Ig genes. The second diversification takes place in dividing centroblasts within the germinal centre during the antigen-dependent phase. This genetic mechanism is known as **somatic hypermutation** – mutations occur at a high rate only within the immunoglobulin V domains of the rearranged genes (mutations do not occur in the C region). Because the mutations accumulate in the V region, antibody affinity for antigen may be altered (lost or increased) or may remain the same.

The fate of the B cell is decided in the adjacent compartment of the gc, the **light zone**, The centroblasts that have undergone hypermutation are known as **centrocytes**, and move into the light zone. The centrocytes are smaller cells with a compact cleaved nucleus: they do not proliferate and are surface Ig^+, $CD19^+$, $CD10^+$, and $CD40^+$. The light zone contains a dense network of $CD23^+$ FDCs that carry antigen in the form of antigen-antibody complexes. This zone of the gc is characterized by the large number of apoptotic cells. Centrocytes with surface Ig that has **lost the affinity for antigen** as a result of the somatic hypermutations undergo apoptosis – i.e. they are not selected for survival by antigen-presenting FDCs. The apoptotic cells are phagocytosed by macrophages (macrophages that engulf the apoptotic centrocytes are known as **tingible body macrophages**).

Centrocytes with surface immunoglobulin that binds antigen with **high affinity** are positively selected for further differentiation, developing into plasma cells or memory B cells.

These final differentiation pathways for effector B cell production depend on interactions with other cells and cytokines. The cells that contribute to the germinal centre reaction are the

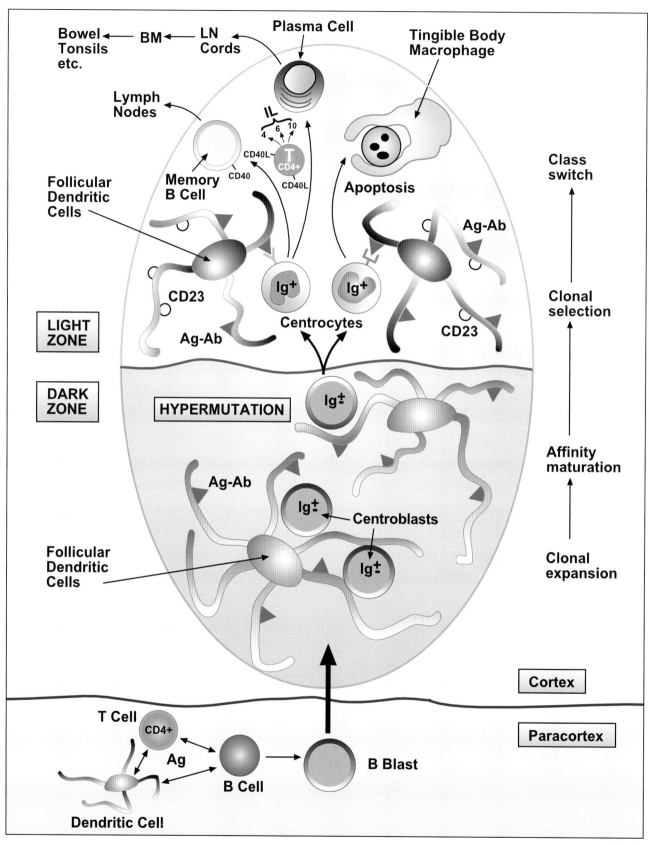

Figure 18-4 Germinal Centre Reaction

FDC (Section 21) and CD4$^+$ T cells (Section 19). When antigen is bound to surface Ig on B cells, it is endocytosed and degraded; the peptides that are returned to the cell surface bound to MHC class II molecules are recognized by the helper CD4$^+$ cells.

B cell activation and differentiation requires **two signals**. One is **antigen specific** and is generated when antigen binds to the membrane Ig of the BCR. This signal alone, however, is not sufficient to support all B cell changes in the germinal centre. Signals generated by cooperating cells and soluble factors in response to the specific antigen are known as **costimulatory signals**. The CD4$^+$ cells within the follicles are known as **follicular B helper T cells (TFH)**. They represent memory T cells which were activated earlier by the same antigen. Their localization within the follicle is due to the expression of the chemokine receptor CXCR5. CXCR5 is not present on naïve T cells, but is upregulated following activation of T cells by antigen; it is the receptor for BCA-1, a chemokine produced by the FDC which also attracts the B cells to the follicles.

Thus chemokines set the stage and regulate T cell-B cell interaction. Helper CD4$^+$ cells that recognize the antigen/MHC class II complex interact with the B cell through two sets of molecules: (1) CD40 on B cells and CD40 ligand (CD154) on T cells, and (2) CD80/CD86 on B cells, and CD28 on T cells. The signals generated by CD40/CD154 interactions are essential for humoral immunity, germinal centre formation, generation of memory cells, and increase of antibody affinity ("affinity maturation") of those antibodies that have switched to other classes from IgM. CD40/CD154 interaction upregulates CD80/CD86 expression on B cells, thus enhancing costimulation. The CD40 is a phosphorylated glycoprotein that belongs to the TNF receptor superfamily. The CD40 ligand (CD154) is homologous to the TNF family; it can be released in a soluble form from activated T cell membranes.

Another important function that takes place in the gc is the **class or isotype switch**, i.e. the change from IgM to IgG, IgA, or IgE antibody production. At the genetic level, class switch involves the translocation of the same V gene to another C gene; as a result, the new class possesses the same antigen specificity as the IgM antibody first produced (Section 17).

The Interleukins

Costimulatory signals for B cell differentiation into plasma cells are provided by soluble factors, including a number of interleukins, IL-2, IL-4, IL-6, and IL-10. Interleukins (cytokines) are not antigen specific. Their characteristic properties are: **pleiotropy** (multiple functions on multiple targets), **redundancy** (the same function provided by more than one cytokine), **synergism** (two or more cytokines required for a particular function), and **antagonism** (interference with the function of another interleukin). Interleukin function is expressed following binding to membrane receptors that are linked intracellularly to various signal transduction pathways.

IL-4 is primarily a B cell growth and differentiation factor. In the presence of CD40/CD154 interaction, it provides a prolonged B cell proliferative stimulus and is a switch factor for IgE production. The IL-4 receptor consists of an α chain and shares the common γc chain with IL-2R (IL-2 receptor: Section 19).

IL-6 is one of the most pleiotropic interleukins and plays a central role in immunity and inflammation. In B cells, it stimulates production of Ig and the growth of plasma cells. It stimulates proliferation of hematopoietic progenitors, and synthesis of acute phase proteins by hepatocytes in response to injury and inflammation. The IL-6 receptor (IL-6R) consists of a unique ligand-binding polypeptide and a common signal transduction polypeptide gp130, shared by several other cytokine receptors. Binding of IL-6 to IL-6R triggers dimerization of gp130, resulting in transduction of a signal that links the gp130 cytoplasmic domain to the JAK kinases and the Ras-MAP kinase pathways.

IL-10 is a dimer of a subunit consisting of four α-helices. It is produced by T cells and macrophages (as well as by EBV infected B cells). IL-10 stimulates proliferation of B cells and induces IgM, IgG, and IgA production following cross-linking of CD40. IL-10 accounts for much of the non-contact help provided by T cells to B cells.

Plasma Cells (Figure 18-1)

The **plasma cell** is round or oval with an eccentrically located nucleus and chromatin arranged in pyramidal blocks that abut against the nuclear membrane and are responsible for the characteristic "cartwheel" appearance. The cytoplasm is intensely basophilic because of the high ribonucleoprotein level. Certain plasma cells stain red to violaceous due to a high carbohydrate content of the Ig in the endoplasmic reticulum (ER). The striking ultrastructural feature of the plasma cell is the elaborate well-organized ER – it consists of membranes studded on one side with ribosomal particles and arranged in parallel arrays.

Circumscribed areas of the ER cisternae are sometimes distended with a homogeneous material composed of Ig; these are the cytoplasmic inclusions known as **Russel bodies** that are seen in chronic inflammation and in malignant disorders. Distension of the plasma cell occurs when there is a large accumulation of Ig throughout the ER cisternae; these cells are referred to as **thesaurocytes**. Both these forms may result from dysfunction in Ig secretion.

Ig synthesis takes place within the ER. H and L chains are synthesized on separate polyribosomes. The complete molecule is assembled from individual chains after release from the ribosomes into the cisternae. The carbohydrate is attached as the molecule passes through the Golgi apparatus. Whether the Ig becomes **membrane-bound** or is **secreted** is determined by its molecular structure. Although the same gene encodes both forms, their role and destination depends on whether there has been: (1) complete transcription of the gene, including the sequences that encode the transmembrane domain and the cytoplasmic tail, with production of membrane Ig, or (2) early termination of transcription that results in absence of the transmembrane and cytoplasmic domains, resulting in production of the secretory protein (secretory Ig).

B Cell Subpopulations

Two B cell subpopulations have been defined on the basis of their CD5 expression. The $CD5^+$ B cells are termed B1, the $CD5^-$ B cells termed B2. The B1 cells are the predominant population during fetal life. After birth, $CD5^+$ B cells are found primarily in the mantle of the lymph node follicles, rarely in the peripheral blood. Because TdT is not expressed during fetal life, the early gene rearrangements lack N nucleotide insertions and therefore the antibodies produced are of limited diversity (Section 17); the V segments generated after birth have a more diverse repertoire. The antibodies produced by B1 cells generally are of low affinity with a broad specificity against common bacterial antigens and autoantigens (**polyspecific**). The $CD5^-$ (or B2) B cells are present throughout adult life. (There are two views concerning the relationship between B1 and B2: they may represent separate lineages or the phenotypic difference may be the result of cell activation).

CLINICAL CORRELATES

B Cell Immunodeficiency

Congenital or acquired immunodeficiency is present when components of the immune system are absent or defective. Susceptibility to infections is determined by the nature of the immunological defect. Congenital immunodeficiency diseases involving B cells include primary defects in B cell development and secondary B cell functional failure as a result of T cell defects. They can be classified as: (1) **defects of antibody production alone, and** (2) **defects of both humoral and cellular immunity.** Immunodeficiency is discussed in Section 19.

B Cell Malignancies (Figure 18-1)

Acute Lymphoblastic Leukemia (ALL) is a proliferative disease of either pro-B or pre-B lymphoid cells. The pro-B group is characterized by arrest at the stage of the early gene rearrangement of the D_H and J_H segments of the H chain. In pre-B ALL, there is complete heavy chain gene rearrangement of V_H D_H J_H C_μ with the production of cytoplasmic but not membrane-associated IgM. Most of these cells display the surface markers CD34 (a stem cell adhesion molecule) and CD10 (a metalloproteinase) known as CALLA - the common acute lymphocytic leukemia antigen.

Chronic Lymphocytic Leukemia (CLL) is characterized by the accumulation of long-lived B cells that carry the marker CD5 (i.e. B1 cells) normally present only on T cells. Other surface markers include: CD20 – a transmembrane protein that regulates B cell activation, CD21 – a receptor for the C3b component of complement, CD22 – an adhesion molecule, and CD23 – a low affinity receptor for IgE. The markers most useful in the differentiation of CLL

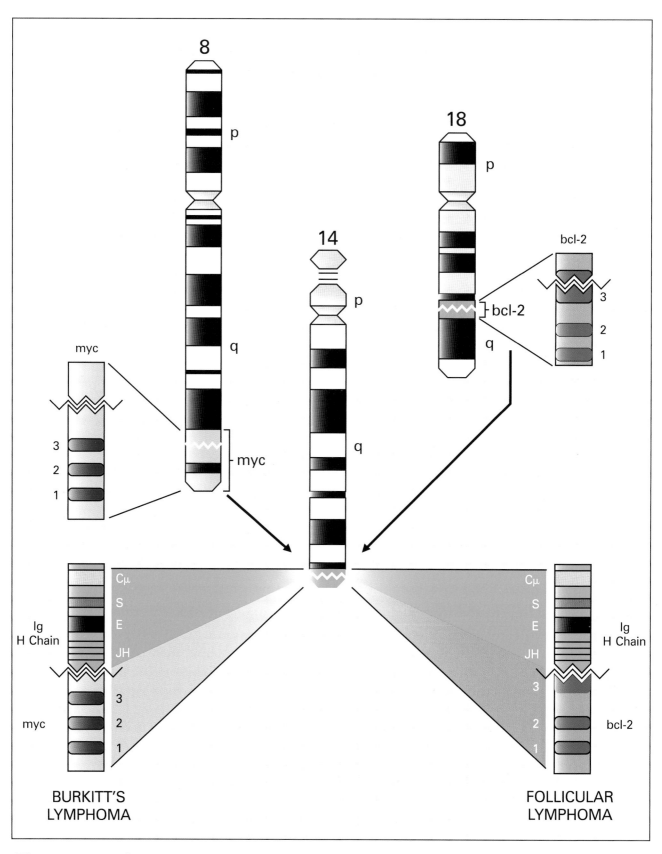

Figure 18-5 Chromosomal Translocations in B Cell Lymphoma

from other B cell lymphomas are CD5/CD23, co-expressed only in B-CLL (Table 18-1). The fact that CD5 B cells can form antibodies against self-antigens may explain the high incidence of autoimmune hemolytic anemia and thrombocytopenia in CLL. Because CLL lymphocytes carry increased levels of Bcl-2, they are resistant to apoptosis; this may be the primary mechanism for the slow accumulation of long-lived lymphocytes that flood the bone marrow, spleen, nodes and peripheral blood in this disease.

Burkitt's Lymphoma (Figure 18-5). This B cell neoplasm exists in two forms: an endemic African form and a sporadic non-endemic American variety. The Epstein-Barr virus (EBV) is associated with 95% of the endemic form and 15% of the non-endemic form. The CD21 marker (receptor for complement C3b) on these cells binds EBV – a potent stimulus for B cell proliferation.

The chromosomal rearrangements in Burkitt's lymphoma and in follicular lymphoma are a study in similarity and contrast. In Burkitt's lymphoma there is a characteristic t(8:14) reciprocal translocation in which the *c-myc* oncogene of chromosome 8 is translocated into the H chain locus on chromosome 14. The *c-myc* oncogene dictates a transcription factor that upregulates gene expression and increases cell proliferation. The breakpoint on chromosome 14 is within the D or J regions of the H chain in endemic Burkitt's and within the μ region in the sporadic form. This brings *c-myc* under the control of the immunoglobulin gene enhancer region, leading to high levels of expression that support rapid cell proliferation.

Follicular Lymphoma (Figure 18-5). In 85% of cases of this low grade lymphoma there is a reciprocal translocation between chromosomes 14 and 18, t(14:18). This translocation moves the oncogene *bcl-2* from chromosome 18 into juxtaposition with the J_H segments of the H chain gene on chromosome 14. The resulting over-expression of *bcl-2* confers a survival advantage and these B cells now defy apoptosis. The continuing accumulation of these cells, rather than their rapid proliferation, is a hallmark of this low-grade lymphoma. In some patients, a subsequent genetic event involving a gene for cell proliferation (eg, *ras*) may transform indolent disease into a more aggressive lymphoma.

Mantle Cell Lymphoma (Figure 18-1). This is another example of a lymphoma associated with a gene translocation into the enhancer region of the Ig heavy-chain gene on chromosome 14. It is an intermediate grade lymphoma associated with gastrointestinal infiltrates and Waldeyer's ring involvement. In this lymphoma, a t(11:14) translocation brings the gene for cyclin D on chromosome 11 into juxtaposition with the H-chain gene enhancer. The overexpression of cyclin D, a regulator of the G_1 phase of the cell cycle, results in cell cycle deregulation (Section 2).

Marginal cell lymphoma (Figure 18-1). The marginal zone is an anatomical site situated between the mantle zone of the follicles and the periphery of the lymph node. The marginal zone also is present in Peyer's patches but is not as distinct as in peripheral lymph nodes and spleen.

Table 18-1   Markers for the Common B Cell Lymphomas

	CD5	CD23	CD10
B-CLL	+	+	−
Mantle Cell Lymphoma	+	−	−
Follicular Cell Lymphoma	−	−	+
Marginal Cell Lymphoma	−	−	−

The marginal zone contains a loose collection of B lymphocytes and macrophages. The B cells differ from those of the adjacent mantle zone: they are large, with a pale irregular nucleus, are IgD⁻, and have mutated Ig-V genes (the result of somatic hypermutation).

Lymphomas arising from B cells of "marginal zones" are called **marginal zone B cell lymphomas (MZBCL)**. There are three types of lymphomas that are included under this term. Generally, the phenotype of all three types is CD19$^+$/CD10$^-$/CD5$^-$/CD23$^-$ which helps to distinguish them from the other lymphomas such as follicular cell (CD10$^+$), mantle cell (CD5$^+$), and B-CLL (CD5$^+$/CD23$^+$).

(1) **Splenic marginal zone B cell lymphoma.** Splenic enlargement and bone marrow involvement are common; villous lymphocytes may be present in the peripheral blood. The disease tends to be indolent. Remission can be induced by splenectomy. The cells are CD19$^+$, CD20$^+$, CD5$^-$, CD10$^-$.

(2) **Lymphomas of mucosa-associated lymphoid tissue (MALT).** These indolent lymphomas involve **extranodal** sites of lymphoid tissue, particularly in the gastrointestinal tract such as Peyer's patches, salivary glands, and stomach – lymphoid sites associated with cuboidal or columnar epithelium. The Ig V$_H$ genes are mutated, consistent with their origin from post-follicular memory B lymphocytes such as the marginal zone B cells. There is a strong association with gastric Helicobacter pylori infection – the gastric lymphomas frequently regress following antibiotic eradication of H. pylori.

(3) **Nodal marginal zone lymphoma.** These non-Hodgkin's lymphomas are proliferations of small and medium-sized B cells (CD5$^-$, CD10$^-$) with an admixture of **"monocytoid B cells"** – this type of cell also may be found in MALT lymphomas. It has been suggested that these lymphomas are due to secondary involvement of the lymph nodes from a disseminating extranodal lymphoma.

The REAL classification has included nodal and extranodal (MALT) lymphomas in a single group under the name mantle zone B cell lymphoma (MZBCL) and, provisionally, assigned splenic marginal zone lymphoma to a separate category. The clinical, morphological, and anatomical heterogeneity of MZBCL probably reflects the equally heterogeneous normal population of "memory" B cells that reside in the marginal zones.

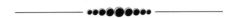

SUGGESTED READING

Craxton A, et al. Signal transduction pathways that regulate the fate of B lymphocytes. Adv Immunol 73:79-152, 1999.

Cyster JG et al. Follicular stromal cells and lymphocyte homing to follicles. Immunol Reviews 176:181-193, 2000.

De Franco AL. B lymphocyte activation pp 225-261 in Fundamental Immunology (4th Ed), W.E. Paul (ed), Lippincott-Raven Publishers, Philadelphia Pa, 1999.

Fearon DT, Caroll MC. Regulation of B lymphocyte responses to foreign and self-antigens by the CD19/CD21 complex. Ann Rev Immunol 18:393, 2000.

Fisher A, Cavazzana-Calvo M, De Saint Basile G, et al. Naturally occurring primary deficiencies of the immune system. Ann Rev Immunol 15:93, 1997.

Harris NL, Jaffe ES, Stein H, et al. A revised European-American classification of lymphoid neoplasms. Blood 84:1361-1392, 1994.

Henderson A, Calame K. Transcriptional regulation during B cell development. Ann Rev Immunol 16:163, 1998.

Hsueh RC et al. Tyrosine kinase activation in the decision between growth, differentiation and death responses initiated from the B cell antigen receptor. Adv Immunol 75:283-316, 2000.

Kishimoto T, Akira S, Narazaki M, Taga T. Interleukin-6 family of cytokines and gp130. Blood 86:1243, 1995.

Küppers R, Klein U, Hansmann M-L, Rajewsky K. Cellular origin of human B-cell lymphomas. N Engl J Med 1520-1529, 1999.

LeBien TW. Fates of human B-cell precursors. Blood 96:9, 2000.

Liu, YJ, Arpin C. Germinal center development. Immunol Rev 156:111, 1997.

Melchers F, RolinkAG, Schaniel C. The role of chemokines in regulating cell migration during humoral immune responses. Cell 99:351, 1999.

Moore KW et al. Interleukin-10 and interleukin-10 receptor. Ann Rev Immunol 19:583-765, 2001.

Paraskevas F. B Lymphocytes pp 464-496, 1999. In Wintrobe's Clinical Hematology (10th Ed), Lee GR, Foerster J, Lukens J, Paraskevas F, Greer JP, Rodgers GM (eds), William and Wilkins, 1999.

Pleiman CM, D'Ambrosia D, Cambier JC. The B cell antigen receptor complex: structure and signal transduction. Immunol Today 15:393, 1994.

Zwiebel JA, Cheson BD. Chronic lymphocytic leukemia: staging and prognostic factors. Semin Oncol 25:42, 1998.

T LYMPHOCYTES

Frixos Paraskevas

*"When the soul has gone to meet its doom,
and here the dust lies, like an empty pod...."*
Peer Gynt
Henrik Ibsen

T lymphocytes are the "soul" of the immune system as the AIDS pandemic has shown. They constitute a diverse group of cells with important regulatory and effector functions.

Within the thymus, T cells are separated into two lineages on the basis of their receptors designated $\alpha\beta$ and $\gamma\delta$. In turn, the $\alpha\beta$-T cells give rise to two functionally and phenotypically distinct sets: those expressing the CD4 marker are regulatory T cells while those expressing the CD8 marker are predominantly cytolytic or killer T cells (Figure 19-1). Outside the thymus, the CD4 $\alpha\beta$-T cells undergo further differentiation which endows them with distinct patterns of cytokine secretion – these are known as **Th1** and **Th2** cells.

Secretion of interleukins (IL-4/IL-6/IL-5/IL-10) by **Th2 cells** provides help to B cells for antibody production **(humoral immunity)**. Antibodies are the main defence against **extracellular bacterial infection**: IgM activation of complement results in cell lysis; IgG is an agglutinin, antitoxin, and opsonin; and IgA blocks adherence of bacteria on mucosal surfaces (Section 17). Th2 secretion of IL-4 and IL-5 regulates eosinophil and basophil production and maturation as well as IgE production. IgE binds to specific Fc receptors expressed by basophils and eosinophils; mediators are released when antigen crosslinks bound IgE. This system constitutes the main defence against **helminths**. **Th1 cells** secrete IL-2 and IFN-γ, inducing macrophage activation for **cell mediated immunity** against intracellular infection. The other arm of cell mediated immunity, i.e. against viral infections and tumor cells, is mediated by the **CD8$^+$ cells**.

ORIGIN (Figure 19-2)

During fetal life, T cell progenitors reside in the yolk sac and liver. After birth, the progenitors, the pre-T cells, are present in the bone marrow. They migrate to the thymus where they mature into functional T cells. The progenitor phenotype is CD34/CD2/CD7; it is not clear whether they are committed to T cell differentiation prior to their migration to the thymus.

The **thymus** is a lymphoepithelial organ found in the superior mediastinum. It consists of two lobes surrounded by a connective tissue capsule from which fibrous bands (trabeculae) extend into the parenchyma, dividing it into the lobules that are the basic anatomical units of the thymus. The lobules have two distinct regions: the peripheral region, called the **cortex**, is divided into the outer **subcapsular cortex** and the inner **deep cortex**; the central region of the

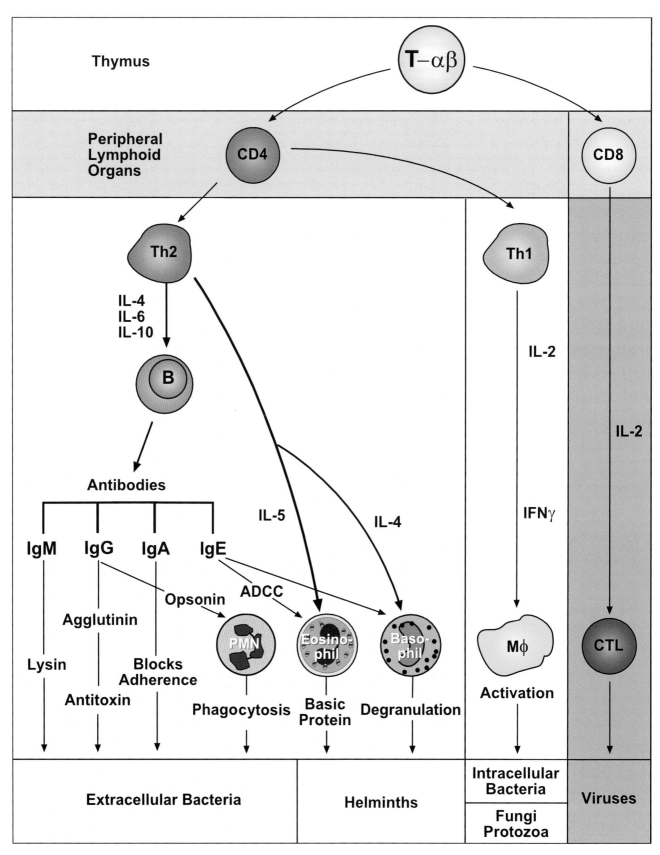

Figure 19-1 T Lymphocytes in Immunity Against Infectious Agents

lobule is the **medulla**. These areas support specific phases of thymocyte differentiation: the subcapsular cortex contains actively dividing blasts; the deep cortex is composed of non-dividing small thymocytes; the medulla contains medium sized thymocytes.

The cortex is composed predominantly of lymphocytes (85-90%). The stroma consists of **dendritic epithelial cells** – named for their long cytoplasmic processes, containing **tonofilaments,** that link to adjacent cells by **desmosomes** to form a **syncytium**; some engulf thymocytes to form lymphoepithelial complexes known as **nurse cells**. These dendritic epithelial cells express MHC class II molecules which play an important role in T cell differentiation. The medullary epithelial cells have short dendritic processes – one subgroup, known as **squamoid,** gives rise to the **Hassall corpuscles** characterized by concentric sheets of keratin and bundles of tonofilaments. Bone marrow derived **macrophages** and **interdigitating dendritic cells** also are present in the thymus: the interdigitating dendritic cells are abundant in the cortcomedullary junction, macrophages reside primarily in the medulla.

T CELL DIFFERENTIATION IN THE THYMUS

Progenitors in the thymus give rise to two T cell lineages, the $\alpha\beta$ and the $\gamma\delta$ T cells. Each lineage is determined by the composition of its T cell receptor (TCR): the TCR of the $\alpha\beta$ lineage consists of α and β chains; the TCR of the $\gamma\delta$ lineage consists of γ and δ chains (Figure 19-2).

(a) Phenotypic Differentiation.

Cell surface markers: Specific T-cell associated antigens or markers define the stages of differentiation and identify functionally distinct mature T cell populations. Some markers are present only during early development, others persist in the mature cell. Expression of some markers is associated with a specific cell function.

Intrathymic differentiation is associated with the rearrangements of the T cell receptor genes which give rise to the two lineages: the $\alpha\beta$-T cells and the $\gamma\delta$-T cells. The $\alpha\beta$ lineage can be described in three phenotypic stages: (1) double negative (DN) dividing blasts; (2) double positive (DP) small thymocytes; and (3) single positive (SP) CD4$^+$ and CD8$^+$ T lymphocytes.

(1) Double negative (DN): Shortly after arrival in the thymus, the large dividing blast cell progenitors are found in the subcapsular cortex. The CD34 marker and the intracytoplasmic CD3 marker are characteristic of these progenitors. The cells are still negative for CD4 and CD8, two important markers of T lineage; for this reason, the cells at this stage are known as **double negatives (DN)**. These cells are TdT (terminal deoxynucleotidyl transferase) positive (Section 17).

(2) Double positive (DP): The second stage of $\alpha\beta$-**T** cell differentiation is characterized by the following phenotypic changes: loss of CD34, the presence of CD3 with the T cell receptor (TCR) on the cell surface, and co-expression of CD4 and CD8 that defines the cells as **double**

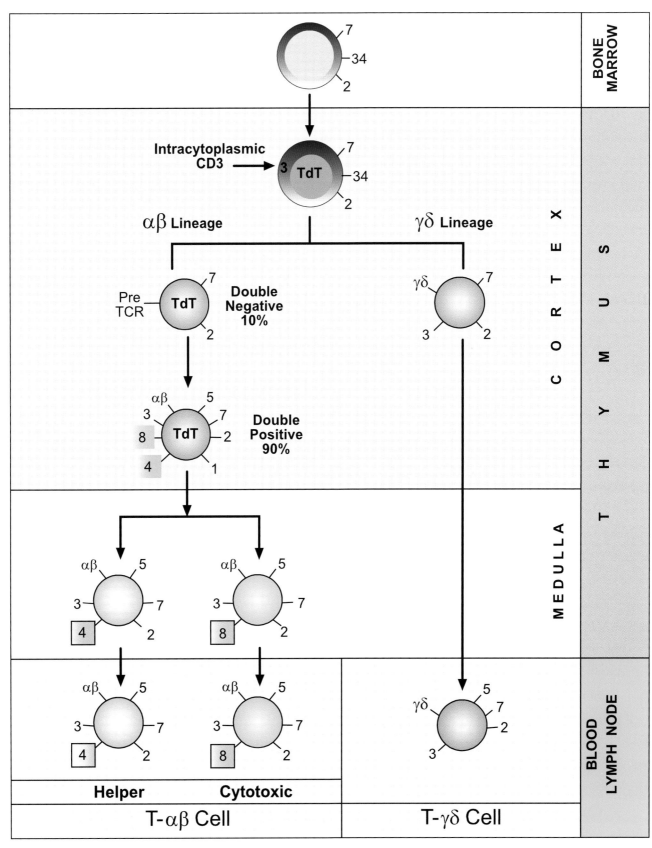

Figure 19-2 T Cell Differentiation in the Thymus

positives (DP). The marker CD1 is characteristic of this stage of differentiation. The cells now move to the inner cortex where they constitute 90% of the thymocytes.

(3) **Single positive (SP)**: The DP cells now commit themselves to either one of the two classes of the αβ-T cell lineage, CD4 or CD8 – **single positive (SP) cells**. The mechanism of lineage differentiation involves the TCR and one of the two markers, either CD4 or CD8, interacting with appropriate ligands on the dendritic epithelial cells.

Normal T cell function depends on TCR recognition of an antigen in the context of (i.e. complexed with) molecules encoded by the **major histocompatibility complex (MHC)**, also known as the **human leukocyte antigens (HLA)**. MHC molecules are divided into class I and class II. The CD4 and CD8 markers act as coreceptors for the TCR: CD4 binds to MHC class II molecules and CD8 to MHC class I. The expression of either one of the coreceptors, CD4 or CD8, must be matched with an αβ-TCR that recognizes antigen in the context of MHC class II or class I, respectively. (When expression of class I MHC (ligand for CD8) is blocked by gene targeting in mice ("knock-out"), the CD8 cells do not develop. Similarly, CD4 cells do not develop in class II knock-out mice). The SP cells are present in the medulla – CD1 has been lost and the typical phenotype of the mature T cell now is fully developed.

(b) T Cell Receptor (TCR) Genes and Gene Rearrangements (Figure 19-3)

The two sets of genes, α/β and γ/δ, generate the two specific TCRs that dictate the T cell lineages: **αβ-T cells and γδ-T cells**. TCRs are generated from random rearrangements of V (variable), D (diversity), and J (junctional) DNA segments.

α gene is located on chromosome 14 at 14q11; it contains approximately 50 Vα, more than 70 Jα segments and one Cα gene, and no D segments. Unique to the structure of the α gene is the presence of the **δ gene** between the Vα and Jα segments – rearrangement of the α gene results in the excision of the δ gene thus blocking generation of γδ-T cells.

β gene is located on chromosome 7q35 and incorporates two Cβ genes; each Cβ has a set of Jβ segments and a single Dβ segment. A common pool of about 57 Vβ segments is used by both Cβ genes.

γ gene is located on the short arm of chromosome 7p14. There are two Cγ genes, each associated with a specific set of Jγ segments. Both use a common set of about 14 Vγ segments, only 8 of which are functional. It has no D segments.

δ gene is located within the α gene complex. One Cδ gene is associated with three segments of each of the Vδ, Dδ, and Jδ components. This limited combinatorial diversity is compensated for by an extensive junctional diversity. (These terms are defined in Section 17).

Successful rearrangement of the γ/δ genes generates the γδ-T cells (Figure 19-2). However, development with production of mature γδ-T cells proceeds only if αβ rearrangements fail. The β gene rearranges concomitantly with the γ/δ genes. If β **gene** rearrangement is successful, the β chain, together with a chain known as **pre-Tα,** forms the **pre-T cell receptor** complex. The pre-TCR promotes cell division, expression of TCR-αβ, and expression of the CD4/CD8 coreceptors, thus directing the cell to the DP stage of differentiation.

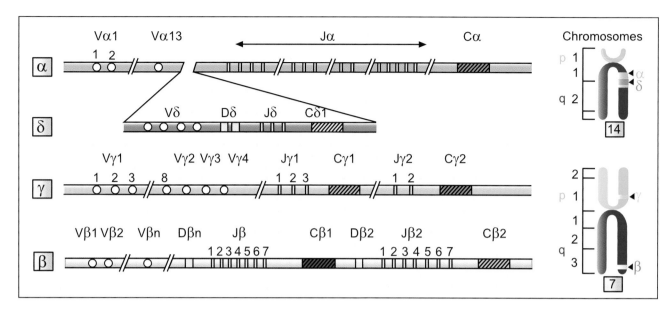

Figure 19-3 T Cell Receptor Genes

These events irreversibly shut down γ/δ T cell differentiation because the δ gene, embedded within the α gene, is excised during this process. In the αβ T cell lineage, rearrangement of the β gene is followed by rearrangement of the α gene – a process that is mediated by the **RAG-1/RAG-2** enzymes (also involved in B cell Ig rearrangements: Section 18). When expression of either RAG-1 or RAG-2 enzyme is absent, there is complete block of both B and T cell development, expressed clinically as a severe combined immune deficiency (SCID).

(c) The Selection of the T Cell Repertoire in the Thymus (Figure 19-4)

Only about 5-10% of thymocytes survive to become mature peripheral T cells, the majority undergo apoptosis within the thymus. An important precept of normal function requires that the thymus generates T cells capable of recognizing foreign antigens but not self antigens. This is achieved by the processes of **positive** and **negative selection**. The molecular interactions that govern these processes involve the TCR of the thymocyte and the MHC/peptide complexes on cells of the thymic stroma (see below).

In the thymus, the MHC molecules are occupied by "self peptides" – these complexes constitute the ligands for "education" of the T cells. During development, these interactions provide the T cell with two choices: **survival** or **death**. Surviving cells are considered to have been positively selected. **Positive selection** is followed by lineage differentiation, either CD4 or CD8. Death may occur under two circumstances: (1) by **neglect** or (2) by **negative selection**. Apoptosis is the generic mechanism of death in both instances. The apoptotic thymocytes are removed rapidly by macrophages through interactions of the macrophage scavenger receptors (Section 21) with the membrane of the apoptotic cell. Although 50 million cells die daily, there is no histological evidence of the thymus as a graveyard.

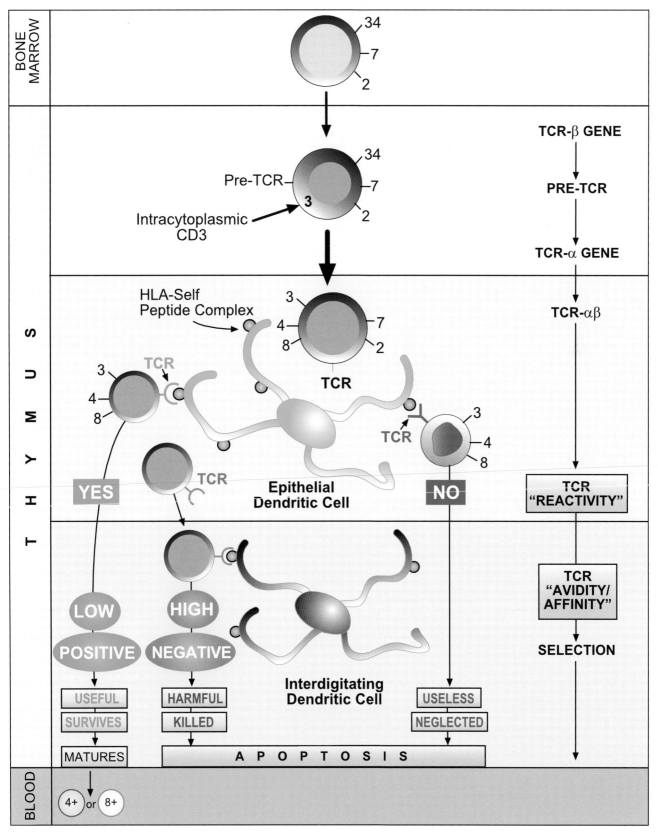

Figure 19-4 Positive and Negative Selection in the Thymus

Two mechanisms have been proposed to explain the choice between survival and death: **avidity (or affinity)** and **differential signaling**. Avidity refers to the binding strength and affinity of the TCR for the MHC-peptide complex that determines the fate of the T cell. Differential signaling implies a "qualitatively" different signal. If the TCR does not recognize the MHC-peptide, the T cell is **"ignored"** and dies by **neglect**. When interaction does take place and the signal delivered by the self-antigens is weak, the cell survives to undergo further differentiation **(positive selection)**. However, if the signal is strong, the cell is deleted **(negative selection)** – this process prevents autoreactive cells from exiting the thymus. Positive selection takes place while the cells are DP and is mediated by cortical epithelial dendritic cells. Negative selection occurs in cells closer to the corticomedullary region, and is mediated by bone marrow derived interdigitating dendritic cells and macrophages (Section 21). This mechanism underlies tolerance, i.e. lack of reactivity against self.

The positively selected cells move from the cortex to the medulla as either CD4 or CD8 cells. Lineage commitment, to either CD4 or CD8, is guided by the interaction of the TCR and the MHC-peptide complex: **the cell with a TCR that recognizes peptides presented by MHC class II becomes CD4; the cell with a TCR that recognizes MHC class I-peptide complexes becomes CD8.**

Thus, T cells exiting the thymus for the periphery carry a **coreceptor (CD4 or CD8) that matches the MHC recognition preference of its TCR.** This correspondence of the coreceptor with the TCR is essential to the function of the mature $\alpha\beta$-T cell: the coreceptors bind to the monomorphic (invariant) part of the same MHC molecule that is recognized by the TCR molecule, CD4 to class II and CD8 to class I. The TCR binds to the polymorphic (variable) region which carries the peptide antigen (see below).

HOMING TO THE PERIPHERAL LYMPHOID ORGANS

Naïve T cells leave the thymus and home to the peripheral lymphoid organs. In the lymph nodes, the cells exit the blood by crossing the high endothelial venules (HEVs) located in the paracortex or deep cortex. T lymphocytes roll along the endothelial surface through interactions of L-selectin with a molecule on endothelial cells known as **peripheral lymph node addressin**. Rolling is followed by tight adhesion mediated by the CD11a/CD18 β_2 integrin (LFA-1: lymphocyte function antigen-1) on T cells which binds to ICAM-1 (intercellular adhesion molecule-1) on endothelial cells (Section 3). This tight adherence requires activation of CD11a/CD18 by the chemokine **SLC (secondary lymphoid tissue chemokine)**, constitutively expressed by the endothelial cells. SLC, a member of the CC group of chemokines, binds to its high affinity CCR7 receptor on naïve T cells, inducing an intracellular signal that results in activation of CD11a/CD18.

Chemokines regulate lymphocyte recruitment to distinct lymphoid compartments and orchestrate the interactions that lead to an immune response. T cells that cross the HEV are retained in the paracortical area as a result of interactions of the chemokine receptor CCR7 with SLC and **ELC (Epstein-Barr virus-induced molecule 1 ligand chemokine)** released by mature dendritic cells. T cells in this area interact with dendritic cells that have carried antigen from the periphery. Antigen-activated CD4 T cells become unresponsive to ELC/SLC signals by downregulating CCR7 while they upregulate CXCR5, the receptor for the B cell attracting chemokine (BCA-1). As a result of this interaction, these activated CD4 cells move to the follicles where they come in contact with the B cells of the germinal centre.

T cells move into inflammatory sites through interaction of the cell surface β_1 integrin VLA-4 (very late antigen-4, $\alpha_4\beta_1$) with the vascular adhesion molecule (VCAM) on endothelial cells.

PERIPHERAL T CELLS

γ/δ T Cells (Figure 19-2)

T cells expressing the γδ TCR constitute about 4% of the peripheral T cells. They share a common progenitor with the αβ T cells but differ significantly in important features that determine their function: (1) The TCR-γδ is limited in its combinational diversity because only a small number of V, D, and J segments are available, especially in the early stages of development. (2) The γδ T cells recognize non-peptide or intact non-processed antigens, a mechanism resembling antigen recognition by antibodies. Some of these non-protein antigens are secreted ubiquitously by bacteria, some are present in edible plants and tea; significantly, most of these antigens contain phosphate groups. Other γδ T cells recognize antigens presented by Class Ib HLA molecules. (3) The cells also respond to antigens released from injured cells (heat-shock proteins) at sites of microbial inflammation. (4) Because γδ T cells secrete epithelial growth factors, they participate in repair of injured epithelial surfaces. This function is facilitated by the unique γδ T cells, generated early in development, which home to the skin – these are known as **epidermal dendritic T cells**. The striking characteristic of this phenotype is that all the cells utilize the same Vγ and Vδ genes. At later stages of development, other γδ T cells populate epithelial surfaces of the intestinal mucosa; these cells have a greater combinatorial diversity and are generated locally, bypassing the thymus.

Thus, the γδ T cells constitute an important link between innate and acquired immunity. This role is determined by their location, TCR specificity, the antigens they recognize, the mechanism of antigen recognition, and their secretion of the cytokines IFN-γ and IL-4.

αβ T Cells (Figure 19-1).

Mature αβ T cells exiting the thymus are of two phenotypically and functionally distinct classes: CD4 cytokine-secreting T cells and CD8 cytotoxic-killer T cells.

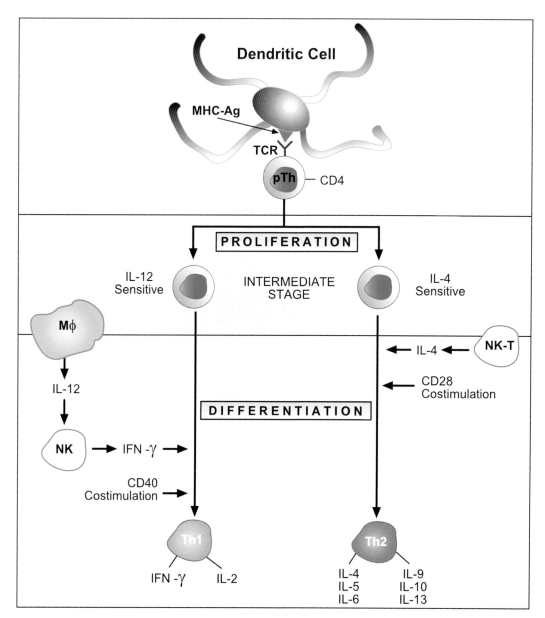

Figure 19-5 Th1 vs Th2 Differentiation

CD4 αβ T Cells: Th1 vs Th2 Differentiation (Figure 19-5)

CD4 naïve T cells in the secondary lymphoid organs receive signals that trigger their activation and proliferation. Under the influence of these signals, the cells undergo further differentiation that determines distinct patterns of cytokine secretion and the emergence of two specific CD4 phenotypes, **Th1** and **Th2**. The primary cytokines secreted by Th1 cells are IFN-γ and IL-2. Th2 cells secrete IL-4, IL-5, IL-6, IL-9, IL-10, and IL-13. These effector T cells regulate the primary immune responses: **Th1 regulates cell mediated immunity, Th2 regulates humoral immunity**.

Both Th1 and Th2 cells derive from a common precursor (known as pTh or Th0).

Differentiation involves two steps: (1) naïve T cells are activated first by antigen presenting dendritic cells to an intermediate stage with the potential to differentiate into either type of effector cell; (2) the factors that regulate differentiation into Th1 or Th2 include: dose of antigen, intensity and duration of the occupation of the TCR by the foreign peptides, nature of costimulatory signals, and the intracellular signaling pathways initiated by TCR activation.

These early events are influenced by the cytokine milieu: IL-12 and IFN-γ stimulate Th1, while IL-4 stimulates Th2 differentiation. The source of the cytokines at this early stage are cells of the innate immunity, such as macrophages, dendritic cells, NK, and the NK-T cells which recognize bacterial lipids. IL-12 released by macrophages stimulates NK cells to secrete IFN-γ, driving Th1 differentiation. IL-4 required for Th2 differentiation is produced by a number of cells – NK-T cell production of IL-4 appears to be of particular importance.

Th1 CD4 effector T cells produce IFN-γ that stimulates **macrophage activation** (Figure 19-1). In addition to IFN-γ, the highly complex process of macrophage activation requires CD40-CD40 ligand interactions as well as the participation of other cytokines and chemotactic factors (Section 21).

The Th2 CD4 T cells regulate humoral immunity (Figure 19-1). The helper cell function of the Th2 cells for B cells is initiated by the TCR recognition of antigen presented by the MHC class II molecules of B cells, and further promoted by a second signal generated by the interaction of the CD40 ligand on T cells with CD40 on B cells; the resultant secretion of IL-4 amplifies helper function. This stimulation triggers B cell proliferation (clonal expansion); subsequent differentiation to plasma cells is regulated by other cytokines released from Th2 cells such as IL-5, IL-6, and IL-10 (Section 18).

CD8 T Cells: Cytotoxic T Lymphocytes (Figure 19-1)

Activation of the naïve CD8 T cells is required for their development into effector cytotoxic or killer T cells. Similar to CD4 cells, this activation requires two signals: (1) the antigen-specific signal provided by the TCR and (2) a second signal by costimulatory molecules, such as CD80/CD86 on the antigen presenting cell (APC) interacting with CD28 on T cells. Dendritic cells are effective activators of naïve CD8 cells, presenting antigen and providing the costimulatory signal that converts the naïve cell to the effector CD8 killer cell; these cells proliferate in response to IL-2 secreted by the CD8 cells themselves (autocrine stimulation). In an alternate pathway, activation of CD8 T cells follows antigen presentation by an APC with IL-2 secreted by CD4 T cells providing the second signal – an example of the "helper" role CD4 cells play in the activation of CD8 cells.

Killing of Target Cells by Cytotoxic T Lymphocytes (CTL) (Figure 19-6)

Killing of target cells involves three successive steps: (1) **adhesion** of the CTL to the target cell; (2) **delivery of the lethal hit**, and (3) **cell death**.

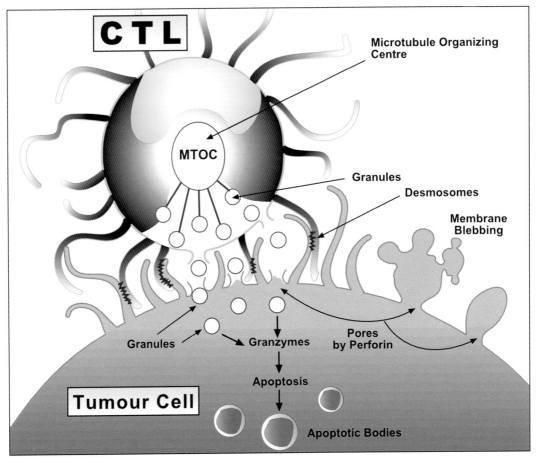

Figure 19-6 CTL Tumour Cell Kill

(1) **CTL-target conjugate** is mediated by two sets of adhesion molecules: (a) CD11a/CD18 (LFA-1) on the CTL interacting with the ICAMs on the target cell, and (b) CD2 on the CTL interacting with CD58 (LFA-3) on the target cell. This initial adhesion allows the TCR to scan for the presence of its specific MHC class I-peptide complex on the surface of the target cell; when an appropriate MCH class I/peptide complex is detected, adhesion is strengthened by CD8 binding to the monomorphic portion of the MHC class I molecule. Fine membrane microvilli provide the sites of contact (desmosomes) between the CTL and the target cell.

(2) **Delivery of the lethal hit:** Specific TCR recognition of the target, supported by interactions between the adhesion molecules, prepares the CTL for delivery of the **lethal hit**. This involves CTL polarization towards the target – the Golgi apparatus, the **microtubule organizing centre (MTOC)**, the cytoskeleton, and the entire complement of **granules** (which normally are found in the back of a motile CTL) move rapidly toward the site of CTL-target contact. Delivery of the lethal hit is initiated by two pathways: (a) the **perforin-granzyme dependent pathway** and (b) the **Fas pathway** – both routes lead to apoptotic death of the target cell (Section 4).

(a) **Perforin-granzyme system (exocytosis):** The CTL granules, 0.5-1 μm in diameter, consist of a homogeneous core surrounded by numerous membrane vesicles. The relative proportion of these components varies – some granules consist entirely of cores, others contain only vesicles. **Perforin, granzymes,** and **proteoglycan** are present in the core. The vesicles contain **lysosomal enzymes.** Exocytosis delivers the granules into the intercellular space between the CTL and its target. Effective killing of targets by the exocytosis pathway requires both perforin and granzymes (Section 4).

Perforin (cytolysin) is a glycoprotein. In the presence of Ca^{2+}, perforin inserts into lipid membranes, polymerizes, and forms pores. On electron microscopy, the perforin pore has a striking structural similarity to the MAC complement pore (Section 20). At the molecular level, perforin consists of two domains: (a) the **complement homology domain,** located near the NH_2 terminal, is related structurally to C9 and the other components of the complement membrane attack complex, and (b) the **C2 domain** that binds to the phospholipid groups of the target membrane in a Ca^{2+}-dependent manner (similar structures are found in membrane-binding proteins such as protein kinase C and Ras activating proteins).

Granzymes are serine proteases that are similar to enzymes present in granules of other cells, such as mast cells, macrophages, and neutrophils. The term granzyme is used exclusively for these lymphocyte proteases. Eight granzymes (A-H) have been described; A and B predominate in human CTLs. Granzyme B has a unique substrate specificity that differs from other mammalian serine proteases: it cleaves a peptide bond that leaves an aspartic amino acid at the carboxy terminal end of the molecule.

Proteoglycans function in the granules as scaffolds to form insoluble stable complexes with perforin and granzymes. This is similar to the role of heparin in mast cell granules (Section 8).

(b) **FasL/Fas Pathway:** This pathway is initiated when the target cell receptor **Fas** is ligated by the Fas ligand **(Fas L)** on CTLs. Binding of Fas to Fas L activates the caspase system, inducing apoptosis (Section 4).

Cell death takes place over a period of 1-7 hours. Both the perforin-granzyme system and the Fas-Fas L pathway contribute to the final event. After the delivery of the lethal hit, the CTL detaches and pursues another target, in the real sense of a "serial killer". In the process of cell kill, the CTL escapes intact – this is achieved by the delivery of the lethal hit in immediate juxtaposition to the target cell membrane.

TCR-αβ: STRUCTURE AND FUNCTION

There are two components of TCR engagement with an APC: **antigen recognition** and **signal transduction.** Generation of functionally diverse TCRs results from unique germline gene rearrangements, similar to the B cell receptor (Section 18).

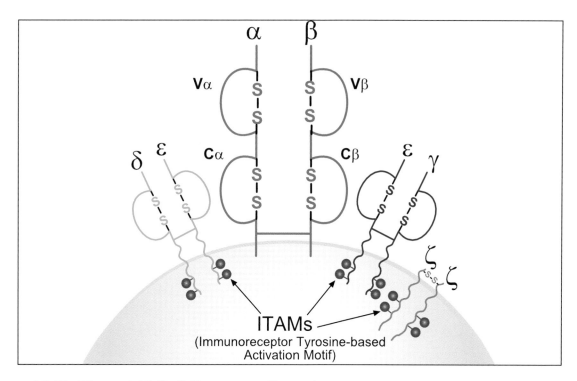

Figure 19-7 The $\alpha\beta$ T Cell Receptor Complex

(a) TCR Structure (Figure 19-7)

The antigen recognition site on the TCR consists of a heterodimer of two chains, α and β, each containing a variable (V_α or V_β) and a constant (C_α or C_β) domain. The V_α is encoded by two DNA segments (V_α and J_α), the V_β from three segments (V_β, D_β, and J_β). The $\alpha\beta$-TCR resembles the Fab fragment of the Ig molecule (Section 17).

The $\alpha\beta$ heterodimer is associated with five other polypeptide chains. Three of them are known collectively as CD3: $CD3_\gamma$, $CD3_\delta$, and $CD3_\epsilon$. A fourth chain, ζ, usually forms a homodimer (ζ-ζ) or, less commonly, a heterodimer with a fifth chain (η). The stoichiometry of the $\alpha\beta$ TCR complex is shown in Figure 19-7. The cluster consists of the α-β heterodimer associated with one ϵ-γ heterodimer, one ϵ-δ heterodimer, and one ζ-ζ homodimer (or ζ-η heterodimer).

(b) Antigen recognition by the TCR (Figure 19-8)

Although the TCR shares many structural features with its counterpart, the B cell receptor, it differs strikingly in the manner of its interaction with the antigen. The B cell receptor interacts with conformational structures of the whole antigen present on the surface of the molecule. In contrast, the TCR recognizes peptides (about 10-20 amino acids long) derived from the **processing** (i.e. **fragmentation**) of the antigen within the antigen presenting cell.

Antigen processing is carried out by dendritic cells, macrophages, and B cells. There are two distinct pathways: (1) **Extracellular antigens** (or bacteria) are endocytosed and digested to

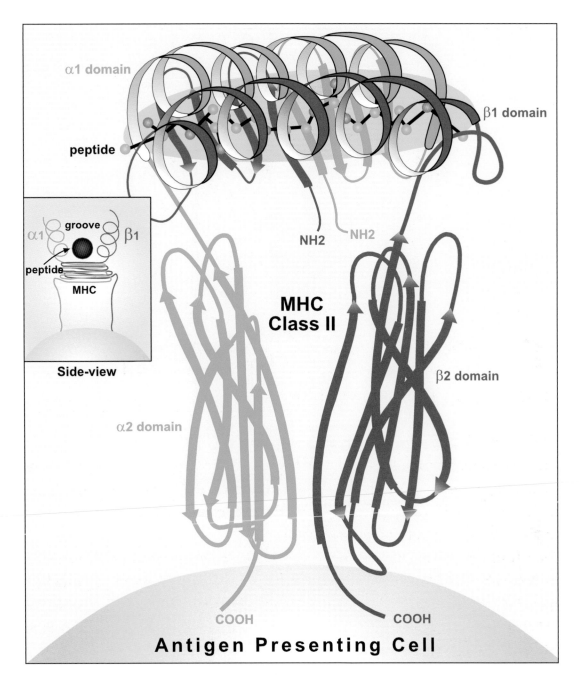

Figure 19-8 MHC Class II – Peptide Complex

small peptides – these are captured within the endocytic vesicles by MHC class II molecules and the MHC/peptide complexes are transported to the cell membrane for presentation to CD4 T cells. (2) Foreign **intracellular antigens** (such as viruses) are fragmented by the cytoplasmic **proteasome** to small peptides. In the endoplasmic reticulum, the peptides form a complex with MHC class I molecules and are transported to the cell membrane for presentation to CD8 T cells.

There are multiple MHC molecules, a property known as **polymorphism** (Greek: polymorphos = multiple forms) that have been generated over evolutionary time to counter an

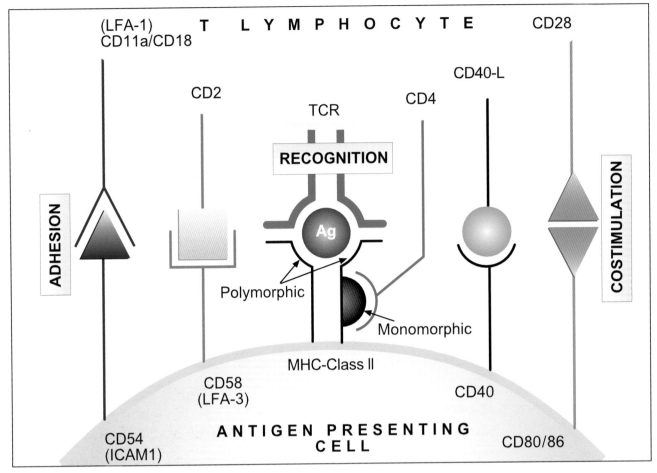

Figure 19-9 CD4 T Cell – APC Interaction

ever diversifying pathogen population. **Class II MHC** molecules are dimers of two chains, α and β. Each chain consists of two domains, α_1/α_2 and β_1/β_2 respectively. The α_1 and β_1 (most distal to the cell membrane) are polymorphic, i.e. they vary in amino acid sequence amongst individuals, while the α_2 and β_2 (proximal to the cell membrane) are invariant or monomorphic. The **class I MHC** molecule is a dimer formed by a large or heavy α chain (encoded by MHC genes) and a small or light β chain (also known as β_2-**microglobulin** or β_2**M**) encoded by a non-MHC gene. The α chain consists of three domains, α_1 and α_2, which are polymorphic, and α_3 which is monomorphic. The MHC molecule of the antigen presenting cell forms a groove: in MHC class I, the groove is formed by the two polymorphic domains, α_1 and α_2 of the α chain; in the MHC class II molecule, the groove is formed by the polymorphic α_1 and β_1 domains of the α and β chains, respectively (Figure 19-8). The peptide lies on the floor of the groove, retained in position by interactions with **anchor residues**.

(c) **Signal transduction**

The α-β chains of the TCR (Figure 19-7) interact with the MHC-peptide complex (antigen recognition) and generate the signal which is transduced by the CD3 and ζ chains, through appropriate pathways to the nucleus. Critical to signal transduction by these associated chains is an important sequence in their intracytoplasmic tails known as the **immunoreceptor tyrosine-based activation motif** or **ITAM**. ITAMs link these chains to **protein tyrosine kinases (PTKs)**, the initial components of the signal transduction pathway. (ITAMs are discussed in Sections 18 and 21).

(d) Coreceptors

Although the $\alpha\beta$-TCR in the two types of $\alpha\beta$-T cells, CD4 and CD8, are structurally the same, they differ strikingly in their function. The TCR on CD4 T cells recognizes antigen presented by MHC class II molecules, while the TCR of CD8 T cells recognizes antigen presented by MHC class I. In addition, CD4 and CD8 associate with the TCR complex and act as **co-receptors** – the CD4 binds to the invariant part (α_2 or β_2) of MHC class II and CD8 to the invariant part (α_3) of MHC class I molecules during antigen recognition.

CD4 is a single chain molecule with four Ig-like domains. It binds to the monomorphic (invariant) domain of the same MHC class II molecule that presents the peptide to the TCR. The intracellular association of the CD4 cytoplasmic tail with PTKs significantly enhances CD4 T cell activation. The **CD8** molecule exists in two isoforms: as a heterodimer of α and β chains, or as a homodimer of two α chains. The association of CD8 with the monomorphic part of the MHC class I molecule enhances CD8 T cell activation.

THE MHC ANTIGEN PRESENTING SYSTEM (Figure 19-9)

Interaction of the TCR with the MHC/peptide complex on an antigen presenting cell (APC) is weak and insufficient to trigger T cell activation. The cell interaction is initiated first by adhesion molecules that allow the T cell to approach the APC – the TCR then scans for MHC/peptide complexes on the APC surface (**adhesion**). For CD4 T cells, engagement of TCR with the MHC/peptide (**recognition**) is strengthened by the binding of the coreceptor CD4 to the monomorphic (invariant) part of the class II MHC molecule (Figure 19-9). CD8 similarly binds to the monomorphic part of the class I MHC molecule. The signal generated by the TCR (signal 1) requires a second signal (signal 2), generated by costimulatory molecules (**costimulation**) for activation. In the absence of signal 2, the T cell becomes unresponsive (tolerance).

T CELL ACTIVATION (Figure 19-10)

Binding of the TCR to the MHC-peptide complex triggers phosphorylation of tyrosine residues on the ITAMs of the CD3 (γ, δ, ϵ) and ζ chains. In signal 1, the protein tyrosine kinases (PTKs) which play a critical role in T cell activation are Lck and Fyn of the **Src** family and

ZAP-70 of the **Syk** family; ZAP-70 is expressed exclusively in T and NK cells. (Mutations in ZAP-70 result in severe combined immune deficiency – SCID). These PTKs interact with ITAMs of the TCR complex. Activation of Lck kinase is dependent upon the **protein tyrosine phosphatase (PTP), CD45** – CD45 dephosphorylates an inhibitory tyrosine in the cytoplasmic tail of Lck. Activated Lck phosphorylates the ITAMs of the CD3 chains. ZAP-70 binds to the phosphorylated ITAMs and is activated (phosphorylated) by Lck. The substrate for ZAP-70 is **LAT (linker for activation of T cells)**, a transmembrane protein with a long cytoplasmic tail. Phosphorylated LAT recruits a number of proteins, resulting in formation of multimolecular complexes. The proteins PLC-γ, Grb2, and PI3-K are crucial to T cell activation. PLC-γ generates second messengers from membrane phosphatidylinositol – diacylglycerol (DAG) and inositol triphosphate (IP$_3$). Grb2 is an adaptor protein linking other proteins that result in Ras activation (Section 1).

Phosphatidylinositol-3 kinase (PI3-K) is recruited to the cell membrane by LAT or by CD28. CD28 on the T cell membrane binds to its ligands B7-1 and B7-2 (CD80 and CD86) on the APC, generating costimulatory signals for T cell activation (Signal 2). PI3-K generates PIP$_3$ from membrane inositol phospholipids; PIP$_3$ recruits a number of proteins to the cell membrane, forming multimolecular complexes that propagate intracellular signaling (Section 1). Proteins bound by PIP$_3$ include members of the TEC family of kinases (eg, Btk in B cells, Akt and Itk), characterized by the presence of the **pleckstrin homology (PH)** domain – these kinases regulate components of the cell cycle and have a role in maintenance of cell survival. PI3-K regulates another group of proteins with PH domains that are involved in the assembly and function of the actin cytoskeleton (i.e. Rac, Rho).

T cell activation is initiated by contact with the APC. The initial contact by adhesion molecules is strengthened by the firm engagement of the TCR and ligation of CD28. Sustained activation is achieved by the aggregation of receptors and signaling molecules in membrane clusters known as **SMACs** (supramolecular activation clusters), floating on lipid rafts (also known as **GEMs**: glycosphingolipid enriched microdomains). This superstructure constitutes the **immunological synapse**. The TCR, CD4, and associated PTKs are clustered at the centre of the SMAC; adhesion molecules with links to actin filaments are found at the periphery. This arrangement maintains the intimate contact between the T cell and the APC that allows the characteristic spreading of the T cell over the APC surface.

Transduction of the signal downstream involves phosphatidylinositol derived second messengers (DAG and IP$_3$), PKC and Ras pathways. Within minutes after initiation of signal transduction, a set of **"immediate activation genes"** synthesize transcription factors. Subsequently, well-regulated waves of activation of **early and late genes** induce a variety of cellular functions, eg, proliferation, expression of new surface molecules required for cell interactions, and migration.

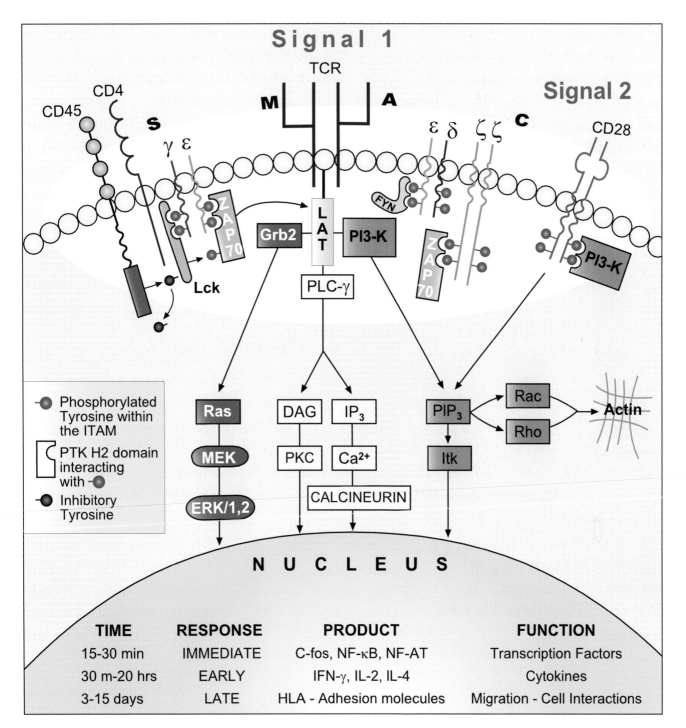

Figure 19-10 CD4 T Cell Activation

CYTOKINES

T cells, particularly CD4 T cells, are a major source of cytokine production. Cytokines regulate T cell development (IL-7), growth (IL-1, IL-2, IL-4), and differentiation (IL-4, IFN-γ, IL-2). These cytokines signal through specific receptors. The IL-2 receptor consists of three transmembrane chains, α, β, and γ, which transmit intracellular signal through JAK3. The IL-2 receptor γ chain is shared by several other interleukin receptors, IL-4, IL-7, IL-9, and IL-15, and therefore is known as the **common γc receptor chain**. Deficiencies of the γc chain or JAK3 are responsible for two forms of severe combined immunodeficiency disease (SCID). Some of these cytokines have been described in Section 18. Others, important for T cell function, are described here.

IL-1: Interleukin-1 is a macrophage-derived cytokine which stimulates a variety of cells that function as effectors of immune and inflammatory responses. There are three distinct but related proteins: IL-1α, IL-1β, and an antagonist known as IL-1 receptor antagonist (IL-1ra). IL-1ra, the only naturally occurring cytokine antagonist, binds to the IL-1 receptor but does not trigger a response.

The biological activities of IL-1 overlap with those of TNF-α and IL-6. It is a pleiotropic mediator of host response to infections and injury. Many of its effects are mediated through its capacity to increase production of other cytokines such as G-CSF, TNF-α, IL-6, and IL-8. It is a mitogen for T cells (originally described as lymphocyte activating factor), upregulating IL-2 production and expression of IL-2 receptors. It also promotes B cell maturation and differentiation.

There are two IL-1 receptors, designated I and II. Type I is found on most cells, including T cells; type II is detected on certain cells, eg, B cells and neutrophils. A receptor accessory protein (IL-1R-ACP) is the component that tranduces the signal although it does not bind directly to IL-1. The functions of IL-1 are mediated only by the type I receptor and the accessory protein. The type II receptor is a "decoy" receptor – it downregulates the activity of bound IL-1. IL-1 binding to receptor type I activates a specific kinase known as IL-1 **receptor-associated kinase (IRAK)** which transduces downstream signaling.

IL-2: Its main function is to stimulate growth of T cells. It stimulates cell proliferation (T as well as B cells), enhances cytokine secretion, and heightens expression of certain surface molecules. The IL-2 receptor consists of three chains - α (ligand binding), β, and γ (signal transduction). The γ chain is shared by several other cytokine receptors (IL-4, IL-7, IL-9, and IL-15) and is now known as the γc (**common**) chain. Binding of IL-2 to the α chain leads to oligomerization of the receptor chains and initiation of signal transduction by the β and γ chains via the JAK/STAT pathway.

IL-7: Interleukin-7 is not a lymphokine per se as it is produced by stromal cells. Its major function is to stimulate growth and differentiation of thymocytes. Its receptor consists of an α chain which binds the cytokine and the γc chain, shared by other cytokines, for signal transduction.

IL-9: Interleukin-9 is produced by activated T cells. It supports the growth of T helper cells but not T cytotoxic cells. The IL-9 receptor consists of a specific IL-9 binding protein and the γc chain.

IL-12: Monocytes, macrophages and dendritic cells are the major producers of IL-12. Endotoxins, intracellular bacteria, and parasites induce IL-12 production. The most physiologically relevant function of IL-12 is stimulation of T and NK cells to produce cytokines, particularly IFN-γ but also TNF-α, GM-CSF, IL-8, and IL-2. IL-12 also enhances T cell and especially NK cell mediated cytotoxicity. It increases the binding of NK cells to targets by upregulating specific adhesion molecules and increases their granularity. IL-12 consists of two polypeptide chains. Its receptor also is composed of two chains, one bearing structural similarities to gp130, a component chain of the IL-6 receptor.

IFN-γ: Interferons (IFN) were discovered by their antiviral activity. They have been distinguished as **type I (IFN-α and IFN-β)** produced by leukocytes and other cells such as fibroblasts, and **type II (IFN-γ)** produced only by NK cells, CD8 and CD4 Th1 T cells. IFN-γ consists of two chains which bind to its receptor. The receptor for IFN-γ is expressed ubiquitously (except on erythrocytes). It consists of two chains: IFNγR-1 required for ligand binding and IFNγR-2 for signaling. Signaling is mediated through the JAK-STAT pathway.

Production of IFN-γ by NK cells is triggered by IL-12, derived from macrophages following phagocytosis of bacteria or stimulation by lipopolysaccharides. IFN-γ has a crucial role in the differentiation of naïve CD4 T cells to effector cells which produce the Th1 type of cytokines, i.e. IL-2 and IFN-γ. Th1 cells through IFN-γ production, stimulate macrophages and induce their activation (Section 21).

NATURAL KILLER (NK) CELLS

NK cells are the major cellular component of innate immunity. They are involved in defence of pathogen invasion and destruction of tumor cells. They are important in the earliest phase of infection by viruses and intracellular bacteria – the cytotoxic activity and production of cytokines are immediate responses, independent of prior stimulation. Morphologically, NK cells are large lymphocytes with prominent granules; the term **large granular lymphocytes (LGL)** refers to these characteristic features and is used interchangeably. NK cells share several markers with T cells, indicative of their common origin. NK cell differentiation, however, is independent of the thymic microenvironment (NK cells are normal in athymic mice). The two most characteristic markers are CD56 and CD57.

NK cells direct Th1 differentiation by secreting large amounts of IFN-γ in response to IL-12 released from infected or activated macrophages (Figure 19-5). They produce additional cytokines, including IL-1β, IL-3, IL-6, TGF-β, and TNF-α, that regulate other functions of the immune system. Their cytotoxic function is similar to that of the CD8 T cells: cytotoxicty involves attachment to the target cell followed by exocytosis of granule contents (perforin and granzymes) that are cytolytic for tumor cells and virus-infected cells. Unlike B and T cells, which express monospecific antigen receptors, NK cells express a number of activating and inhibiting receptors which determine their function. Presentation of peptides by MHC class I molecules is not required – indeed, expression of MHC class I molecules confers resistance to killing by NK cells. NK cells display **killer cell immunoglobulin (Ig)-like receptors (KIRs)** for polymorphic MHC class I molecules. KIR members are divided into two subfamilies with either inhibitory or activating function. Inhibitory KIRs are receptors for self-MHC class I molecules that prevent killing of normal self cells. When inhibitory KIRs recognize self MHC, they send an inhibitory signal to the NK cell. (Inhibitory KIRs are dominant over the activating receptors). Loss or alteration of MHC class I molecules, due to malignant transformation or viral infection, abolishes the inhibitory signal, leaving an unopposed default activating signal that results in the killing of the transformed or infected cell. This interpretation of target recognition by NK cells is known as the **"missing self" hypothesis**.

The best-defined activating receptor of NK cells is the CD16 or Fcγ receptor III, a low affinity Fc receptor for IgG. When the CD16 Fc receptor on an NK cell binds to antibody attached to a cellular target (i.e. an infected cell), activation of the cytotoxic mechanism results in killing of the infected cell. This is known as **antibody-dependent cell cytotoxicity (ADCC)**, a cell defence mechanism against tumor or infected cells. In addition to its crucial role in innate immunity and as an important link to adaptive immunity (Th1 differentiation), NK cells have a role in tumor surveillance, regulation of hematopoiesis (both inhibitory and stimulatory effects), and bone marrow engraftment (early NK cell development may control viral infections and stimulate hematopoiesis).

NK-T CELLS

NK-T cells are a population of $\alpha\beta$-T cells in peripheral blood that share characteristics with NK cells. The TCR of the NK-T cell is encoded by a limited number of β genes, and it recognizes antigen presented by CD1, an MHC class I-like protein. They are either $CD4^+$ or double negatives ($CD4^-/CD8^-$). NK-T cells primarily recognize glycolipids. A distinctive feature of NK-T cells is the rapid production of high levels of IL-4 when the TCR is engaged. The cytokine IL-4 directs Th2 differentiation (Figure 19-5). NK-T cells may be involved in the control of tissue damage in autoimmune disease and play a major role in defence against mycobacteria and malaria.

CLINICAL CORRELATES

THE IMMUNODEFICIENCIES (Table 19-1)

Selective Deficiencies of Immunoglobulin Subtypes.

Isolated **IgA deficiency** may be inherited in an autosomal dominant or recessive manner. Patients may lack both serum and secretory IgA; they may be asymptomatic or suffer from recurrent respiratory and gastrointestinal infections. The defect is due to failure of terminal differentiation of IgA^+ B cells (Section 17). Selective **IgM deficiency** is rare and associated with severe recurrent infections. A defect in synthesis of the IgG2 subclass is the commonest form of **IgG deficiency**. It is manifest by recurrent respiratory infections and the inability to generate antibodies to polysaccharides.

Failure of antibody synthesis.

Pure B cell deficiency (**Bruton's X-linked agammaglobulinemia**) is due to a defective *btk gene* that encodes the Bruton tyrosine kinase (Btk) (Section 17). Maturation arrest occurs at the pro-B stage of cell development. There is marked depletion of peripheral B cells, but an increased number of pro-B and pre-B cells in the bone marrow. Serum Ig is low or undetectable. Germinal centres are absent from the secondary lymphoid organs. A non X-linked panhypogammaglobulinemia also has been described.

The X-linked hyper-IgM syndrome is due to a point mutation of the T cell CD40 ligand, resulting in the loss of CD40:CD40L interaction. Although B cell expression of IgM is normal, in the absence of CD40 (B cell):CD40L (T cell) interaction the B cells fail to undergo class switch. These patients have high levels of IgM, but IgG and IgA are not synthesized. Clinically, there is an increased incidence of autoimmunity, malignancy, and a propensity for *P carinii* pneumonia.

Severe combined immunodeficiency disease (SCID)

SCID comprises a phenotypically and genotypically heterogenous group of diseases associated with profound defects of both cellular and humoral immunity. SCID may be classified on the basis of the presence or absence of B and T cells: B+ or B- and T+ or T-.

X-linked (T-, B+) SCID is the most common form of SCID. There is a profound defect in cellular and humoral immunity. It is uniformly fatal within 1-2 years of age unless treated by bone marrow transplantation. The disease is due to mutations of the common γc chain, a component of the interleukin receptors for IL-2, IL-4, IL-7, IL-9, and IL-15. The γc gene is located on chromosome Xq13. The patients have markedly reduced or absent T/NK cells. Although B cell numbers are normal, there is a profound impairment of B cell maturation in response to antigens and, as a result, there is failure of B cell differentiation and proliferation. IgG and IgA are low; IgM is present in variable concentration.

Janus kinase 3 (JAK 3) deficiency (T-, B+). This is an autosomal recessive SCID due to a mutation in JAK3. It is characterized by low numbers of T and NK cells; B cell numbers are normal or elevated. JAK-3 is the only member of the JAK family that interacts with the γc chain of the interleukin cytokine receptors. The cytological and functional manifestations are similar to the X-linked γc deficiency described above.

Adenosine deaminase (ADA) deficiency (T-, B-). Although the defect affects all body cells, it is particularly damaging to lymphoid development in the thymus. ADA is a ubiquitous enzyme that deaminates adenosine and deoxyadenosine to inosine and deoxyinosine, respectively. In the absence of ADA, the accumulation of deoxyadenosine and deoxyadenosine triphosphate (dATP) inhibits ribonucleotide reductase and blocks synthesis and repair of DNA strand breaks. The depletion of T cells and B cells results in a combined immunodeficiency syndrome.

RAG1 or RAG 2 deficiency (B-, T-). This is an autosomal recessive SCID due to nonsense, missense, or deletional mutations of the RAG1/RAG2 genes. Patients lack both B and T cells, but NK cells are normal. There is complete failure of the VDJ gene rearrangements for the B cell receptor (BCR) and for the T cell receptor (TCR). As a result, B and T cell differentiation is blocked (Section 17).

Major histocompatability complex (HLA) class II deficiency. Deficiency of (MHC)

HLA class II molecules (**bare lymphocyte syndrome**) is an autosomal recessive disorder characterized by the lack of expression of surface molecules, such as HLA-DR, DQ, and DP, on B lymphocytes, monocytes, and activated T cells. The CD4 T cells are decreased: with lack of expression of class II molecules on thymic epithelial dendritic cells, positive selection of CD4 T cells is absent. Furthermore, the few CD4 T cells that do develop cannot be stimulated by antigen presenting cells in the periphery because they also lack class II HLA molecules. The defect manifests as a SCID syndrome. **HLA class I deficiency** also has been described; these patients lack CD8 T cells.

Other T Cell Deficiencies

Di George syndrome (DGS). DGS is due to defective development of the third and fourth pharyngeal pouches, resulting in thymic and parathyroid hypoplasia or aplasia, anomalies of the great vessels, esophageal atresia, and congenital heart disease. T cells are decreased, and B cell function is impaired due to lack of T helper cells.

Omenn's syndrome. This is a severe immunodeficiency with failure to thrive that resembles graft-versus-host disease. Patients present with diarrhea, splenomegaly, eosinophilia, and elevated IgE levels. Tissues are infiltrated by activated T cells that produce high levels of IL-4 and IL-5 (explaining the eosinophilia and high IgE levels). Evidence suggests that this is a Th2-mediated disease.

Wiscott-Aldrich syndrome (WAS). WAS is a complex X-linked recessive syndrome characterized by the classical triad of eczema, immunodeficiency, and thrombocytopenia. The immunodeficiency consists of defective antibody production to polysaccharides, a T cell deficiency with low CD4 T cell counts, and depletion of the T cell zone of paracortical areas. Patients suffer from severe opportunistic bacterial infections, indicative of B and T cell deficiencies, as well as autoimmune disease and lymphomas.

The WAS gene, mapped to Xp11-13, encodes the WAS protein (WASP) which belongs to a family of proteins involved in transduction of signals from the cell membrane to the actin cytoskeleton. Normally, T cell activation through the TCR involves a dramatic change in cytoskeletal organization that effectively clusters TCRs on membrane "rafts" ("capping"), and focuses cytokine secretion and cytotoxicity on the target. WASP deficiency interferes with these cytoskeletal changes and blocks the downstream signaling essential for T cell proliferation (Section 30).

Acquired Immune Deficiency Syndrome (AIDS). This syndrome was recognized in 1981. In 1983, the causative agent of AIDS was isolated: the **human immunodeficiency virus (HIV)**. There are two types of HIV: HIV-1 and HIV-2. The virus most commonly is spread by sexual contact and contaminated needles during intravenous drug use. It belongs to the category of retroviruses called **lentiviruses**. The virion structure consists of an **envelope** which encloses the **core** containing the genomic structure of HIV. The genome contains three genes common to all retroviruses: gag encodes core proteins, pol encodes reverse transcriptase, and env encodes envelope proteins. Six additional genes encode accessory proteins. The principal targets of HIV are the CD4 T cells, dendritic cells, and macrophages. Isolates of HIV show special affinity for specific cells, a feature known as **tropism**: some isolates grow only in macrophages and monocytes **(M-tropic),** others grow in T cells but not macrophages **(T-tropic).**

The viral envelope glycoprotein gp120 binds to CD4 which acts as the receptor for the virus. Subsequently, there is fusion of the lipid bilayer of the viral envelope with the host cell plasma membrane, mediated by the viral gp41 protein, that allows the virus to enter the cell cytoplasm. Entry of the virus depends upon coreceptors that function in concert with CD4. These coreceptors are members of the **chemokine** receptor family. For viral entry into macrophages, the coreceptor is CCR5; for T cell entry, CCR5 and CXCR4 are required, although some strains use CXCR4 exclusively.

Primary infection is associated with a vigorous host response (antibody, CD8 T cell cytotoxicity, ADCC, and NK cells) which inhibit HIV replication but are insufficient to clear the virus. A vicious cycle is established as the immune system is activated with enhanced release of several cytokines; a number of these cytokines, such as TNF-α, IL-1β, IL-2, the interferons, and GM-CSF, are potent activators of HIV replication. Furthermore, HIV diversification leads to disease progression associated with depletion of CD4 T cells. The measurement of cell-associated HIV mRNA in peripheral blood serves as an independent predictor of disease progression. The CD4 T cells, the principal targets of HIV infection, are gradually depleted. The loss of CD4 T cells probably is due to multiple mechanisms. Direct killing cannot be the only factor because, even during the advanced stages of the disease, fewer than 1% of T cells are infected by HIV. Indirect mechanisms have been implicated, such as formation of T cell syncytia, enhancement of apoptosis, and inhibition of T cell production.

T Cell Malignancies

T-ALL constitutes approximately 15% of childhood acute lymphoblastic leukemia (ALL). T-ALL arises from precursors of the T lineage with the phenotype of early thymocyte development. The cells express intranuclear TdT. The phenotype is usually CD34$^+$, CD7$^+$, CD2$^+$, CD3$^-$/TCR$^-$, CD4$^-$/CD8$^-$ (double negative or stage I). Another phenotype may be present: CD34$^-$, CD7$^+$, CD2$^+$, CD1$^+$, CD3$^+$/TCR$^+$, CD4$^+$/CD8$^+$ (double positive or stage II). Expression of CD4 or CD8 with loss of CD1 corresponds to stage III. The phenotype, however, may not fall precisely into these categories, suggesting that there is a continuum of differentiation.

Malignancies of Peripheral T Cells (Table 19-2)

Peripheral T cell lymphomas are a highly heterogeneous group – some are associated with well-defined clinical syndromes and morphologic subtypes of T cells. The specific variants include the following:

Angioimmunoblastic T cell lymphoma. The phenotype is $CD4^+$ with clonal TCR gene rearrangements. There is a proliferation of small HEVs and a mixture of small cells and immunoblasts. There frequently is an associated polyclonal hyperglobulinemia and a Coombs' positive immune hemolytic anemia.

Adult T cell lymphoma/leukemia. This is a rapidly progressive T cell leukemia caused by HTLV-1 (human T cell leukemia virus 1). The cells are $CD2^+/3^+/5^+$ and, most often, also $CD4^+$ and $CD25^+$ with clonal TCR gene rearrangements.

Anaplastic large cell lymphoma ($CD30^+$). The majority of these tumors are of T cell origin (a small number involve B cells). The phenotype is $CD30^+$, EMA^+ (epithelial membrane antigen), and $CD3^+$ (mainly $CD3$-ϵ^+). These tumors are associated with a 2/5 chromosomal translocation, which juxtaposes the **nucleophosmin (NPM) gene** (5q35) to the gene encoding the receptor for tyrosine kinase, the **anaplastic lymphoma kinase (ALK)** at 2p23. NPM is a phosphoprotein which shuttles between nucleolus and cytoplasm as a carrier of newly synthesized proteins. The translocation results in the coding of a fusion protein, NPM-ALK, which constitutively activates the catalytic domain of ALK, generating signals that induce mitogenesis and may be involved in the neoplastic transformation.

Cutaneous T-cell lymphomas. These include **mycosis fungoides** and the **Sézary syndrome**. The Sézary cells in the peripheral blood have a characteristic cerebriform nucleus. They infiltrate the epidermis and paracortex of lymph nodes. They arise from CD4 helper cells. The phenotype is $CD2^+/3^+/5^+$, and most are $CD4^+$.

T-CLL. This comprises 2-5% of CLL and up to 20% of prolymphocytic leukemias (T-PLL). The cells are small with irregular nuclei and prominent nucleoli; the phenotype is $CD2^+/7^+/3^+/5^+$. T-PLL is associated with mutations and deletions of the ATM gene (Section 1) in ataxia telangiectasia.

Large granular lymphocyte (LGL) leukemia / lymphoma. Lymphoproliferative disease of LGLs (NK cells) is a heterogeneous group. Diagnosis depends on the demonstration of a homogeneous pattern of reactivity with monoclonal antibodies. The most important markers are CD56, CD57, and CD16. The $CD56^+$ cells are usually $CD3^-/CD8^-$ while the $CD57^+$ cells are positive for both these markers. The presence of $CD57^+$ frequently is associated with rheumatoid arthritis.

Table 19-1   The Immunodeficiency Diseases

	Ig	B Cells	T Cells	Pathogenesis	Gene Defect
A. PREDOMINANTLY Ig DEFICIENCY					
Bruton's agammaglobulinemia	↓↓↓	↓↓↓	N	btk gene mutation	XL
Selective deficiency of IgG classes	One or more IgG isotypes ↓	N	N	Defects in isotype differentiation	
IgA deficiency	IgA↓	N	N	Failure of terminal differentiation of IgA and B cells	Variable
Hyper IgM (failure of class switch)	IgM↑ IgA, IgG, IgE ↓	¹IgM+N ²IgG+↓↓	N	Mutation of CD40 ligand on T-cells	XL
B. SEVERE COMBINED IMMUNODEFICIENCY DISEASE					
X-linked SCID	↓	N	↓↓↓	γc mutations	XL
JAK 3 deficiency	↓	N	↓↓↓	JAK 3 mutations	AR
Rag1/Rag 2 mutations	↓	↓↓↓	↓↓↓	Rag 1/2 mutations	AR
ADA deficiency	↑	↓	↓	Toxic metabolites (dATP)	AR
MHC-class II deficiency (Bare lymphocyte syndrome)	N/↓	N	CD4↓	Mutation of transcription factors	AR
ZAP-70 deficiency	N	N	CD8↓	Mutation ZAP-70 gene	AR
C. OTHER T-CELL DEFICIENCIES					
Wiskott-Aldrich	IgM↓	N	↓	Mutation in WASP	XL
Ataxia telangiectasia	IgM↑ IgG↓	N	↓	Mutations of ATM gene (cell cycle checkpoint)	AR
Di George Syndrome	N or ↓	N	↓	Thymus development	22q11

Adapted from the report by WHO Scientific Group, Clin Exp Immunology 109: Suppl 1, 1997.

XL: X-Linked   ¹B cells expressing surface IgM
AR: Autosomal recessive   ²B cells expressing surface IgG

N   - Normal
↓   - Decreased
↑   - Increased

Table 19-2   Structure and Function of the Main T Cell Markers

CD	Structure	Function	Marker on Normal Cells	Diagnostic Applications
CD1	Class Ib HLA H chain = a-e L chain = β_2 microglobulin	Antigen presentation (lipid)	Thymocytes (CD4$^+$/CD8$^+$) B cells (CD1c) Not on mature T cells	T-ALL
CD2	Two Ig domains	Adhesion (T-APC)	T cell (all stages) B cell (fetal)	T-ALL T lymphoma Rare B-ALL and B cell lymphoma
CD3	Three proteins: γ, δ, ϵ	Members of TCR signaling	T cells	T-ALL and T-lymphoma Intracellular detection = T lineage
CD4	Glycoprotein Four Ig domains	Interacts with HLA class II Coreceptor for TCR T cell activation Adhesion (T-APC)	Thymocytes Peripheral T cells Hemopoietic stem cells Monocytes Macrophages	T-ALL (some) T lymphoma AML: M_4 and some M_2
CD5	Three scavenger receptor domains	T-B interactions Signaling	T cells B1 cells	T-ALL T-lymphoma B-CLL Mantle lymphoma
CD7	One Ig domain	–	T cells Stem cells Fetal B cells Myeloid cells at certain stage	T-ALL T lymphoma CD7$^+$ AML
CD8	Two polypeptides α-β or α-α One Ig domain each	Interacts with HLA class I Coreceptor for TCR T cell activation	Thymocytes Peripheral T cells	T-ALL T lymphoma Rare B-CLL
CD25	Two complement control domains	α chain of IL-2 receptor	T cells	T lymphoma
CD28	Homodimer with an Ig domain in each chain	T cell activation Costimulatory molecule Counter receptor for CD80/CD86	T cells	–
CD154 (CD40 ligand)	Trimer of α chain with similarities to TNF	Member of TNF family T-B interactions: generation of memory B cells	T cells	CD154 mutation – Hyper IgM syndrome

SUGGESTED READING

André P, Biassoni R, et al. New nomenclature for MHC receptors. Nature Immunol 2:661, 2001.

Buckley RH. Primary immunodeficiency diseases due to defects in lymphocytes. N Engl J Med 343:1313-1324, 2000.

Chambers CA, Allison J. Costimulatory regulation of T cell function. Curr Opin Cell Biol 11:203-210, 1999.

Delves PU, Roitt IM. The immune system. N Engl J Med 343:37-61 and 108-117, 2000.

Gately MK, Renzetti LM, Magram J, et al. The interleukin-12/interleukin-12 receptor system: role in normal and pathologic immune responses. Ann Rev Immunol 16:495, 1998.

Godfrey DI, Hammond JL, Poulton LD, et al. NKT cells: facts functions and fallacies. Immunol Today 21:573, 2000.

Hayday AC. γδ cells: a right time and a right place for a conserved third way of protection. Ann Rev Immunol 18:975, 2000.

Henkart PA. Cytotoxic T lymphocytes. In: Fundamental Immunology, 4th Ed. W.E. Paul, Ed. p:1021, 1999.

Kamradt T, Mitchison NA. Tolerance and autoimmunity. N Engl J Med 344:655-664, 2001.

Kimbrell Da, Beutler B. The evolution and genetics of innate immunity. Nature Rev Genetics 2:256-267, 2001.

Klein J, Sato A. The HLA system. N Engl J Med. 343:702-709 and 782-786, 2000.

Lanier LL. NK cell receptors. Ann Rev Immunol. 16:359, 1998.

Paraskevas F. T cells and NK cells. p:497-593. In: Wintrobe's Clinical Hematology, 10th Ed. Lee GR, Foerster J, Lukens J, Paraskevas F, Greer JP, Rodgers GM, Eds. William and Wilkins, 1999.

Parkin J, Cohen B. An overview of the immune system. Lancet 357:1777-1789, 2001.

Report of a WHO scientific group. Primary Immunodeficiency diseases. Clin Exp Immunol 109:S1:1-28, 1997.

Seder RA, Mossmann TM. Differentiation of effector phenotypes of CD4+ and CD8+ T cells. In: Fundamental Immunology, 4th Ed. W.E. Paul, Ed. p:879, 1999.

Snapper SB, Rosen FS. The Wiskott-Aldrich syndrome protein (WASP): roles in signaling and cytoskeletal organization. Ann Rev Immunol 17:905, 1999.

Spits H, Lanier LL, Phillips. Development of human T and natural killer cells. Blood 85:2654, 1995.

Von Andrian, MacKay CR. T cell function and migration. N Engl J Med 343:1020-1034, 2000.

Yokoyama WM. Natural killer cells. In: Fundamental Immunology, 4th Ed. W.E. Paul, Ed. p:575, 1999.

Complement

Frixos Paraskevas

"We shall not seriously err if we ascribe to this 'complement' a ferment-like character."
– Paul Erlich (1900)[7]

Antibodies do not lyse bacteria or cells directly but do so by sequential activation of a series of plasma proteins collectively known as **complement**. Complement plays a major effector role in defense against infectious agents, constituting an important component of innate immunity. It kills invading bacteria directly, i.e. in the absence of antibodies, but it also "complements" antibody lytic activity (thus the name). Complement recruits phagocytes to sites of infection and, as an opsonin, markedly enhances their phagocytic activity. The beneficial biological effects of complement may be compromised by some deleterious consequences: lysis of red cells (innocent bystanders), tissue necrosis by potent inflammatory mediators (anaphylatoxins), and the action of recruited and activated phagocytes. Regulatory mechanisms limit complement activation and prevent destruction of host cells.

Complement activity depends on a complex cascade of interactions that involves more than 30 proteins. Complement activation is initiated by three pathways: **classical, lectin,** and **alternative**; all lead to the final common pathway that results in the formation of the membrane attack complex (MAC), a rigid cylinder that penetrates the membrane of the target cell. The classical cascade is initiated by antigen-antibody complexes; the lectin and alternative pathways can be activated in the absence of an immune response.

THE CLASSICAL PATHWAY

The components of the classical pathway are designated by the uppercase C followed by a number denoting their order of participation in the cascade reaction – the exception is C4 that acts before C2 and C3. Functionally, the components may be grouped into three main categories: 1) **serine proteases**, 2) **cell surface binding proteins**, and 3) **cell membrane penetrating proteins**.

The first component of the classical pathway (C1) consists of three proteins: C1q, C1r, and C1s. C1q is the "linker" to the antibody, interacting with the Fc domain of the immunoglobulin. C1q has six subunits, each subunit composed of 3 different polypeptide chains; these chains have an amino acid composition that is similar to collagen (an unusual feature for a plasma protein). Each of the six subunits has a helical N-terminal structure joined by a filamentous segment to a globular C-terminal end. The globular ends form a configuration

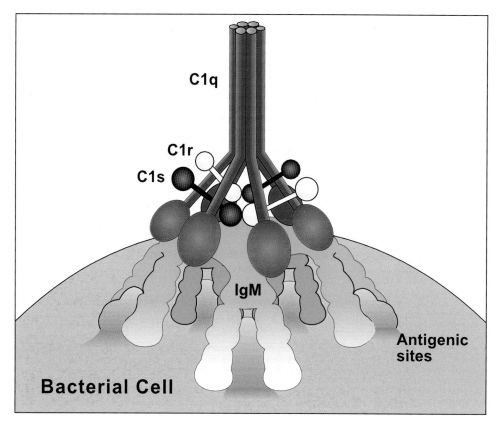

Figure 20-1 C1 Esterase

resembling a "bouquet of flowers"; the "stem" consists of the N-terminal helical structure (Figure 20-1). The globular C-terminal contains the site that interacts with antibody. (IgM binds more strongly than IgG: Section 17).

In the presence of Ca^{2+}, the components of C1 form a pentameric complex consisting of one C1q, two C1r, and two C1s, known collectively as **C1 esterase** (Figure 20-1). Formation of C1 esterase results from a series of sequential molecular actions. When an IgM antibody molecule binds to specific antigens on the surface of an infectious agent, it assumes a "crab" or "staple" configuration (Figure 20-1: IgM bound to a Salmonella flagellum). The exposed Fc domain of the antibody is bound by a C1q molecule through its globular heads, forming a cone. The two C1r and two C1s molecules interact within the arms of C1q at a site between the globular heads and the stem. (C1r and C1s are proenzymes). A conformational change of C1q, brought about by its binding to the antigen-antibody complex, allows C1s to approach the catalytic site of C1r which then cleaves and activates C1s, resulting in the appearance of the **C1 esterase** activity of the complex. (Activated C1s provides the enzymatic activity of the C1 esterase complex: Figure 20-2)

The C4 component of complement consists of three chains, α, β and γ. C1 esterase cleavage of the alpha chain releases a small fragment designated C4a (Figure 20-2). The remaining molecule (C4b) binds covalently to the cell surface. This binding depends upon an unusual and highly reactive internal **thioester bond**, formed between the thiol group of a cysteine and the carbonyl group of a glutamyl residue. The thioester bond is present only in C4 and C3; upon cleavage activation of C3 or C4, the bond opens and allows these molecules to bind covalently to the cell surface.

In the presence of Mg^{2+}, C2 binds to the surface-bound C4b and then is cleaved by C1 esterase into two fragments, C2a and C2b. The C2a, which remains bound to C4b, expresses the enzymatic activity. The C4b-2a complex is known as **C3 convertase** (Figure 20-2).

C3 is the most abundant component of complement in plasma; it is composed of an alpha and a beta chain linked by a disulfide bond. C3 convertase removes a small fragment (C3a) from the alpha chain. As a result of conformational changes, the **internal thioester bond** is broken, allowing the covalent binding of C3b to the cell membrane. Deposition of multiple C3b fragments on the membrane in the vicinity of the C3 convertase complex (C4b-C2a) converts this complex to the enzyme complex **C5 convertase** (C4b-C2a-C3b). The enzymatic activity of C5 convertase continues to reside in C2a. The small fragments split from the C components possess anaphylatoxin (C3a, C4a) or kinin (C2b) activity. C3b and a cleavage fragment iC3b are important complement opsonins.

THE LECTIN PATHWAY (MANNOSE-BINDING LECTIN PATHWAY)

The **mannan-binding lectin (MBL)**, also known as mannose-binding lectin, is a protein of the **collectin** family. (Other members of the collectin family include the surfactant proteins, SP-A_1, SP-A_2 and SP-D, important in the early neonatal period). MBL consists of a collagenous region and a lectin domain – the lectin domain is the **carbohydrate recognition domain (CRD)**. MBL can activate complement directly in the absence of antibody, bypassing the C1q/antibody step (Figure 20-2).

Binding of multiple MBLs to various carbohydrate moities on the surface of a bacterial cell activates two serine proteases MASP-1 and MASP-2 (MBL-associated serum protease). These enzymes have structural homology to the C1r and C1s of the classical pathway. Activation of MASP results in cleavage of C4 and C2 with the generation of **C3 convertase** and cleavage of C3. The subsequent generation of C5 convertase proceeds through the same steps as in the classical pathway.

THE ALTERNATIVE PATHWAY

The alternative pathway is, phylogenetically, the oldest of the complement-activating pathways. It is activated in the absence of an immune response, thus constituting an important

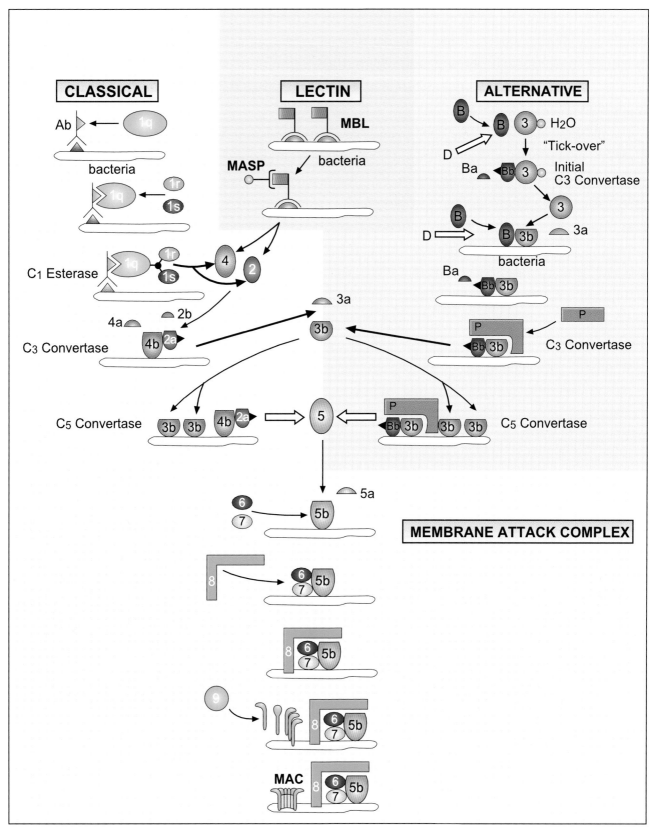

Figure 20-2 Complement Cascades

component of innate immunity. A number of substances activate this pathway, including: endotoxins, lipopolysaccharides, aggregated IgA or IgE, and collagen. The initiating mechanism is the spontaneous hydrolysis of the internal **thioester bond** of C3 by one molecule of H_2O, resulting in the formation of C3(H_2O) that is comformationally similar to C3b although it is uncleaved (Figure 20-2).

The formation of **C3(H2O)** takes place continuously in the plasma at a very low rate (in a process referred to as "tick-over"). This hydrolyzed form of C3 possesses all the properties of C3b. C3(H_2O) associates with **factor B**, which then is cleaved by the serine protease **factor D** into a small (Ba) fragment and a large (Bb) fragment. (Factor B is structurally and functionally homologous to C2 of the classical pathway; both molecules are encoded by genes located in close proximity to the class III region of the MHC complex). Bb remains associated with C3(H_2O) and, in the presence of Mg^{2+}, forms a **C3 convertase** [C3(H_2O)•Bb•Mg^{2+}]. This C3 convertase is present only briefly in the plasma (Figure 20-2). During this brief period, this **initial C3 convertase** cleaves C3, resulting in the deposition of several C3b fragments on the cell surface. The subsequent fate of C3b depends on the nature of the surface, i.e. whether it is a host cell membrane or a foreign cell membrane, eg, bacteria (Figure 20-3).

Activation of the alternative pathway is a continuous ongoing process (C3 tick-over). Consequently, the [C3(H_2O)Bb] complex is readily available to form an active stable C3 convertase upon contact with appropriate activating surfaces such as bacteria. It is remarkable that the alternative complement system, a component of innate immunity (non-specific), possesses self versus non-self discriminating properties characteristic of adaptive (specific) immunity.

Host (self) cell surfaces are non-activating – on this surface, C3b preferentially binds **factor H** rather than factor B. Factor H acts as a cofactor for the enzyme **factor I**, which degrades C3b, effectively terminating complement activation. In contrast, when C3b is deposited on a **bacterial surface (activating)**, it has a higher affinity for factor B. Factor B bound to C3b is cleaved by factor D; the Ba fragment is released and Bb remains bound to C3b. This bacterial cell bound complex [C3b•Bb•Mg^{2+}], known as **amplification C3 convertase,** is stabilized by the large protein molecule, **properdin (P)**. Multiple C3b fragments cluster on the cell membrane in the vicinity of C3 convertase and, as in the classical pathway, generate the specific enzyme **C5 convertase**.

MEMBRANE ATTACK COMPLEX: CELL LYSIS (Figure 20-2)

The key enzyme **C5 convertase** acts on C5 which is composed of an alpha and a beta chain linked by a disulfide bond. C5 convertase cleaves a small fragment (C5a) from the alpha chain. The larger fragment, C5b, forms a trimolecular complex with C6 and C7; this complex binds to the membrane and forms the base whereby the C8 component is inserted deeply into the phospholipid bilayer. The C5b, 6, 7, 8 complex generates transmembrane channels; however,

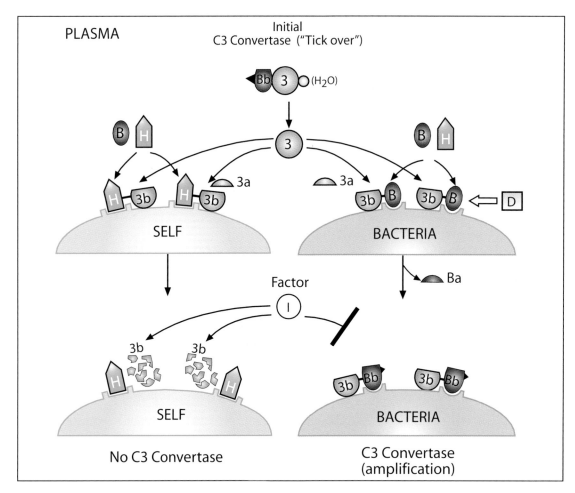

Figure 20-3 Self-Nonself Discrimination by Complement

cell lysis is slow and requires high concentrations of C8.

Lysis is achieved more efficiently by the participation of C9, the last component in the cascade. C9 is a single polypeptide chain that, in the native state, has a globular configuration and displays two domains, one hydrophilic (C9a) and one hydrophobic (C9b). Upon interaction with the C5b, 6, 7, 8 complex, C9 elongates and polymerizes through formation of disulfide bonds with other C9 molecules. The polymerized C9 forms a cylindrical structure that penetrates the membrane but also projects above its surface. The tubular structure, formed of several (up to 18) C9 molecules, remains in contact with the C5b, 6, 7, 8 complex. The entire C5b, 6, 7, 8, 9 macromolecular grouping is the **membrane attack complex (MAC)**. Cell lysis results from the free communication of the interior of the cell with the external environment.

REGULATORS OF COMPLEMENT ACTIVATION (Table 20-1)

In the process of complement activation, there is release of biologically active fragments that are potent mediators of the inflammatory response. The majority of activated C3 and C4 molecules escape interaction with the surface of the target cell and are deposited on neighbouring host cells. In addition, the persistent low turnover of the alternative pathway ("tick-over") continuously deposits activated complement components on host cells. Within 5 minutes of complement activation, several million C3b fragments are deposited on the target cell and an equal number of C3a anaphylatoxin molecules are liberated into the surrounding fluids. Because C3b molecules bind not only to foreign cells but also to host cells, mechanisms for limiting the duration of complement activation are essential. Regulators of complement activity function throughout the complement cascade, during initiation, activation, and assembly of the membrane attack complex.

I. Control of the initiation step

C1 esterase inhibitor (C1-INH) functions early in the classical pathway. It is a plasma protein that belongs to the family of **ser**ine **pro**tease **in**hibitors (**serpins**). C1-INH inhibits C1 esterase by reacting with the catalytic sites of activated C1r and C1s, preventing C1 esterase activation both in the fluid phase and on the cell membrane. C1-INH also has a regulatory role outside the complement system: it inactivates kallikrein, and coagulation factors XIa and XIIa, and interacts with plasmin. Deficiency of C1-INH is responsible for **hereditary angioedema,** an autosomal dominant disorder that presents with subcutaneous and submucosal edema, most prominently in skin, gastrointestinal and respiratory tracts; pharyngeal edema may be life threatening. The increased vascular permeability is due to the excess bradykinin produced through kallikrein cleavage of high molecular-weight kininogen – as a result of C1-INH deficiency, kallikrein activity is unopposed (Section 24).

II. Control of C3/C5 convertases (Figure 20-4)

Protection of normal cells from C3 and C5 convertases is afforded by six proteins: three plasma proteins (C4bBP, factor H, and factor I), and three cell surface proteins (MCP, DAF and complement receptor 1 – CR1). Factor I is a serine esterase. The other five proteins belong to a structurally and functionally related group known as **regulators of complement activation (RCA);** their genes are clustered on the long arm of chromosome 1. Each protein is composed of multiples of a cysteine-rich module known as **complement control protein repeats (CCPR).** Control of convertase activity is accomplished by two mechanisms: (a) decay accelerating activity, and (b) proteolysis in which the regulator acts as a cofactor for the proteolytic enzyme Factor I.

(a) Decay accelerating activity (Figure 20-4)

Decay accelerating factor (DAF, CD55), an inhibitor of classical C3 convertase, is a glycoprotein that contains four CCPR modules. It is attached to the cell membrane by a glycosylphosphatidylinositol (GPI) anchor that provides it with the mobility to patrol the cell surface for deposited C components. The GPI anchor consists of three components:

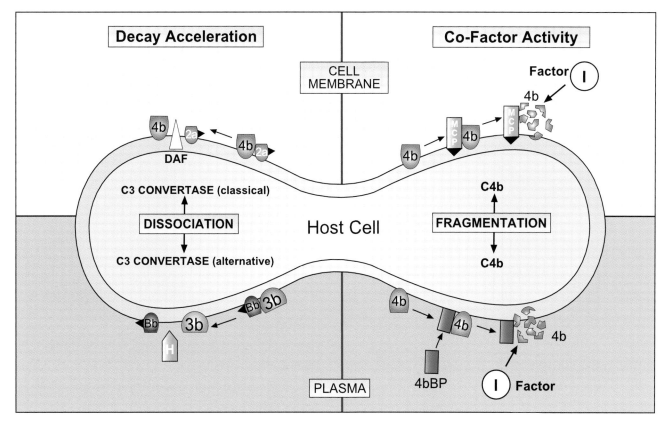

Figure 20-4 Decay and Co-factor Activities

phosphoethanolamine, a **glycan core**, and **phosphatidylinositol** (Figure 20-5). The glycan core consists of three mannose molecules and one N-acetylglucosamine. N-acetyl glucosamine transferase, the product of the **PIG-A** gene (**P**hosphatidyl **I**nositol **G**lycan complementation class **A**), is involved in the first step of GPI-anchor biosynthesis. The second step involves the addition of three mannose molecules; the addition of phosphoethanolamine is the final step. DAF inhibits C3 convertase by mediating the rapid release of C2a from its binding site on C4b thus dissociating the C3 convertase complex. The GPI anchor is shared by several proteins, including another regulator of complement activation, **CD59** (see below). Deficiency of DAF and CD59 is associated with paroxysmal nocturnal hemoglobinuria (PNH): erythrocytes deficient in DAF and CD59 are exquisitively sensitive to lysis by complement (Section 10).

    Factor H is a plasma protein that consists of 20 CCPRs. It is the single most important regulator of the complement cascade. Factor H accelerates the decay of the alternative C3 convertase by displacing factor Bb from the C3bBb convertase, thereby destroying C3 convertase activity (Figure 20-4).

    Complement receptors. Only the CR1 complement receptor plays a role in the regulation of C activation. (The other complement receptors, CR2 and CR3, do not participate in this regulatory function). CR1 has decay accelerating activity, and also functions as a cofactor for factor I.

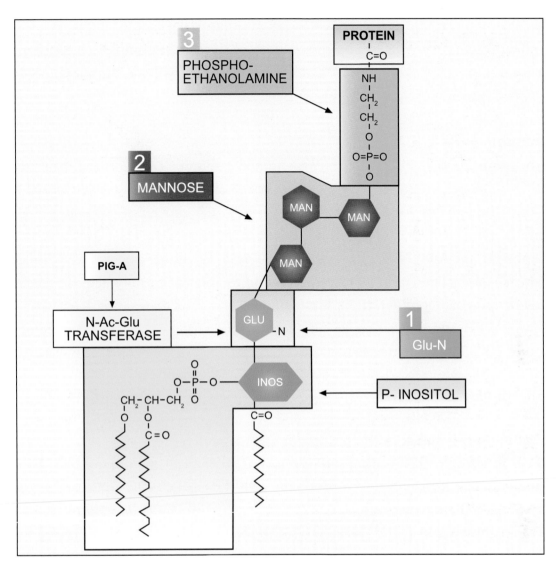

Figure 20-5 Three Steps in GPI Synthesis

(b) Cofactor Activity (Figure 20-3)

Factor I is a regulatory enzyme that degrades C3b and C4b with the participation of cofactors such as factor H, MCP, C4bBP and CR1. Factor I cleavage degrades C3b to iC3b, and a second cleavage converts iC3b to C3dg. CR1 is the primary cofactor for Factor I cleavage of iC3b. C3dg remains bound to the cell surface. (C3d is a proteolytic fragment of C3dg – anti-C3d antibodies are used in the direct Coombs test to determine the presence of complement on the surface of red blood cells: Section 11).

Membrane Cofactor Protein (MCP, CD46), expressed on all cells except erythrocytes, is composed of four CCPR modules. MCP is a cofactor for factor I. MCP and DAF activities are complementary – functioning together, they efficiently inhibit the complement convertases.

C4b-binding protein (C4bBP) is a plasma protein. It consists of seven α chains and one β chain linked by disulfide bonds; there are 8 CCPRs in each α chain and 3 CCPRs in the β chain. The chains are arranged in a "spider" configuration with flexible "tentacles". C4bBP has decay accelerating activity, accelerating dissociation of the C4b2a complex. It also functions as a cofactor for factor I. (Appoximately 50% of C4bBP in plasma is bound to protein S, a cofactor in the protein C pathway: Section 25).

(c) Other regulators

Properdin consists of non-covalently linked subunits that form dimers and larger polymers. It functions to stabilize the formation of alternative C3 convertase (C3bBb): it increases the affinity of factor B for C3b, and protects C3 convertase from factor H/factor I proteolysis.

Nephritic factors (NeF) are non-physiological Ig autoantibodies that bind to and stabilize the C3 convertase enzyme C3bBb, resulting in abnormal prolonged cleavage of C3. In some cases of membranoproliferative glomerulonephritis, NeFs are associated with depleted plasma levels of C3 and deposition of complement on renal glomeruli. The etiology of the production of NEF autoantibodies is unclear.

III. Control of MAC

(a) Regulators on cell surfaces

CD59 is a single chain glycoprotein attached to the cell membrane by a GPI anchor, present on all circulating blood cells, endothelial cells, epithelial cells, and spermatozoa. It has two binding sites, one for the α chain of C8 and another for the β domain of C9. It inhibits MAC formation: following C5b-7 insertion into the cell membrane, CD59 is incorporated into the evolving MAC, inhibiting incorporation of the first C9 molecule and subsequent C9 polymerization. Its absence on red blood cells is associated with PNH.

(b) Regulators in body fluids

S protein (site-specific protein) is identical to vitronectin. It is a plasma protein synthesized primarily in liver and platelets. S protein binds to the metastable C5β-7 complex and prevents its insertion into the membrane; it also inhibits C9 polymerization.

Clusterin is a plasma protein composed of an α and a β chain. It inhibits the terminal stages of C activation: following formation of the C5b-7 complex, clusterin binds with high affinity to C7, the β chain of C8, and the β domain of C9. Clusterin is present in high concentrations in the epididymis where it may be important in immune protection of sperm.

IV. Removal of products of complement activation

The circulating anaphylatoxins, C3a, C4a and C5a, released during complement activation are inactivated rapidly by the plasma enzyme **carboxypeptidase N** which removes the carboxyl-

Table 20-1   Regulators of Complement Activation

SITE OF ACTION	REGULATOR	TARGET
I. C1 esterase	C1 esterase inhibitor	Inhibits C1 esterase

II. C3 / C5 convertases	(a) on cell surfaces
	     MCP (CD46)
		Cofactor for factor I
		     cleavage of C3b/C4b

	DAF (CD55)	Inhibits C3 convertase

	Complement receptor 1	Decay and cofactor activities
		Promotes further fragmentation
		     of C3b
		Carries immune complexes on
		     RBC to spleen for disposal

	(b) in fluids Factor I	Degrades C3b and C4b

	Factor H	Prevents formation of C3
		     alternative convertase
		Dissociates the formed
		     alternative convertase

	C4bBP	Cofactor for factor I: cleavage
		     of C4b
		Decay accelerating activity for
		     C3 convertase (C4b2b)

	Properdin	Stabilizes C3 alternative convertase
	Nephritic factors	Stabilize C3 convertase
III. Control of MAC	(a) on cell surfaces CD59	Inhibits MAC formation

	(b) in fluids
	     S protein
	     Clusterin
		Inhibits MAC formation
		Inhibits MAC formation

terminal arginine residue of these molecules. **Carboxypeptidase R** exists in plasma as a precursor (proCPR); this molecule has been identified as the thrombin-activatable fibrinolysis inhibitor (TAFI) described in Section 29. CPR has two roles: one as an inhibitor of fibrinolysis, and the other as a regulator of the inflammatory response by inactivation of C3a and C5a.

V. Factor H in self / non-self discrimination (Figure 20-3)

The main function of factor H is the control of tick-over in the alternative pathway. On **host cell surfaces** ("non-activating"), factor H competes successfully with factor B in binding to C3b – this results in fragmentation of C3b by factor I due to factor H **cofactor activity**. In

contrast, on foreign surfaces ("activating"), carbohydrate rich polymers prevent binding of factor H to C3b; this allows the generation of the alternative convertase (C3bBb), leading to the kill of micro-organisms by the MAC complex.

COMPLEMENT RECEPTORS

Receptors for the activated components of complement are expressed on many cells and tissues. Receptor binding mediates the various effector functions of complement.

C1q receptors are present on cell surfaces as well as within the cytoplasm. The C1q receptor known as C1qRp is a typical transmembrane protein; it is expressed on the surface of macrophages/monocytes – binding of C1q enhances phagocytosis. A second C1q binding protein, gC1qR, is located intracellularly within the mitochondrial matrix; it binds to the globular heads of C1q (as well as to kininogen and factor XII). A third C1q binding protein, cC1qR, binds to the collagen-like regions of C1q; it is indistinguishable from calreticulin, a Ca^{2+} binding protein in the endoplasmic reticulum. C1q binding to cC1qR may interfere with the removal of immune complexes.

Complement receptor type 1 (CR1, CD35) is expressed on all peripheral blood cells (except platelets), and on follicular dendritic cells (Section 21). Cell membrane expression of CR1 is upregulated by chemotactic peptides such as C5a, endotoxin, and cytokines. There are about 500 CR1 molecules on the erythrocyte; leukocytes display about 50,000 per cell. CR1 cooperates with the Fc receptors and CR3 in enhancing phagocytosis of opsonized particles. CR1 possesses both decay accelerating activity and cofactor activity for Factor I. It is the primary receptor for C3b; it also binds C4b and iC3b. CR1 is upregulated on activated neutrophils and monocytes. Antigen-antibody complexes opsonized by complement (C3b/C4b) bind to CRI receptors on circulating erythrocytes; these immune complexes subsequently are removed by the monocyte/macrophages in the spleen and liver without red cell lysis.

Complement receptor 2 (CR2, CD21) is expressed on B lymphocytes, on follicular dendritic cells, and on some epithelial cells. It forms a trimolecular complex with CD19 and CD81, which acts as an activating receptor on B cells. **Antigen-antibody-complement** complexes cross-link CR2 with surface IgM (as complement binds to CR2 and antigen binds to IgM), enhancing Ig production 100-1000 fold (Section 18). CR2 is a weak cofactor for factor I. Its primary ligands are iC3b and C3dg. EB virus has a high affinity for B cells expressing CR2.

Complement receptor 3 (CR3, CD11b/CD18) belongs to the family of leukocyte integrin adhesion molecules (Section 3). CR3 is expressed on the surface of activated neutrophils, monocytes, and NK lymphocytes. It is a receptor for iC3b and C3d.

Complement receptor type 4 (CR4, CD11c/CD18) is an integrin adhesion molecule with a cellular distribution similar to CR3. It is a receptor for iC3b.

Factor H receptor is present on B lymphocytes, monocytes, and polymorphonuclear leukocytes. Binding of factor H to this receptor results in cellular release of factor I.

C3a receptor reacts with both C3a and C4a. Binding of C3a to the receptor on mast cells and basophils results in degranulation with release of histamine.

C5a receptor, like the C3a receptor, is a G protein-coupled receptor. Binding of C5a results in degranulation of mast cells and basophils. Receptor binding of C5a on the surface of neutrophils initiates intracellular signaling that results in an inflammatory response: upregulation of surface adhesion molecules, and migration into inflammatory sites (Section 7).

CLINICAL CORRELATES

Paroxysmal Nocturnal Hemoglobinuria (PNH)

PNH is an acquired hematopoietic stem cell disorder manifest by intravascular hemolysis, venous thrombosis, aplastic anemia, myelodysplasia and leukemia. The defect is the result of somatic mutations consisting of deletions, insertions, or point mutations of the **PIG-A** gene. Pig-A encodes an N-acetylglucosamine transferase which acts in the first step of glycosylphos-phatidylinositol (GPI) synthesis (Figure 20-5).

In PNH, proteins dependent on the GPI anchor, including CD59 and CD55 (DAF), are absent in all hematopoietic cell lines. As a result, the red cells in PNH are sensitive to lysis by complement activation (classical or alternative) – absence of CD59 is more critical than CD55 in red cell lysis. The GPI defect explains the red cell hemolysis but does not account for the other manifestations of PNH, such as bone marrow failure (aplastic anemia) or the proliferative advantage of this clone over normal stem cells. The diagnosis of PNH may be confirmed using flow cytometry to demonstrate the absence of red blood cell CD55 and CD59 (Section 10).

Role in Innate Immunity and Humoral Immunity

Complement plays an essential role in defense against infections. It is an important component of non-specific innate immunity: it acts immediately and directly as a lysin in the killing of bacteria (alternative and lectin pathways) and also as an opsonin for phagocytosis before the adaptive immune response comes into play.

Complement also enhances the adaptive immune response. It increases antigen-specific immune responses by two mechanisms: (a) it is instrumental in the trapping of antigen-antibody complexes by follicular dendritic cells within the follicles of the lymphoid organs (Section 21), and (b) it enhances B cell response to antigen by several orders of magnitude as antigen/ antibody/ complement complexes bind to the surface complement receptor-2 (CR2) and to surface IgM (antigen receptor) on the same B cell.

Role in Pathogenesis of Infections and Chronic Diseases

Proteins of the complement system may be involved in the pathogenesis of certain infectious diseases. MCP is the receptor for measles virus as well as for Staphylococcus pyogenes. HIV activates complement even in the absence of antibodies; activated complement enhances its infectivity, facilitating deposition of the virus within lymph node follicles. HIV avoids virolysis by absorbing control proteins (CD59) on its envelope.

Complement activation plays a critical role in the pathogenesis of a number of human diseases such as vasculitis and glomerulonephritis that are due to deposition of immune complexes on cell surfaces. During relapse in **systemic lupus erythematosus** when circulating antigen-antibody complexes are present, there is a marked decrease in the plasma level of C3. Levels of C3 provide a means of monitoring disease activity. Individuals with hereditary homozygous deficiency of C1q or C4 are predisposed to development of SLE.

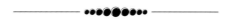

SUGGESTED READING

Barrington R, Zhang M, Fischer M, Carroll MC. The role of complement in inflammation and adaptive immunity. Immunol Rev 180:5-15, 2001.

Campbell W, Okada N, Okada H. Carboxypeptidase R is an inactivator of complement-derived inflammatory peptides and an inhibitor of fibrinolysis. Immunol Rev 180:162-167, 2001.

Carroll MC. The role of complement receptors in induction and regulation of immunity. Annu Rev Immunol 16:545-568, 1998.

Carroll MC. The role of complement in B cell activation and tolerance. Adv Immunol 74:61-88, 2000.

Colten HR, Rosen FS. Complement deficiencies. Annu Rev Immunol 10:809-834, 1992.

Liszewski MK, Post TW, Atkinson JP. Membrane cofactor protein (MCP or CD46): newest member of the regulators of complement activation gene cluster. Annu Rev Immunol 9:431-455, 1991.

Liszewski MK, Farries TC, Lublin DM, Rooney IA, Atkinson JP. Control of the complement system. p. 201-283. In Advances in Immunology 61:201-283, 1996.

Muller-Eberhard HJ. Molecular organization and function of the complement system. Ann Rev Biochem 57:321, 1988.

Paraskevas F. Cell interactions in the immune response. p:544-614. In Wintrobe's Hematology, Lee GR, Foerster J, Lukens J, Paraskevas F, Greer JP, Rodgers GM, Eds. Williams-Wilkins, 10th Ed, 1999.

Prodinger WM, Würzner R, Erdei A, Dierich MP. Complement. p:967-995. In Fundamental Immunology, Paul WE, Ed. Lippincott-Raven Publishers, 1999.

Sahu A, Lambris JD. Structure and biology of complement protein C3, a connecting link between innate and acquired immunity. Immunol Rev 180:35-48, 2001.

Walport MJ. Complement. N Engl J Med 344:1058-1066 and 1140-1144, 2001.

DENDRITIC CELLS AND MACROPHAGES

Frixos Paraskevas
Esther Israels

"Then Prometheus gave wisdom, which is strength to Jupiter, clothed him with the dominion of wide Heaven"
"Prometheus Unbound"
Percy Bysshe Shelley

DENDRITIC CELLS

In Greek mythology, Jupiter won the battle against the Titans with the help of Prometheus and, thus, became the ruler of the universe. In the immunological universe, dendritic cells (DCs) play a "Promethean" role in initiating and regulating the functions of the immunological ruler, the T cell. In 1868, Langerhans identified these cells in the skin; they were "rediscovered" in 1973 in mouse spleen. Their distribution is ubiquitous, present in most tissues with the exception of brain.

DCs are the primary initiators of lymphocyte activation and regulators of self-tolerance – they are referred to as "nature's adjuvants" because of their potency in stimulating the immune response. They constitute a highly diversified lineage in terms of origin, function, and phenotype, but all members of the family share the **dendritic morphology** which describes their arborescent appearance (Greek: dendron = tree). Cytoplasmic extensions vary from spiny fillipodia to large sheets of lamellipodia and veils, structures well suited to capturing and presenting antigen to T cells – the expanded surface increases the probability of DCs contacting the rare antigen-specific T cells. DCs are the most effective of the antigen presenting cells (APCs); the term "potency" applied to DCs indicates that relatively low doses of antigen are sufficient to initiate a rapid T cell response.

Ontogeny

DCs originate from pluripotent $CD34^+$ hematopoietic stem cells in the bone marrow. Stem cell differentiation proceeds through intermediate precursors that give rise either to a **lymphoid** progenitor capable of T- or B-lymphocyte lineage commitment or to a **myeloid** progenitor capable of differentiation into cell lines that include granulocytes and macrophages. A distinct DC subtype develops from the myeloid lineage; a second DC subtype is linked to the lymphocyte lineage. *In vitro*, immature $CD34^+$ progenitors in the presence of GM-CSF, IL-4, and TNF-α give rise to DCs considered to be myeloid because they express CD14 (transiently), CD13, and CD33, markers that also are present on macrophages and myeloid cells; in the presence of M-CSF these progenitors may differentiate into macrophages. *In vitro*, lymphoid DCs develop from thymic-derived precursors upon stimulation with IL-3. The Langerhans cells (LCs) in the

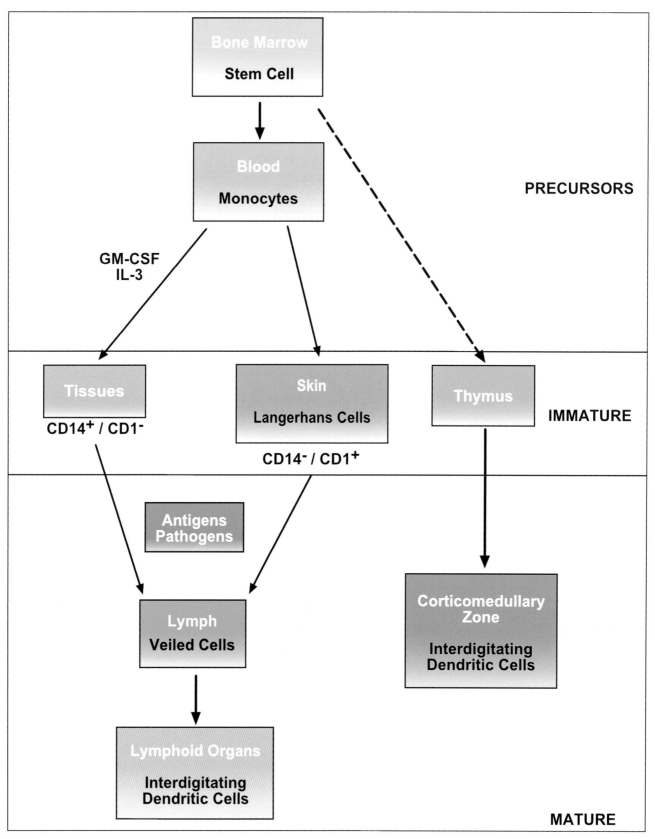

Figure 21-1 Dendritic Cell Differentiation

epidermis probably originate from the myeloid progenitor; TGF-β is the major cytokine required for LC differentiation. The characteristic LC markers are CD1α and CD11c.

DCs migrate out of the bone marrow into peripheral tissues and, finally, into lymph nodes (Figure 21-1): (1) **Precursors** of DCs move out of the bone marrow, circulate through blood and lymphatics and migrate into tissues in response to chemokines constitutively expressed or induced by inflammatory stimuli. Two potent chemotactic chemokines for DCs are SDF-1 (stromal-derived factor-1) and MDC (macrophage derived chemokine) – the corresponding receptors expressed on DCs are CXCR4 and CCR4, respectively. (2) **Immature DCs** infiltrate peripheral tissues and are found at body surfaces and in interstitial spaces – immune sentinels positioned to engulf foreign proteins. (3) After capturing antigen, the cells migrate to secondary lymphoid organs where they become **mature DCs**, capable of activating antigen-specific naïve T lymphocytes to initiate the immune response. Terminal differentiation of DCs is augmented by stimuli arising from: (a) inflammatory cytokines such as IL-1, IL-6, TNFα, as well as IL-4 and IL-13; (b) costimulatory signals delivered by CD40/CD40 ligand interaction; and (c) foreign substances such as lipopolysaccharides, viruses, and phagocytosed bacteria.

Function

The sequential activities in which DCs are engaged include: (1) antigen capture, (2) migration, (3) antigen presentation, (4) cell interactions, and (5) activation of lymphocytes. DC maturation is a continuous process, initiated in the periphery by exposure to antigen and/or cytokines and completed in lymphoid organs during DC-T cell interactions. The transition of immature antigen-capturing DCs to mature antigen-presenting DCs is marked by phenotypic changes as the cells adapt to their new roles.

Antigen capture. The immature DC captures antigens by endocytosis via a number of pathways: (1) soluble antigens are taken up by **macropinocytosis,** an endocytotic process by which large volumes of extracellular fluid enter the cell; (2) receptor-mediated endocytosis via **Fcγ receptors** (that mediate internalization of Ag-Ab complexes or opsonized particles) and two C-type lectin receptors, the **mannose receptor (MR)** and **DEC-205**; and (3) **phagocytosis** of particles and pathogens. Once the DC has captured antigen, its ability to take up additional antigen is reduced as the expression of surface receptors is downregulated.

Migration. Traffic of DCs is regulated by cytokines (IL-1, TNFα), chemokines, and pathogen-derived lipopolysaccharides. These modulators regulate the expression of surface adhesion molecules. Following antigen capture, the membrane adhesive properties are lost, the cytoskeleton is reorganized and the cells become mobile – changes that enable DCs to migrate through the afferent lymph channels to specific T cell areas of lymph nodes and spleen where they trigger activation of naïve T cells.

Chemokine interaction with DC receptors plays a critical regulatory role during migration. DC maturation is accompanied by an alteration in the expression of chemokine receptors. An example of this are Langerhans cells (LCs), a specific DC subtype. Immature LCs express the chemokine receptor CCR6 which directs them to the skin where the CCR6 ligand MIP-3α (macrophage inflammatory protein-3α) is constitutively produced by keratinocytes, providing homing signals for the positioning of immature LCs in the suprabasal layer of the epidermis. The LCs are connected physically to keratinocytes by homotypic bonds of E-cadherin (Section 31), a cell adhesion molecule expressed by both the LC and the keratinocyte. Contact allergens and inflammatory cytokines reduce E-cadherin expression, resulting in LC detachment from the keratinocytes. Concomitantly, the CCR6 chemokine receptor is downregulated, while the chemokine receptor CCR7 is upregulated – this allows the now mobile LCs to move towards the lymphatic vessels in response to the chemokine **SLC (secondary lymphoid tissue chemokine)** which binds to the CCR7 receptor. The basement membrane of the skin, however, stands as a barrier to their migration. LCs penetrate the lamina densa, which consists of type IV collagen, by releasing **matrix metalloproteinase (MMP)**, an enzyme with substrate specificity for collagen IV. Thus, under the guidance of SLC, LCs cross the labyrinthine space of the dermis and reach the abluminal side of the vessels. Entry into the lymphatic vessels is poorly understood, but P-glycoprotein, a mediator of cell membrane transport (Section 23), may be involved. LCs now move into the T cell areas in the lymph node where SLC and MIP-3β, the other CCR7 ligand, are expressed.

In areas of tissue injury, immature DCs expressing CCR6 are recruited by the ligand MIP-3α. Following antigen loading and as these cells mature, the downregulation of CCR6 allows them to leave the local environment. Concomitant or subsequent upregulation of the chemokine receptor CCR7 allows the maturing DC to home to T cell areas where the CCR7 ligand, MIP-3β, is expressed.

Antigen presentation. Upon arrival in the lymph nodes, DCs present the antigens captured in the periphery to naïve T cells. Antigen presentation is preceded by **antigen processing**, i.e. the breakdown of large, complex antigens to simple peptides no larger than 10-15 amino acids. These peptides are "loaded" onto class II or class I MHC molecules (depending on the site of origin of the antigens) and ultimately presented on the plasma membrane where they serve as ligands for antigen-specific T cell receptors (TCRs). Expression of class I and class II molecules is upregulated during DC maturation.

Exogenous antigens, i.e. those present outside the cell, such as pathogens or their products, enter the DC by endocytosis and are incorporated into endosomes rich in MHC class II molecules **(MHC II compartments)**; antigens are degraded in these compartments by lysosomal enzymes and the peptides are loaded onto class II MHC molecules for transport to the cell surface. Endogenous antigens that are present in the cytosol of the cell (i.e. viral antigens), are degraded in proteasomes and the peptides are transported to the endoplasmic reticulum where they are loaded on MHC class I molecules.

MHC class II-antigen presentation is critical for CD4 T cell activation; MHC class I presentation is required for activation of CD8 T cells (Section 19). It had been accepted that exogenous antigens located within endosomes could not be transported to the cell membrane by MHC class I molecules and, therefore, could not be presented to CD8 T cells. Recently, however, it has been shown that, in contrast to other antigen presenting cells (macrophages, B cells), DCs possess the unique ability to divert endocytosed antigens to the cytosol to follow the class I pathway – a process that is referred to as **cross-priming**. This allows exogenous antigen to be presented by MHC class I to CD8 T cells – thus, DCs do not have to be infected in order to activate CD8 T cells. This endosome-to-cytosol pathway operative in DCs allows a larger range of antigens to be presented to CD8 T cells.

Cell interactions. Mature DCs that carry foreign antigens form clusters ("rosettes") with naïve T cells. The **initial contact** is mediated by a DC specific molecule known as **DC-SIGN** (**DC-**Specific **ICAM-3 G**rabbing **N**on-integrin), a mannose-binding membrane protein with a C-lectin domain. The interaction of DC-SIGN with ICAM-3 on T cells establishes the initial adhesion to the naïve T cell. This proximity allows the T cell receptor to search the DC surface and bind specific MHC-peptide complexes. This specific DC-T cell interaction delivers the antigen-specific signal (signal-1) to the T cell. Simultaneously, strong costimulatory signals (signal-2) are generated by binding of CD40 on the dendritic cell to the CD40 ligand on the T cell and CD80/CD86 binding to its T cell ligand CD28. Adhesion is strengthened by additional adhesive protein interactions (eg, CD58 (LFA-3) with CD2 (T cells), and CD54 (ICAM-1) on DCs with CD11a/CD18 (LFA-1) on T cells (Section 19).

The term "**immunological synapse**" describes the molecular clustering at specific physical sites on opposing membranes where the interaction between DCs and T cells takes place. Mobile microdomains of the plasma membrane, called lipid rafts, may facilitate the clustering of cell receptors, costimulatory proteins, and adhesion molecules in areas of cell-cell contact. Some of the molecules that are present at this site include: MHC/peptide complexes, CD86, and CD40 on DCs; T cell receptors (TCRs), CD28, and CD40 ligand on T cells.

T cell activation and differentiation. DCs initiate T cell activation as a result of the molecular interactions described above. These interactions are reciprocal, i.e. T cells activate and promote DC maturation, enhance their viability, and upregulate the expression of costimulatory molecules; CD40/CD40L has a significant role in this process. This intimate DC-T cell cross-talk is facilitated by cytokines (eg, TNFα and IL-1) and chemokines produced by both cells. In addition to activation of T cells, DCs regulate early differentiation of CD4 T cells: IL-12 produced by activated DCs directs CD4 T cells to the Th1 differentiation pathway (Section 19).

DCs present antigen, in the context of the MHC/peptide complex, to prime the immune response of naïve T cells. Once primed, these memory T cells have the capacity to recognize the same antigen when presented subsequently by other antigen presenting cells (APCs) such as macrophages and B cells. Thus the priming of resting naïve T cells establishes immunological memory; activated (memory) T cells do not interact with DCs.

Types of Dendritic Cells

DCs constitute a heterogeneous group of cells derived from CD34$^+$ stem cells, although the precise differentiation pathways have not been defined. There are likely multiple differentiation pathways that involve both **myeloid** and **lymphoid** DC lineages. Cytokines such as GM-CSF and TNFα are important in this process, as well as IL-2, IL-3, and IL-7. The anatomical location of DCs frequently is associated with specific functional and phenotypic differentiation.

Langerhans Cells (LC), Veiled Cells, and Interdigitating Cells (IDC). It appears that LCs (skin), veiled cells (highly motile DCs seen in lymphatics), and lymph node IDCs (paracortical areas) are closely related. The first two are representative of DCs at an earlier stage of functional differentiation that are capable of capturing and transporting antigen to the T-cell rich lymph node paracortical areas. LCs are located in the epidermis; at a density of about 400-1000 cells/mm^2 they constitute 3-8% of the epidermal cell population (Plate 21-1). The

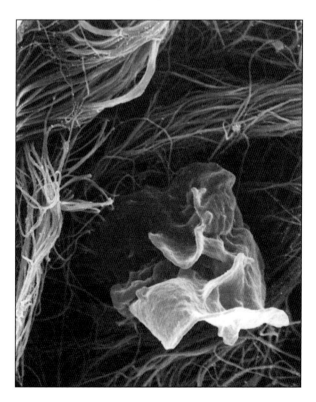

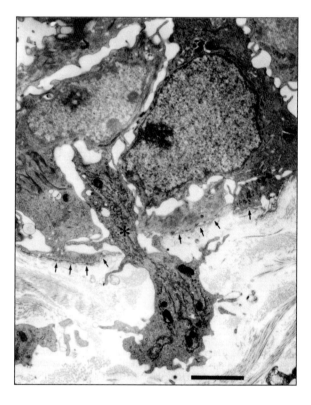

Plate 21-1   A Murine Dendritic
Cell within the Dermis

Plate 21-2   A Migratory Murine
Dendritic Cell

Reproduced from Romani et al. Int Rev Cytol 207: 237, 2001. Courtesy of Academic Press.

morphologic marker of the cell is the **Birbeck granule** identified by specific stains and electron microscopy. The specific marker for LCs is CD1a; they also are positive for Fcγ and C3 receptors. LCs capture antigens that enter the skin (such as contact allergens and microbial antigens) and immigrate to the paracortical areas of draining regional lymph nodes, where they present antigen to T cells (Plate 21-2). (When contact allergens are applied to the skin, the afferent lymphatics contain LCs identifiable by the Birbeck granule). **Veiled cells**, large DCs with an irregular shape and large motile sheets of lamellipodia (veils), are present in the afferent lymphatics that connect the periphery to the T cell paracortical areas (Plate 21-2). Veiled cells (and probably LCs) represent precursors of the **interdigitating dendritic cell (IDC)** of the nodal paracortical areas. The IDCs are mature DCs and potent stimulators of T cell activation. They express, at high density, MHC class I and class II molecules, adhesion and costimulatory molecules, and their characteristic marker CD83. IDCs form a physical network, their cytoplasmic extensions "interdigitating" between the other cellular components of the deep cortex where T cells reside.

Follicular Dendritic Cells (FDC) are crucial to the formation and organization of primary lymph node follicles, forming a stromal network which constitutes the B lymphocyte settlement area; a few CD4 T cells also are present. FDCs contain one or more nuclei with dispersed chromatin and numerous small cytoplasmic vesicles; their characteristic morphological feature is the display of prominent "filiform" or "beaded" dendrites. They express Fcγ receptors, complement receptors, several adhesion molecules (eg, ICAM-1, VCAM-1, and VLA 3-6), and costimulatory molecules (CD40). The FDCs are distinct from other DCs in their origin, mechanism of maturation, and phenotype. There is evidence that, although FDCs are not bone marrow-derived, their maturation requires stimulation by specific bone marrow-derived cells.

FDCs carry antigen-antibody-complement complexes on their dendrites. These complexes, captured in the periphery, are brought to the follicles by DCs that are referred to as antigen transport cells (ATC). The Ag-Ab complexes on the surface of the DC dendrites form small spherical beads known as "**iccosomes**" which are endocytosed by B cells, processed, transported to the cell surface in a complex with MHC class II molecules, and presented to CD4 helper T cells.

Thymic Dendritic Cells (TDC). The interdigitating dendritic cells of the thymus constitute about 0.1% of the cells in the medulla and corticomedullary junction. The TDC are considered to be "lymphoid" DCs that are generated from bone marrow $CD34^+/CD10^+$ precursors and undergo maturation in the thymus upon stimulation by IL-3. TDC are responsible for negative selection of the maturing thymocytes, i.e. thymocytes that have too high an affinity for self antigens are considered to be autoreactive and are eliminated – thereby, DCs regulate self-tolerance. This process is known as **central tolerance** to distinguish it from peripheral tolerance that takes place in lymphoid organs outside the thymus (Section 19).

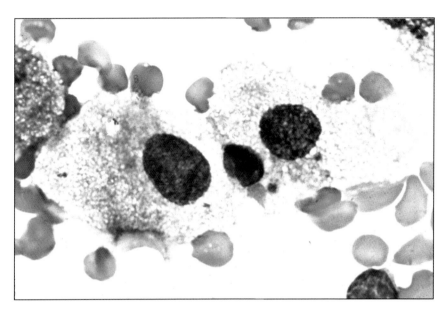

Plate 21-3   Tissue Macrophages

MACROPHAGES

Macrophages (Mφs) represent the tissue component of the mononuclear phagocytic system. They are extremely versatile cells, present in practically every tissue, with the potential to develop into an array of phenotypically and functionally diverse effector cells. These phagocytic cells initiate cellular immunity that results in the killing of invading microorganisms and tumor cells, and they play a key role in tissue remodeling essential to development and repair.

Morphology (Plate 21-3)

The tissue Mφs are a heterogeneous population with widely varying morphology. They can be identified by cytochemical staining for lysosomal enzymes and by monoclonal antibodies for Mφ specific markers. Membrane lamellipodia and villi can be seen on electron microscopy (Plate 21-3). In the activated cell, the cytoplasm contains abundant endosomes and phagosomes, the Golgi apparatus is large, and microfilaments are abundant under the membrane at sites of contact with particles targeted for phagocytosis.

Ontogeny

The Mφ represents a continuum of the monocyte-derived cell line (Section 5). The monocyte/Mφ line arises from the bone marrow stem cell through CFU-GEMM and CFU-GM precursors. The CFU-GM can commit to two lineages: under the influence of G-CSF to myeloid cells, and under M-CSF to monocytes. The monocyte circulates in the peripheral blood for one to three days before marginating and exiting into the extravascular space to take on its Mφ role.

Monocytes contain a single type of granule that has the appearance of a lysosome. In the tissues, the cell becomes larger and the cytoplasm stains blue (indicative of its high RNA content) as the features characteristic of Mφs appear and become more abundant: lysosomes, mitochondria, and endoplasmic reticulum. Changes indicative of the functional role of Mφs also appear: endocytic competence (phagocytosis) marked by expression of cell surface Fc and complement receptors, development of the NADPH-oxidase complex, and an abundant vesicular system that serves the secretory function. Mφs primarily produce metalloproteases and metalloprotease inhibitors. (Hydrolases are produced by monocytes but not by Mφs). With completion of the differentiation pathway, these cells become the **tissue Mφs**. Upon stimulation by foreign substances, these cells are transformed into **inflammatory Mφs** and, with further stimulation by immunologically-mediated inflammation (cytokines and chemokines), to **activated Mφs**. Within the tissues, Mφs are long-lived and, in some sites, they are self-replicating. Mφs have the ability to adapt to local environments through phenotypic alterations that affect their function, eg, alveolar Mφs, Kupffer cells, peritoneal Mφs, osteoclasts, and synovial type A cells – cells sometimes referred to collectively as the **reticuloendothelial system**.

Mφ Receptors

Responses to stimuli depend upon the nature of the cell surface receptors engaged and the type of pathogen or particle internalized.

Fc Receptors (FcR) interact with the Fc portion of immunoglobulins (antibodies). The FcRs for IgG are the best characterized – FcγR-I, II and III. These mediate the uptake of immune complexes and Ig-opsonized particles. FcγR-I (CD64) is a high affinity receptor that binds only monomeric IgG. FcγR-II (CD32) is a low affinity receptor for IgG and does not bind monomeric IgG; it is present in three isoforms, A, B and C:FcγR-IIA effectively induces the intracellular signal that leads to phagocytosis via the two ITAM sequences in its cytoplasmic tail. FcγR-IIB has an ITIM motif, therefore is unable to transmit a phagocytic signal – it functions as an inhibitory receptor. FcγR-III (CD16) is also of low affinity. Both FcγR-I and FcγR-III lack ITAMs, but interact with two γ chains that contain the ITAMs necessary for the transduction of the intracellular phagocytic signal. Ligand binding to FcR triggers phagocytosis that is tightly coupled to the production and secretion of pro-inflammatory molecules, eg, reactive oxygen intermediates, arachidonic acid metabolites, and TNF-α. (The ITAM and ITIM motifs are discussed in Sections 18 and 19).

Complement Receptors. Two types of complement receptors (CR) are present on Mφ: CR1 (CD35) binds C3b/C4b, CR3 (CD11b/CD18) binds the inactivated form of C3b (iC3b). These receptors identify pathogens opsonized by complement fragments. Because complement-mediated uptake does not elicit the release of inflammatory mediators, these receptors provide a portal of entry for such organisms as Mycobacteria and Leishmania that enhances the possibility of their intracellular survival.

Mannose Receptor (MR) is a type I membrane glycoprotein with an extracellular region that has eight C-type lectin domains ("C-type" indicates that binding to carbohydrate ligands is Ca^{2+}-dependent). The MR recognizes carbohydrates containing mannose oligosaccharides; MR binding to microorganisms with cell walls that contain these carbohydrates mediates phagocytosis and generation of pro-inflammatory signals. MR expression is upregulated by IL-4 and downregulated by IFN-γ. The pro-inflammatory molecules released when MR is ligated include IL-6, TNF-α, and IL-12. The other lectin receptor **DEC 205** has ten C-type lectin domains with a molecular organization similar to MR.

Scavenger Receptors (SR-AI, SR-AII) are alternatively spliced products of the same gene – they are trimers of either type I or type II chains. Both are type II glycoproteins (i.e. the amino terminal is within the cytoplasm). Their expression on tissue Mφs is upregulated by inflammatory stimuli. SR recognition of bacterial cell wall lipopolysaccharides (LPS) results in phagocytic clearance of microorganisms. SRs also mediate the uptake of oxidized low density lipoproteins (LDL) and scavenge cholesterol from high-density lipoprotein (HDL) – excessive accumulations in Mφs give rise to the "foam cells" in atherosclerotic plaques. SRs have a major role in the uptake of apoptotic cells, recognizing ligands that are not present on healthy cells: phosphatidylserine in the outer leaflet of the plasma membrane (Section 4), changes in glycosylation of cell surface proteins, and changes in surface charge. Mφs that have ingested apoptotic bodies actively suppress the release of inflammatory cytokines.

Cytokine Receptors include: the interferon γ receptor IFN-γR that mediates Mφ activation, the receptor for the monocyte-specific cytokine M-CSF that stimulates growth, and tissue necrosis factor receptors TNF-RI and TNF-RII that mediate the pleiotropic effects of the TNF-α cytokine. TNF-α, in synergy with IFN-γ, activates Mφs and enhances their resistance to intracellular bacteria.

Other receptors include: **α2-macroglobulin-R** (α2-macroglobulin is a protease inhibitor); **transferrin-R** for iron transport; **lipoprotein-R** for endocytosis of lipoproteins; **chemotactic-R** for chemotactic bacterial peptides such as N-formyl-Met-Leu-Phe; **endotoxin-R**, a low affinity receptor for bacterial endotoxin (lipopolysaccharides – LPS). At low concentrations of LPS, binding is to the high affinity receptor, **CD14** – binding is facilitated by an acute-phase serum protein, the LPS-binding protein. Because CD14 is attached to the membrane through a GPI anchor, it cannot transmit signals to the cell interior and therefore must interact with other receptors to initiate intracellular signaling. CD14 also may be involved in recognition and internalization of apoptotic cells.

Tissue factor is a membrane receptor that binds factor VII and VIIa to initiate the coagulation process; it is expressed constitutively on tissue Mφs. It is not expressed constitutively on circulating monocytes but appears when these cells are activated, contributing to disseminated intravascular coagulation associated with malignancies and systemic infections (Section 24). Fibrin deposition at sites of delayed hypersensitivity is largely the result of Mφ procoagulant activity.

Adhesion Receptors and their ligands allow Mφs to home to specific tissues, to migrate to sites of infection and injury, and to interact with other immune cells. Cell-cell adhesion receptors include the β_1 and β_2 integrins and L-selectin on Mφs and members of the immunoglobulin superfamily, ICAM-1 and PECAM, on endothelial cells. β_1 integrins mediate binding of Mφs to extracellular matrix. The β_2 integrins are CD11a/CD18, CD11b/CD18, CD11c/CD18. L-selectin is expressed on Mφs as are the ligands for P- and E-selectin. The ligand CD11a/CD18 mediates monocyte attachment to ICAM-1 on endothelial cells and lymphocytes. Monocyte migration across the endothelium into subendothelial tissues is mediated by PECAM at inter-endothelial cell junctions (Section 3).

Phagocytosis and Antigen Processing

Endocytosis is the process by which cells take up macromolecules. Material to be ingested is enclosed by the plasma membrane and pinched off to form an intracellular vesicle. Mφs internalize particles and solutes through a variety of processes: pinocytosis, receptor-induced endocytosis, and phagocytosis. Pinocytosis (cellular drinking) is a constitutive endocytic process that involves ingestion of fluid and solutes – Mφs ingest 25% of their volume of fluid every hour. Receptor-mediated endocytosis is closely related but is a specific process that involves receptor/ligand binding. Both these processes are based on formation of clathrin-coated pits and do not induce actin polymerization.

In receptor-mediated endocytosis and phagocytosis, recognition and binding of an extracellular macromolecule (the ligand) results in receptor activation and initiation of an internal signal. In phagocytosis, the Mφ is induced to extend pseudopods that engulf the particle to form a phagosome. Maturation of the phagosome and fusion with a lysosome results in formation of the phagolysosome – the low pH and the presence of a variety of enzymes are critical to the degradation of the ingested material. Small peptides that are produced by this proteolytic processing bind to MHC class II molecules and are transported to the cell membrane for presentation to T cells. (Receptor-induced endocytosis similarly involves degradation of the internalized particles and presentation of peptide/MHC class II complexes). Highly reactive oxygen radicals produced by membrane-associated NADPH oxidase (the respiratory burst – Section 7) are released into the phagosome to kill microorganisms. Reactive nitrogen intermediates derived from nitric oxide may participate. Paradoxically, some pathogens, such as Salmonella typhimurium, Legionella pneumophila, and Mycobacterium tuberculosis, may escape degradation and continue to multiply intracellularly. When M. tuberculosis gains entry into the body, complement binding to the surface (opsonization) results in recognition and binding by complement receptors; the internalized pathogen interferes with phagosome maturation, a strategy that provides a privileged compartment for survival: fusion with lysosomes is suppressed and there is only mild acidification.

Phagocytosis of apoptotic cells is a fundamental biological process essential for development and homeostasis. Mφs are the principal cells responsible for their clearance; the degradation of apoptotic cells takes place without activating pro-inflammatory responses (Section 4). This scavenger function of Mφs is quantitatively more significant than the engulfment of invading pathogens – more than 10^{11} senescent blood cells are removed daily.

The Cytoskeleton and Phagocytosis

Phagocytosis is the classical function of Mφs and is the property that led to Metchnikoff's discovery of these cells. Actin-dependent changes in the cytoskeletal organization of the component microfilaments and microtubules are essential for particle internalization. **Actin,** the primary constituent of microfilaments, regulates the extension of pseudopodia – it is present in two forms, **G-actin** (globular or monomeric) and **F-actin** (filamentous or polymeric). Actin filaments are assembled from monomers with energy provided by ATP and regulated by a number of other proteins that contribute to both polymerization and disassembly:**profilin** binds actin monomers, **gelsolin** binds at the end of the filament, and other proteins cross-link filaments to form bundles or networks. Phagocytic engulfment of a foreign particle is carried out through an orchestrated extension of pseudopodia and the change of G-actin to F-actin. The engulfment of an antibody-opsonized bacterium involves sequential binding of Fc receptors to the Fc domains of antibodies distributed over the surface of the pathogen. The two ends of the pseudopodia, advancing around the particle, meet and fuse in a **"zippering"** process that results in the engulfment of the microorganism within the newly created "phagosome".

Toxic Effector Functions

Activated Mφs produce toxic oxygen and nitrogen metabolites, important for parasiticidal and bactericidal effects and for the killing of malignant cells.

Reactive O_2 intermediates are produced when membrane NADPH oxidase (Section 7) is activated through intracellular signals induced by IFN-γ and ligand-bound Fc receptors. Superoxide anions (O_2^-), hydroxyl radicals with a free electron (•OH), and singlet O_2 ($^1O_2$) are powerful oxidants with high bactericidal activity. Unlike neutrophils, Mφs do not possess myeloperoxidase, and therefore are unable to produce hypochlorous acid (HOCl) from H_2O_2 and Cl^-, a highly effective toxic radical which mediates halogenation of bacterial cell walls. With the exception of alveolar Mφs, all Mφs depend on anaerobic glycolysis for phagocytosis.

Reactive nitrogen intermediates (RNI): Nitric oxide (NO) is produced by oxidation of L-arginine through the action of nitric oxide synthase (NOS). Both constitutively expressed and inducible NOS isoforms are present in Mφs. NO functions poorly as a free radical, but its derivatives (nitrosonium ion, nitroxyl radical, and peroxynitrite) are profoundly cytotoxic. The primary cytotoxic effects of RNI are due to inhibition of iron/sulfur containing enzymes and disruption of non-heme iron enzymes, as well as mitochondrial inhibition and suppression of ribonucleotide reductase. In mice, production of RNI is the major mechanism for protection against M. tuberculosis; the relatively low production of RNI in humans may account for the high susceptibility to tuberculosis.

Secretory Functions

Mφs have an extensive secretory repertoire that includes over one hundred biologically active substances.

Enzymes: Stimulated Mφs release a number of enzymes, including lysozyme and neutral proteases (i. e. collagenase, elastase, plasminogen activator). Lysozyme can destroy gram positive bacteria. Degradation of extracellular matrix by neutral proteases produces tissue damage.

Complement factors: Mφs synthesize all complement components except C6-9.

Arachidonic acid metabolites include prostacyclin (PGI_2), thromboxane A_2, prostaglandin E_2, leukotriene C_4 (slow reacting substance of anaphylaxis), and leukotriene B_4 (potent mediator of chemotaxis). Mφs are a major source of these molecules; there is increased secretion by inflammatory Mφs.

Cytokines and the Acute Phase Response

Mφs produce a plethora of cytokines and chemokines. In response to microbial stimuli (LPS), cytokine secretion takes place within hours and, depending on the intensity and duration of the stimuli, the effects may be either **local** or **systemic**. Local effects include IL-8 mediated recruitment of leukocytes that access the inflammatory site through increased blood vessel permeability (TNF-α). Activation of neutrophils (TNF-α), lymphocytes (IL-1, IL-6), and NK cells (IL-12) leads to phagocytosis by neutrophils and initiation of adaptive immune responses by T and B cells.

The systemic effects, known as the **acute phase response (APR)**, are mediated by IL-1/IL-6/TNF-α. APR is characterized by general symptoms such as fever induced by hypothalamic stimulation (IL-1 and IL-6 are endogenous pyrogens), release of ACTH and leukocytosis. Hepatic stimulation by IL-6 results in the production and release of a number of proteins known as **acute phase reactants**, including C-reactive protein, mannan-binding lectin (MBL), fibrinogen, ferritin and factor VIII. C-reactive protein binds to the phosphorylcholine on the bacterial cell wall, thus opsonizing bacteria for phagocytosis; it also interacts with C1q to activate the classical complement cascade. MBL triggers complement activation through the MBL complement pathway (Section 20).

Macrophages and Chronic Inflammation

Mφs are the effector cells of the delayed type of hypersensitivity and they constitute a key cellular component of the chronic inflammatory response. **Mφ activation** is induced by endogenous (eg, cytokines) and exogenous (eg, bacterial) stimuli. Mφ secreted C-C chemokines recruit T cells and monocytes. Microorganisms are eliminated through enhanced phagocytosis and the cytotoxic action of reactive oxygen and nitrogen intermediates. Certain intracellular bacteria may reside comfortably within "resting" Mφs for prolonged periods of time and can be eliminated only by Mφ activation. Occasionally, the release of proteolytic enzymes by activated Mφs with its concomitant tissue destruction may result in bacterial dissemination. More often, the release of bacteria that have been sequestered in inaccessible sites exposes them to destruction by the arrival of additional activated Mφs.

Upon ingestion of bacteria, activated Mφs release IL-12 which stimulates NK cells to produce IFN-γ. This generates conditions for the differentiation of CD4 T cells to the Th1 phenotype. In a feedback process, Th1 cells also produce IFN-γ that augments Mφ activation and degradation of ingested organisms. A second signal is delivered by the costimulatory molecular couple of CD40 (Mφ) and CD40 ligand (Th1). Mφ activation is downregulated by Th2 cell release of IL-4 and IL-10. As activation of large numbers of Mφs may result in significant tissue destruction, the process is regulated and limited to the Mφs that are engaged with antigen-specific Th1 cells (whose TCRs recognize the specific antigens presented by the Mφs): these antigen-specific interactions between Th1 and Mφs are enhanced with increased expression of both MHC class II molecules and the costimulatory molecules CD80 and CD86.

Granulomata are present in many chronic inflammatory states. Multinucleated giant cells that result from the fusion of macrophages and/or monocytes are common, accompanied by T cells and epithelioid cells. In M. tuberculosis infections, mycobacteria may be sequestered within macrophages in the granulomata where they are able to avoid killing, although their proliferation is restricted by fibrosis and calcification, and the reduced supply of nutrients and O_2. IFN-γ (Mφ activation) and TNF-α are instrumental in granuloma formation. The granulomata increase in size by the influx of additional activated monocytes with formation of new multinucleated giant cells. With a change in immune status of the host, the granuloma undergoes caseation and spills viable bacilli into the tissues – in the case of pulmonary tuberculosis, entry of bacilli into the airways facilitates aerosol spread of the disease.

Site-Specific Macrophages

Mφs, with distinct roles in health and disease, exhibit phenotypical differences that are dependent on their tissue location.

Lung alveolar Mφs are present just beneath the pulmonary epithelium at the tissue-air interphase where they encounter and trap inhaled pollutants. They also are found as free cells within the alveolar surfactant film. Because they reside in a high O_2 environment, expression of some metabolic pathways is reduced, eg, the respiratory burst and the hexose monophosphate shunt. Mφ secretion of elastase and collagenase plays a significant role in tissue destruction in emphysema that is amplified in α1-antitrypsin deficiency.

Spleen Mφs are present in all areas. Within the red pulp, they cull old red cells, spherocytes, parasitized cells, and "pit" red cells containing inclusions. They also act as scavengers in the marginal zone. Mφs present antigen to B cells in the white pulp germinal centres.

Bowel Mφs are located along the base of the mucosal epithelial cells. They have a role in both the disposal of dead enterocyes and generation of an immune response. In Crohn's disease, Mφ release of proteolytic enzymes may contribute to bowel injury.

Liver Mφs that line the sinusoidal walls are designated Kupffer cells. These cells are in an optimum location to capture blood borne particles, microorganisms, and opsonized red blood cells. They regulate the synthesis of various hepatic proteins including fibrinogen and cytochrome p450. Kupffer cell production of NO influences hepatic metabolic function.

Brain Mφs are the microglia. They are refractory to most inflammatory signals, a feature that serves to protect surrounding neurons. Microglia phagocytose dying cells, debris, and foreign material, but do not secrete cytokines or other inflammatory mediators. Their numbers increase following brain injury.

Peritoneal Mφs are increased in response to local inflammatory or malignant disease. The Mφs at this site have a major respiratory burst mechanism that can be elicited by bacteria and some tumor cells.

Synovial Mφs are known as the synovial type A cells. These phagocytic cells display MHC class II molecules and Fc receptors. Their numbers are increased in rheumatoid arthritis; the secreted proteases and pro-inflammatory cytokines play a major role in the initiation and propagation of inflammation and joint destruction.

Bone. The multinucleated osteoclast is derived from the monocyte/macrophage lineage. It is responsible for bone resorption and remodeling.

CLINICAL CORRELATES

THE ROLE OF DENDRITIC CELLS IN DISEASE

The role of DCs in diseases is based on their ability to capture and transport antigen from the periphery to the lymph nodes, resulting in T cell activation and initiation of an immune response.

DCs have been implicated in a variety of diseases characterized by intense T cell activation, such as rheumatoid arthritis, psoriasis, contact allergy and asthma. In organ transplantation, donor DCs that are present as passenger cells contribute to primary rejection; depletion of DCs from donor organs increases organ acceptance even in the presence of an MHC mismatch. However, when host DCs invade the graft, their presentation of graft peptides to T cells induces a chronic inflammatory response.

Langerhans Cell Histiocytosis

The Langerhans cell histiocytoses are a group of clinical disorders that most commonly present in childhood. (Historically, the term histiocytosis X was used to encompass a number of the clinical syndromes: Hand-Schüller-Christian disease, eosinophilic granuloma, and Letterer-Siwe disease). The histological lesion is a histiocytic granuloma consisting of dendritic cells, eosinophils, and lymphocytes along with varying numbers of neutrophils, plasma cells, and giant cells. There is marked cell proliferation and accumulation in various organs, including skin, bone, lymph nodes, liver, lung, and the central nervous system. The definitive histological diagnosis depends on the identification of the Langerhans cell's Birbeck granules and the CD1 marker. The clinical manifestations depend upon the site(s) and extent of disease. The presence of lesions associated with primary bone erosion in the skull producing exophthalmus and diabetes insipidus is referred to as Hand-Schüller-Christian disease. General system involvement, including skin, lymph nodes, liver, spleen, bone marrow, and lung, is referred to as Letterer-Siwe disease. Lesions may regress spontaneously, and bone lesions may regress following curettage. In some cases of rapidly advancing disease, combination chemotherapy has been successful.

DCs and HIV

Large numbers of HIV particles can be detected on the dendrites of DCs in lymph nodes; DCs do not internalize the virus. *In vitro*, explosive HIV replication occurs when DCs and naïve T cells are co-cultured, although T cells alone in the resting state do not support HIV replication.

HIV that penetrates mucosal surfaces encounters tissue DCs, binds to the DC-SIGN receptor, and is presented to local T cells or transported to regional lymph nodes. DC-SIGN positive DCs are present beneath the vaginal and rectal mucosa, potential sites of HIV entry. HIV attached to DC-SIGN remains viable for several days, increasing the possibility that infectious viruses will be delivered to $CD4^+$ lymphocytes. In contrast to antigens that are internalized and processed prior to presentation, DCs present whole unprocessed infectious virions to T cells. DCs facilitate the initial steps of HIV infection, first by stabilizing the virus during transport and, secondly, by activating T cells – activated T cells are more permissive than naïve T cells for HIV replication.

THE ROLE OF MACROPHAGES IN DISEASE

Lysosomal Storage Disease

Gaucher Disease is a congenital lysosomal storage disease due to deficiency of β-glucocerebrosidase. The multiple gene mutations are classified clinically as: type 1 (adult, non-neuropathic), type 2 (infantile, neuropathic), and type 3 (juvenile, neuropathic). Type 1 disease is the most common: macrophage lysosomes are loaded with non-degraded glucocerebroside derived from membranes of phagocytosed erythrocytes and leukocytes; the "stuffed" macrophages (Gaucher cells) accumulate in bone marrow, liver, and spleen, resulting in splenomegaly, hepatomegaly, bone marrow replacement, and bone erosion. In type 2 disease, there is neurological involvement at birth and death within one to two years. Type 3 manifests as organomegaly with later (adolescent) development of neurological pathology. Diagnosis is made by the identification of the Gaucher cell and biochemical confirmation of the missing enzyme. Progressive type 1 disease has been treated by enzyme replacement therapy.

Niemann-Pick Disease (NPD) describes a group of autosomal recessive disorders that are characterized by the accumulation of sphingomyelin or low density lipoprotein (LDL)-derived cholesterol in the cells of the monocyte/macrophage system. NPD is subclassified into two groups based on biochemical and molecular criteria: (1) types A and B are due to mutations in the acid sphingomyelinase gene on chromosome 11, resulting in deficiency of lysosomal acid sphingomyelinase; (2) types C and D are due to mutations in the *NPC-1* gene on chromosome 18 – deficiency of the NPC-1 (Niemann-Pick type C-1) protein results in defective processing and transport of LDL-derived cholesterol from the lysosome to the cytosol. All types are associated with macrophage foam cells. In types A and B, sphingomyelin accumulates in the lysosomes of the macrophages, producing lipid-laden Niemann-Pick foam cells that are present in the bone marrow, liver, and spleen. Type A is associated with rapid central nervous system involvement and early death. Type B is manifest by progressively increasing hepatosplenomegaly, pancytopenia, and pulmonary infiltrates. In types C and D, neurological degeneration progresses more slowly.

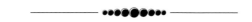

SUGGESTED READING

Aderem A, Underhill DM. Mechanisms of phagocytosis in macrophages. Annu Rev Immunol 17:593-623, 1999.

Banchereau J, Steinman RM. Dendritic cells and the control of immunity. Nature 392:245-252, 1998.

Banchereau J, Briere F, Caux C, et al. Immunobiology of dendritic cells. Annu Rev Immunol 18:767-811, 2000.

Charrow J, Esplin JA, Gribble J, et al. Gaucher disease. Arch Intern Med 158:1754-1760, 1998.

de Villiers WJS, Smart EJ. Macrophage scavenger receptors and foam cell formation. J Leukocyte Biol 55:740-746, 1999.

Fong L, Engleman EG. Dendritic cells in cancer immunotherapy. Ann Rev Immunol 18:245, 2000.

Fraser IP, Koziel H, Ezekowitz RAB. The serum mannose-binding protein and the macrophage mannose receptor are pattern recognition molecules that link innate and adaptive immunity. Sem Immunol 10:363-372, 1998.

Gordon S. Macrophages and the immune response. In: Fundamental Immunology, 4th Ed. W. E. Paul, Ed. pp:533, 1999.

Kolodny EH. Niemann-Pick disease. Curr Opin Hematol 7:48-52, 2000.

Martin JC, Bandrés JC. Cells of the monocyte-macrophage lineage and pathogenesis of HIV-1 infection. JAIDS 22:413-429, 1999.

Reid CDL. Dendritic cells and immunotherapy for malignant disease. Br J Haematol 112:874-887, 2001.

Romani N, Ratzinger G, Pfaller K, et al. Migration of dendritic cells into lymphatics - the Langerhans cell example: routes, regulation, and relevance. Int Rev Cytol 207:237-251, 2001.

Roncarolo MG, Levings MK, Traversari C. Differentiation of T regulatory cells by immature dendritic cells. J Exp Med 193:F5-F9, 2001.

Satthaporn S, Eremin O. Dendritic cells (I): biological functions. J R Coll Surg Edinb 46:9-20, 2001.

Steinman RM. Dendritic cells. In: Fundamentals in Immunology, 4th Ed. W. E. Paul, Ed. pp:547-573, 1999.

Steinman RM. DC-SIGN: a guide to some mysteries of dendritic cells. Cell 100:491-494, 2000.

Steinman RM. Dendritic cells and the control of immunity: enhancing the efficiency of antigen presentation. Mt Sinai J Med 68:160-166, 2001.

Watts C. Dendritic cells spill the beans. Nature Cell Biol 1:E152-E154, 1999.

THE MYELOID LEUKEMIAS

"Weisses Blut" (white blood) — Virchow — 1845
"The presence of purulent matter in the blood" — Bennett — 1845

The acute and the chronic myeloid leukemias are morphologically and clinically different entities, and usually are not considered as a unit. However, both are included in this Section because of the similarity in their basic biological and molecular mechanisms. Chronic myeloid leukemia is a rather homogenous entity; the acute myeloid leukemias exhibit major biological, molecular, and clinical heterogeneity.

THE ACUTE MYELOID LEUKEMIAS (AML)

AML is characterized by maturation arrest of the malignant clone early in myeloid cell differentiation. One clinical/morphological working description – the French American British (FAB) classification – is shown in Table 22-1. This classification is based on the morphology and cytochemistry of the cells correlated, in so far as possible, with normal maturational counterparts; the original classification has been expanded to include the surface markers (the cluster differentiation antigens - CDs) most commonly found on these cells. The majority of cases of AML do not conform rigidly to these categories as there is considerable overlap in morphology, cytochemistry and CD markers. Certain karyotypic anomalies, CD markers and morphology are prognostic indicators.

AML may arise *de novo* in the absence of an obvious predisposing risk factor, or it may occur in the presence of pre-existing genetic defects, or following exposure to known carcinogens or environmental agents. The cell of origin is probably the $CD34^+$ /$CD38^-$ stem cell, not the lineage-specific progenitors of the sub-populations; the exception is acute promyelocytic leukemia (M3) which probably arises at the level of promyelocytic differentiation. Congenital predisposing diseases include: Bloom syndrome (defective DNA repair), Fanconi anemia (a familial autosomal recessive stem cell disorder), Down syndrome (trisomy 21), as well as Kostmann syndrome (severe congenital neutropenia), Wistkott-Aldrich (immunodeficiency) syndrome, and Li-Fraumeni syndrome (germline p53 mutation). Acquired hematological diseases that frequently terminate in AML include the myelodysplastic syndromes characterized by refractory anemia, bone marrow hyperplasia, and abnormalities in myelopoiesis. AML may follow exposure to ionizing radiation, to toxic chemicals such as benzene, or to antineoplastic drugs – particularly the alkylating agents and inhibitors of topoisomerase II (anthracyclines, epipodophylotoxins). Most cases, however, arise *de novo*.

In the acute leukemias, there is a high rate (up to 85%) of somatically acquired chromosomal translocations and inversions. The majority of the translocated genes encode transcription factors that regulate blood cell development. Abnormal activation of transcription factor genes takes place by two mechanisms: (1) The translocation may insert a gene into juxtaposition with and subject to the control of a promoter or enhancer in a major synthetic pathway (eg, the gene for an immunoglobulin molecule or T-cell receptor), leading to overexpression of the translocated gene. This type of translocation is seen most frequently in B-cell malignancies. (2) Balanced reciprocal translocations with formation of fusion genes that transcribe unique chimeric proteins – resulting in transcriptional deregulation and, sometimes, suppression of normal gene expression. Reciprocal translocations frequently are present in AML.

Numerous structural chromosomal abnormalities have been identified in AML, including translocations, deletions and inversions. Some of the more common abnormalities that can be linked to cell dysfunction or growth deregulation are described.

Table 22-1   FAB Classification of Acute Myelogenous Leukemia
(Plus commonly observed surface markers)

FAB	Subtype	Morphology	Myeloperoxidase	Surface Markers
M0	Acute Myeloblastic No maturation	Myeloblasts No granules	-	CD13 CD33 CD34
M1	Acute Myeloblastic Minimal maturation	Myeloblasts Few granules	+/-	CD13 CD33 CD34
M2	Acute Myeloblastic With maturation	Myeloblasts Promyelocytes Auer Rods +/-	+ +	CD13 CD15 CD33
M3	Acute Promyelocytic	Promyelocytes Granules prominent Auer Rods +/-	+ + +	CD13 CD15 CD33
M4	Acute Myelomonocytic	Myeloblasts, Monoblasts, Promonocytes, Monocytes	+	CD11b CD13 CD14 CD15 CD33
M5	Acute Monoblastic	Monoblasts, Promonocytes Monocytes	+/-	CD11b CD13 CD14 CD15 CD33
M6	Acute Erythroleukemia	Megaloblasts Myeloblasts	+/-	CD33 CD36
M7	Megakaryocytic	Megakaryoblasts	-	CD41 CD61

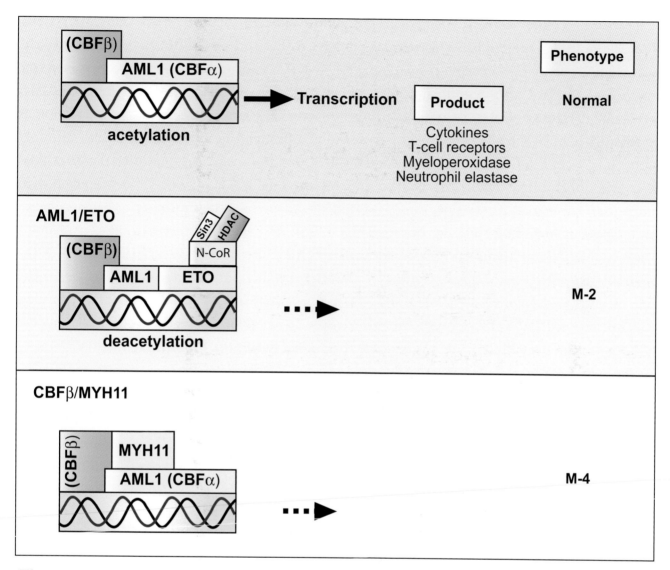

Figure 22-1 Acute Myeloblastic Leukemia

Translocations and Inversions

In AML, the translocations frequently are associated with dysfunction or abrogation of normal transcription. The translocation may give rise to a fused gene that either is not itself transcribed or that transcribes a non-functional or alternate transcription factor.

AML1/ETO. Core-binding factor (CBF) is a transcription factor essential to normal hematopoiesis. CBF up-regulates expression of a number of genes: cytokines (GM-CSF, IL-3), T-cell antigen receptor, neutrophil myeloperoxidase and elastase. It is a heterodimer consisting of α and β units. CBFα (also known as AML1) is the DNA-binding subunit, and CBFβ facilitates the DNA binding. The gene for CBFα (AML1) is located on chromosome 21; the gene for the β component is on chromosome 16. (High expression of AML1 is restricted primarily to cells of the hemopoietic lineage). Both CBF components are breakpoint sites in AML: CBFα (AML1) in M2 and CBFβ in M4 disease.

One of the most frequent chromosomal translocations in AML is AML1/ETO, [t(8;21)(q22;22)], present in 15-20 percent of cases. AML1 codes for CBFα; it is fused with the ETO (eight twenty one) gene on chromosome 8q22. ETO binds the nuclear receptor co-repressor (N-CoR). The N-CoR/mSin3/histone deacetylase complex (HDAC) mediates transcriptional repression. (Histone deacetylation is a strong inhibitor of gene transcription). Juxtaposition of the AML1 gene to the ETO gene results in a chimeric protein that includes the amino-terminal portion of AML1 and almost the full length of ETO. In the fusion protein, the transcriptional activation domains of AML1 are deleted and replaced by ETO sequences that interact with nuclear co-repressors. As a result, there is diminished expression of a number of hematopoietic specific genes including those for cytokines (GM-CSF, and IL-3), myeloperoxidase, neutrophil elastase and T-cell antigen receptor. In addition to failure of normal transcription, AML1/ETO increases expression of the anti-apoptotic protein Bcl-2. The result is a transformed cell that has lost its ability to differentiate while transcribing a gene that inhibits its destruction. Following therapy, the AML1/ETO fusion protein has been used as a molecular marker of residual disease, although it is detectable in some patients who have been in complete clinical remission for many years (Figure 22-1).

CBFβ/MYH11 is due to an inversion in chromosome 16 – inv(16)(p13q22). CBFβ (16q22), the heterodimeric partner of CBFα (AML1), is fused to MYH11 (16p13), a smooth muscle myosin heavy chain gene. This chimeric protein disrupts AML1 transcriptional activity. It is manifest clinically as AML-M4 with characteristic dysplastic bone marrow eosinophilia (Figure 22-1).

MLL 11q23 – There are some 30 reciprocal translocations at this site. MLL encodes a large protein whose normal function is unclear. These translocations frequently develop following chemotherapy with topoisomerase II inhibitors (epipodophylotoxins and anthracyclines).

t(15:17) PML/RARα – In contrast to the other forms of AML, the defect in acute promyelocytic leukemia (APL) is not at the level of the stem cell but at the point of promyelocytic differentiation. The balanced reciprocal translocation between the long arms of chromosomes 15 and 17 is present in 95% of cases of APL (FAB M3). The breakpoint on chromosome 17 is within the retinoic acid receptor (RARα) gene.

Retinoids have a significant role in normal myeloid development and differentiation. The retinoic acid receptor RARα (a member of the steroid-thyroid family of nuclear transcription factors) is expressed in normal hematopoietic cells. It is a transcription factor with binding domains for both retinoic acid (RA) and DNA. RARα normally forms a heterodimer with other retinoid receptors (RXRs). The heterodimer binds to specific DNA sequences, the retinoic acid response elements (RARE), located in the promoter region of a number of retinoic acid responsive genes. Gene transcription is initiated when the RA ligand binds to the dimers (Figure 22-2).

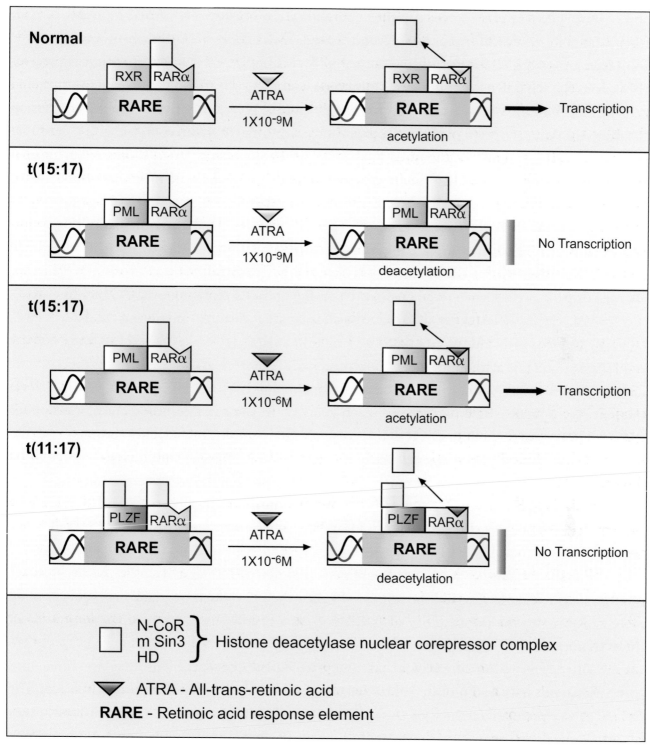

Figure 22-2 Role of ATRA in PML

Promyelocyte maturation is regulated by the binding of these normal RXR/RARα heterodimers. In the absence of RA, the retinoic acid receptors down-regulate transcription through recruitment of a protein complex containing the nuclear receptor co-repressor N-CoR (or its homologue SMRT), plus mSin3 and histone deacetylase (HD). (Gene transcription is inhibited by histone deacetylation and activated by histone acetylation). When RA is present, it binds to the RXR/RARα complex, causing dissociation of the N-CoR repressor complex and concomitant binding of co-activator proteins with histone acetylase activity; histone acetylation is followed by transcription of genes necessary for promyelocyte maturation.

The PML (promyelocytic leukemia) gene on chromosome 15 is expressed in normal hematopoietic cells. The PML protein is a transcription factor located in discrete areas of the nucleus referred to as the PML oncogenic domains (PODs). Its function as a growth- and tumor-suppressor includes interactions with p53, Rb and Bax. PML is a mediator of immune surveillance: the PODs increase during viral infection or following treatment with interferon. (In APL, the PML-RARα translocation is associated with a breakdown of the PODs that now appear as small speckles within the nucleus. Upon RA-induced remission, the PODs reassemble).

APL is associated with four distinct translocations involving RARα: PML [t(15;17)(q22;q21)], PLZF [t(11;17)(q23;q21)], NPM [t(5;17)(q32;q21)] and NuMA [t(11;17)(q13;q21)]. Although these four proteins are not related structurally, they all are nuclear proteins that contain a dimerization domain for RARα. APL probably results from interference of RARα function by the fusion protein. In the most common translocation, the PML-RARα chimeric protein binds the repressor N-Cor complex more tightly than normal and does not dissociate at physiological concentrations of RA, thereby inhibiting promyelocyte maturation; at pharmacological doses of RA, the N-Cor complex dissociates, suppression is lifted and maturation proceeds (Figure 22-2). All four of these translocations fail to respond to physiological concentrations of RA. However, with the exception of PLZF/RARα, pharmacological doses of RA will induce dissociation of the repressor and degradation of the fusion protein. In contrast to the other chimeric proteins, PLZF-RARα contains two N-CoR binding sites: one on RARα and the other on PLZF – the site located on PLZF maintains binding to N-CoR even in the presence of excess RA and, as a result, the block to transcription is not lifted (Figure 22-2).

All-transretinoic-acid (ATRA), at pharmacological concentrations that are three logs greater than physiological requirements, induces promyelocyte differentiation both *in vitro* and *in vivo* in the presence of three of these translocations. ATRA combined with chemotherapy (As_2O_3) induces remission and is potentially curative in a number of patients with M3 leukemia. APL often is accompanied by a life-threatening coagulopathy with clinical and laboratory findings indicative of DIC (Section 24). ATRA downregulates the expression of procoagulants present in the undifferentiated promyelocyte – its use has reduced the incidence of DIC as well as successfully terminating DIC in patients who present with this coagulopathy.

t(6:9) dek/can – This translocation is found most frequently in FAB M2 and FAB M4. **Dek** is probably a regulator of transcription, **can** regulates DNA-binding domains.

Deletions

Chromosome 5 – Deletions in this chromosome are found most commonly in AML developing subsequent to chemotherapy for other malignancies. The deletions range from loss of a portion of 5q, all of 5q, or the entire chromosome. This site is of particular significance because genes encoding several hematopoietic growth factors (GM-CSF, IL-3, IL-4) are located on 5q. The most frequent deletion is 5q31.1, the region of the interferon regulatory factor (IFR-1); because interferons are negative growth regulators, this may represent the loss of a tumour suppressor gene.

Chromosome 7 – Loss of chromosome 7 occurs in AML subsequent to myelodysplastic syndromes or exposure to alkylating agents. The loss may involve the entire chromosome or deletion of all or part of 7q. It has been suggested that this represents a loss of one or more tumor suppressor genes, although these have not been identified.

Gene Mutations

Overexpression of a number of proto-oncogenes, including *myc, fos,* and *fms,* have been described. The most common abnormalities are mutations of *ras* and *p53.*

Ras – The ras family of small GTP-binding proteins includes H-ras, Ki-ras and N-ras. These plasma membrane-associated 21 kD proteins ($p21^{ras}$) induce cell activation and proliferation by relaying signals from membrane receptor tyrosine kinases to the nucleus. Normally, the system is activated by the binding of GTP to $p21^{ras}$, and deactivated when GTP is hydrolyzed to GDP by the intrinsic GTPase activity of $p21^{ras}$ in concert with a cytosolic GTPase-activating protein (GAP). Transforming activity of Ras is associated with various point mutations of $p21^{ras}$ that prolong the active GTP-bound state or are resistant to the GTPase activity of GAP; mutations resulting in reduction or loss of GAP have a similar effect. As a result, the system remains in an activated state with unregulated cell stimulation and proliferation (Section 1). Mutations of N-ras are present in about 25% of AML patients.

p53 – The p53 gene is located on chromosome 17. Mutations in p53 or 17p monosomy are present in 7-10% of cases of AML. p53 is a normal transcription factor that mediates cell cycle arrest in G_1 allowing time for DNA repair; when the damage to DNA exceeds the potential for repair, p53 guides the cell into apoptosis. Mutations or loss of p53 remove this control mechanism for the elimination of genotoxic damage. In the absence of this genomic monitor, the accumulation and propagation of mutant events facilitates evolution of the leukemic clone (Sections 2 and 4).

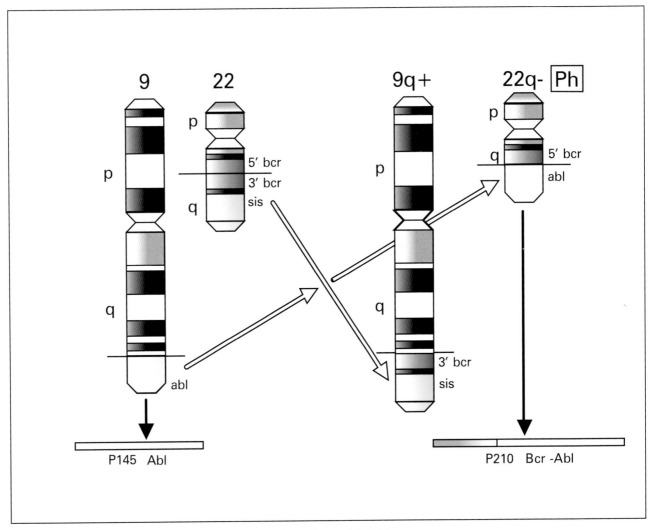

Figure 22-3 Chronic Myeloid Leukemia - t(9:22)

CHRONIC MYELOID LEUKEMIA

Chronic myeloid (myelocytic) leukemia (CML) is manifest by the accumulation of myeloid cells of all stages, from blasts to mature granulocytes, in the peripheral blood. The chronic phase of this disease averages 35 to 45 months, eventually transforming into an acute terminal blast phase. The chronic phase is characterized by a specific karyotype: the reciprocal translocation between the long arms of chromosomes 9 and 22, [t(9;22) (q34;q11)], that generates a longer chromosome 9 and a shorter chromosome 22 (Figure 22-3). The truncated chromosome 22, the Philadelphia or Ph chromosome, can be identified in 90% of CML patients. Ph also is present in approximately 20% of adults and 5% of children with acute lymphoblastic leukaemia (ALL).

This translocation moves the major part of the *abl* **proto-oncogene** from 9q to 22q. The c-abl gene codes for a 145 kD nonreceptor tyrosine kinase – the homologue of the v-abl oncogene of the Abelson murine leukemia virus. The normal Abl protein is a regulator of the cell cycle, integrin signaling, and apoptosis. Under physiological conditions, there is tight regulation of Abl. Translocation deletes its negative regulator domain. The insertion breakpoint on 22q is confined to a small area designated the major **breakpoint cluster region** (bcr); it is part of a larger *bcr* gene that encodes a 160 kD protein. The role of the normal Bcr protein is as yet unclear although it has several tyrosine residues and encodes a serine-threonine kinase. (Bcr-1-knockout mice are viable – it appears that most Bcr-1 pathways are redundant). The new *bcr/abl* gene generates a 210 kD Bcr/Abl fusion protein with increased SH2 binding sites (Section 1) and enhanced tyrosine kinase activity. (The ALL patients have a somewhat shorter fusion protein of 190 kD). The chimeric protein activates Ras, PI3 kinase, Myc and Fak (focal adhesion kinase), and the Bcl-2 pathway. This results in increased cell proliferation (Ras, Myc, PI3-K), decreased apoptosis (Bcl-2), and defective stromal cell adhesion and signaling (Fak).

When CML transforms into the accelerated phase, additional chromosomal abnormalities appear. Although there are no specific karyotypic changes characteristic of this acute transformation, a number of chromosomal abnormalities commonly are observed, including the disappearance or duplication of the Ph chromosome, trisomy 8, trisomy 19, or loss of the Y chromosome. The response to treatment can be monitored by PCR for residual Bcr/Abl transcripts; these may regress or disappear following chemotherapy or bone marrow transplant, providing a sensitive index of molecular / biological remission.

Therapeutic approaches include bone marrow transplant, interferon-α, alkylating agents, hydroxyurea and, more recently, specific inhibitors of the Bcr/Abl tyrosine kinase. In the chronic phase and during early transformation, the <u>s</u>ignal <u>t</u>ransduction <u>i</u>nhibitor 571 (STI571) has been effective in eliminating the Ph chromosome and the Bcr/Abl transcript. STI571 (phenylaminopyrimidine) blocks the ATP-binding site of the Bcr/Abl tyrosine kinase, preventing phosphorylation of proteins involved in Bcr/Abl signal transduction. This highly selective inhibition of the Bcr/Abl kinase has resulted in clinical remission in the chronic phase and in some patients with acute transformation and blast crisis.

— •••●●●••• —

SUGGESTED READING

Baer MR, Bloomfield CD. The clinical significance of biological characteristics of the cells in acute myeloid leukemia. Annu Rev Med 42:381-389, 1991.

Barbui T, Finazzi G, Falanga A. The impact of all-trans-retinoic acid on the coagulopathy of acute promyelocytic leukemia. Blood 91:3093-3102, 1998.

Boxer LM. The role of oncogenes in hematological malignancies. Annu Rev Med 45:1-11, 1994.

Deininger MWN, Goldman JM, Melo JV. The molecular biology of chronic myeloid leukemia. Blood 96:3343-3356, 2000.

Downing JR. The AML1-ETO chimaeric transcription factor in acute myeloid leukemia: biology and clinical significance. Br J Haematol 106:296-308, 1999.

Druker BJ, Lydon NB. Lessons learned from the development of an Abl tyrosine kinase inhibitor for chronic myelogenous leukemia. J Clin Invest 105:3-7, 2000.

Druker BJ, Talpaz M, Resta DJ, et al. Efficacy and safety of a specific inhibitor of the BCR-ABL tyrosine kinase in chronic myeloid leukaemia. N Engl J Med 344:1031-1037, 2001.

Enright H, McGlave PB. Chronic myelogenous leukemia. Curr Opin Hematol 2:293-299, 1995.

Faderl S, Talpaz M, Estrov Z, O'Brien S, Kurtzrock R, Kantarjian HM. The biology of chronic myelocytic leukemia. N Engl J Med 341:164-172, 1999.

Gotoh A, Broxmeyer H. The function of BCR/ABL and related proto-oncogenes. Curr Opin Hematol 4:3-11, 1997.

Grignani F, De Matteis S, Nervi C, et al. Fusion proteins of the retinoic acid receptor-α recruit histone deacetylase in promyelocytic leukaemia. Nature 391: 815-818, 1998.

Guo A, Salomoni P, Luo J, Shih A, et al. The function of PML in p53-dependent apoptosis. Nature Cell Biol 2:730-736, 2000.

He LZ, Merghoub T, Pandolfi PP. In vivo analysis of the molecular pathogenesis of acute promyelocytic leukemia in the mouse and its therapeutic implications. Oncogene 18: 5278-5292, 1999.

Kogan SC, Hong SH, Schultz DB, Privalsky ML, Bishop JM. Leukemia initiated by PMLRARα: the PML domain plays a critical role while retinoic acid-mediated transactivation is dispensable. Blood 95:1541-1550, 2000.

Lin RJ, Egan DA, Evans RM. Molecular genetics of acute promyelocytic leukemia. Trends Genet 15:179-184, 1999.

Marcucci G, Caligiuri MA, Bloomfield CD. Molecular and clinical advances in core binding factor primary acute myeloid leukemia: a paradigm for translational research in malignant hematology. Cancer Invest 18:768-780, 2000.

Melnick A, Licht JD. Deconstructing a disease: RARα, its fusion partners, and their roles in the pathogenesis of acute promyelocytic leukemia. Blood 93:3167-3215, 1999.

Russell NH. Biology of acute leukemia. Lancet 349:118-122, 1997.

Sawyers CL. Molecular genetics of acute leukaemia. Lancet 349:196-200, 1997.

Wang J, Hoshino T, Redner RL, et al. ETO, fusion partner in t(8;21) acute myeloid leukemia, represses transcription by interaction with the human n-CoR/mSin3/HDAC1 complex. Proc Natl Acad Sci 95:10860-10865, 1998.

Zhong S, Salomoni P, Pandolfi PP. The transcriptional role of PML and the nuclear body. Nature Cell Biol 2:E85-E90, 2000.

CHEMOTHERAPEUTIC ANTINEOPLASTICS

Asher Begleiter
Lyonel Israels

"Arsenic has a positive value in Hodgkin's disease – the results in many instances have been striking."
The Practice of Medicine (4th ed) 1901
Sir William Osler

Chemotherapeutic agents used in the treatment of hematological malignancies interfere with cell replication by either deregulation of cell division or promotion of cell death. Most agents function at more than one metabolic site; the inter-relationships are complex and, for many agents, the relative contribution of each to the overall biological activity remains unresolved. As these drugs also are used in combination to improve the therapeutic effect and avoid the emergence of drug resistance, it is even more difficult to determine the principal event(s) leading to cell kill in individual human tumours. The metabolic effects produced by these chemotherapeutic agents are not confined to the population of malignant cells; normal cells also are affected – particularly those with rapid turnover such as bone marrow progenitors and gut mucosal cells – accounting for the frequently observed side effects of bone marrow suppression and gastrointestinal toxicity.

The effect of many chemotherapeutic agents is dependent on their interruption or disruption of the cell cycle (Figure 23-1). The cell cycle, leading to mitotic division, may be separated into four phases; the relative duration of each phase varies with the cell type and the rate of proliferation. In a model system, the times would approximate the following: G_1 (gap 1) following mitosis is the longest phase, 12 to 96 hours; **S**, DNA synthesis requires 2-4 hours; G_2 (gap 2), the post DNA synthetic phase, 2-4 hours; (**M**), mitosis occupies about 1-2 hours. Cells may move out of cycle for prolonged periods (G_0) before re-entering the replicative cycle. The subset of cells in active cycle is termed the **growth fraction.** Cells may die either in or out of cycle (Section 2).

The ability of many chemotherapeutic agents to restrict growth or induce cell kill depends on their site of action and relationship to the cell cycle. **Phase specific agents** are effective only during a specific phase of the cycle. Examples are agents that interfere with DNA synthesis (S phase) such as the antimetabolites, or those that inhibit mitosis (M phase) such as the vinca alkaloids. Other drugs, although not restricted to a specific phase, more actively target cycling cells rather than cells in G_0. Some agents have a major effect on non-cycling cells, probably by the induction of apoptosis. The toxic events alone may not be sufficient to cause cell death, but metabolic dysfunction may generate an intracellular signal that sets the apoptotic process in motion. In some cases, this may be mediated through the p53 tumor supressor gene: tumors expressing wild-type (normal) p53 frequently are more sensitive to chemotherapy than tumors with absent or mutant p53 (Sections 2 and 4).

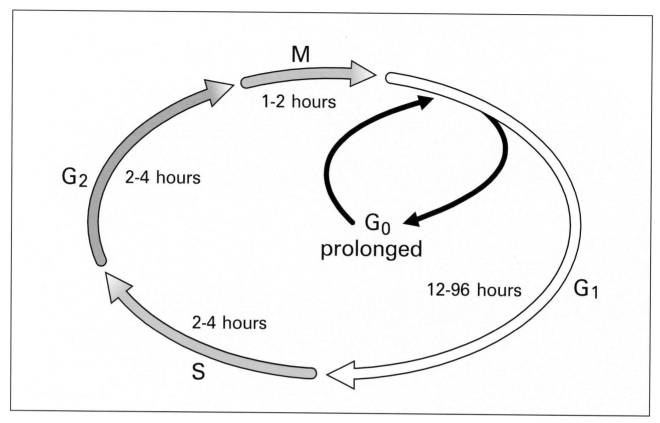

Figure 23-1 Cell Cycle

Although the leukemias, lymphomas and solid tumours are described as clonogenic (indicating that they arise from a single clone), cells with a high mitotic and proliferative rate undergo additional mutations that result in a heterogenous population with various drug sensitivities. As many chemotherapeutic agents are most effective during S phase, and as the cells of this heterogenous population are asynchronous and some are in G_0 (non-cycling cells), cell kill will vary with the mode and duration of drug administration. Although many tumour cells may be killed by any one drug in any one course of chemotherapy, this heterogeneity and asynchronous growth often necessitates the use of combination chemotherapy, i.e. administration of multiple drugs, together or in sequence.

Classifications of chemotherapeutic agents attempt to define the critical site(s) of cell damage, the metabolic consequences, or the mechanisms triggering apoptosis. The following description is confined largely to agents in common use. The bracketed numbers appearing as a superscript refer to the primary targets of the agent, as shown in Figure 23-2.

ANTIMETABOLITES

Because the structures of the antimetabolites closely resemble normal metabolic substrates, they can be incorporated into the metabolic sequence of cell function and replication.

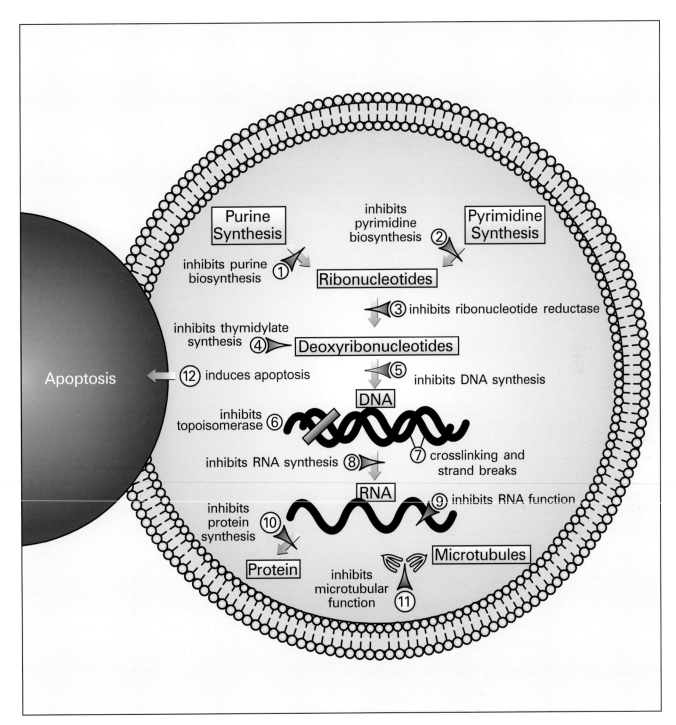

Figure 23-2 Mechanisms of Action of Chemotherapeutic Agents

They interfere with the synthesis of DNA and RNA by: (a) inhibiting production of nucleoside or nucleotide precursors, (b) competing for the anabolic enzymes of DNA and RNA synthesis, or (c) incorporation into DNA and RNA as substitutes for the normal nucleotides. The antimetabolites may inhibit both de novo purine and pyrimidine synthesis as well as the salvage pathways for recycling these bases or their nucleosides.

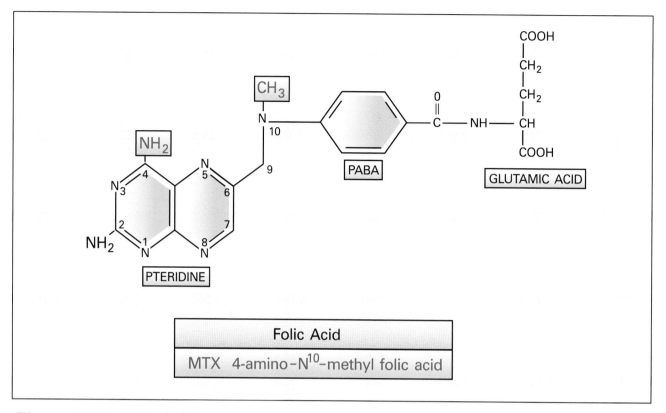

Figure 23-3 Folic Acid and Methotrexate (MTX)

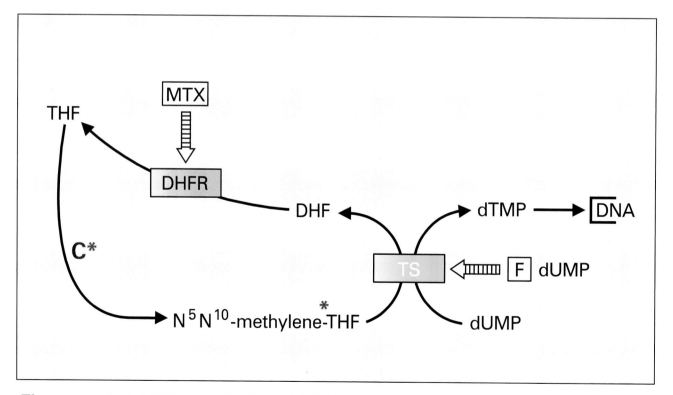

Figure 23-4 Inhibition by MTX and 5-FU

FOLATE ANTAGONISTS (Figure 23-3 and 23-4)

Methotrexate (MTX) - 4-amino-N^{10}-methyl folic acid [1] [2] [4]

    MTX is the prototype and the most widely used folate analogue. It enters cells on the folic acid transport carrier and binds to and inhibits **dihydrofolate reductase (DHFR)**, the enzyme that converts dihydrofolate (DHF) to tetrahydrofolate (THF) – thus interfering with one-carbon transport and blocking de novo synthesis of both purines and pyrimidines. MTX, like folic acid, forms polyglutamates that are held within the cell by decreased efflux and by their high affinity for DHFR (Section 14). The primary block produced by MTX is the denial of one-carbon groups in the synthesis of thymidylate (dTMP) from deoxyuridylate (dUMP). The metabolic block and cytotoxicity can be by-passed by N^5-formyl tetrahydrofolate (leukovorin) – this agent is used therapeutically to rescue normal cells following a period of MTX exposure. MTX is used in combination with other agents in the treatment of the acute leukemias and lymphomas and in a number of solid tumours including breast, bowel, bone, testis, and choriocarcinoma.

PURINE ANALOGUES (Figure 23-5)

6-Mercaptopurine (6-MP) [1] [5] [8] [9]

    6-MP is a sulfur (S) substituted analogue of the natural purine, hypoxanthine. 6-MP is converted *in vivo* to the ribonucleotide derivative 6-MP-ribose phosphate, a competitive inhibitor of *PRPP (phosphoribosyl-pyrophosphate) transferase* – the enzyme that catalyzes the initial reaction in the synthesis of the purine ring. In addition, the incorporation of the ribonucleotide into DNA and RNA interferes with DNA and RNA synthesis and function.

6-Thioguanine (6-TG) [1] [5] [8]

    6-TG, a sulfur (S) substituted analogue of guanine, reduces purine synthesis by inhibiting *PRPP transferase*. It also is incorporated into DNA, impairing its function and thereby interfering with the synthesis of messenger RNA.

    The purine analogues are used primarily in the treatment of the acute leukemias.

PYRIMIDINE ANALOGUES (Figure 23-5)

5-Fluorouracil (5-FU) [4] [5] [9]

    The halogenated pyrimidine analogue, 5-FU, is converted *in vivo* into the monophosphate nucleotide analogue FdUMP and the triphosphate analogue FdUTP. FdUMP binds tightly to thymidylate synthetase (TS), inhibiting the synthesis of thymidylate (dTMP) from dUMP, blocking DNA synthesis. In addition, FdUTP is incorporated into RNA, compromising RNA processing and function. As both 5-FU and MTX are inhibitors of dTMP synthesis, they frequently are used together in combination chemotherapy (Figure 23-4). 5-FU is used primarily in the treatment of non-hematological malignancies such as bowel and breast.

PURINE NUCLEOSIDE ANALOGUES (Figure 23-5)

2'-Deoxycoformycin (DCF) (pentostatin) [3] [5] [12]

This adenosine analogue functions as an inhibitor of adenosine deaminase, allowing the accumulation of toxic levels of deoxyadenosine triphosphate (dATP) in the cell. dATP inhibition of ribonucleotide reductase results in interference with DNA synthesis and repair. The drug also promotes apoptosis.

2-Chlorodeoxyadenosine (2-CdA) [3] [5] [12]

This chlorine analogue of deoxyadenosine is phosphorylated intracellularly to the triphosphate, 2-CdATP. 2-CdATP inhibits ribonucleotide reductase and, incorporated into DNA, it inhibits DNA synthesis and repair in replicating cells. It is a promoter of apoptosis.

Fludarabine [3] [5] [8] [12]

Fludarabine is the monophosphate of F-Ara A (2-fluorodeoxyadenosine arabinoside). Prior to entry into the cell, fludarabine is dephosphorylated to the active metabolite F-Ara A; intracellular phosphorylation converts F-Ara A to the triphosphate. The triphosphate incorporated into DNA and RNA inhibits DNA synthesis and repair, and RNA transcription. It is also an inhibitor of ribonucleotide reductase and a promoter of apoptosis.

These purine nucleoside analogues are used in the treatment of low-grade lymphomas, hairy cell leukemia and chronic lymphocytic leukemia.

PYRIMIDINE NUCLEOSIDE ANALOGUES (Figure 23-5)

Cytosine Arabinoside (Cytarabine) (Ara-C) [5]

This is a structural analogue of 2'-deoxycytidine. It is activated *in vivo* by conversion to the 5' monophosphate nucleotide, Ara-CMP, then phosphorylated to Ara-CTP. Ara-CTP is incorporated into DNA, interrupting DNA synthesis and inhibiting DNA polymerase, DNA ligase, and DNA repair. It is a useful agent in the treatment of acute leukemia.

Gemcitabine [3] [5] [12]

This analogue of 2'-deoxycytidine contains two fluorine atoms in the sugar group. It is phosphorylated *in vivo* to the di- and triphosphate which interrupt DNA synthesis and repair by

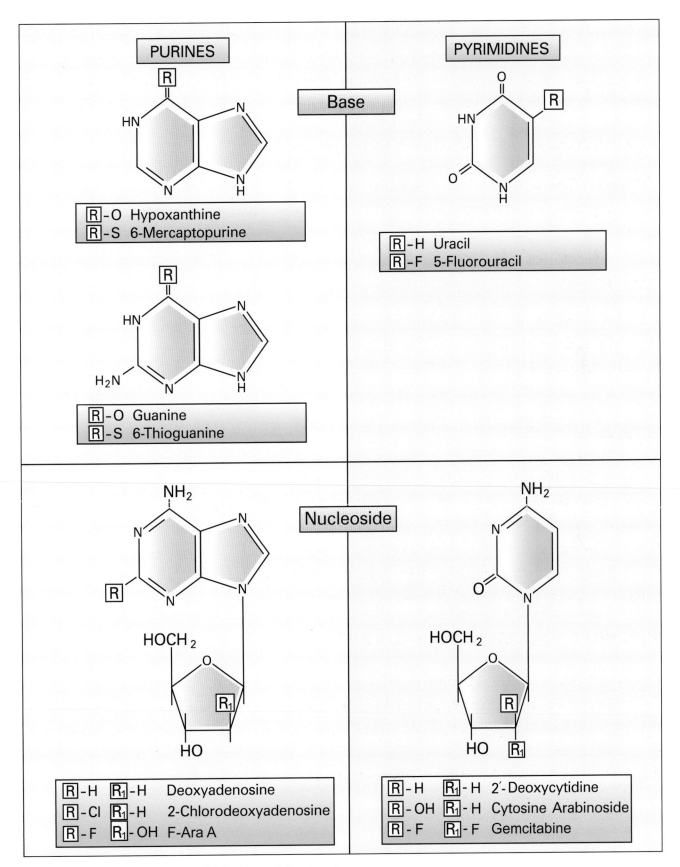

Figure 23-5 Base and Nucleoside Analogs

inhibition of ribonucleotide reductase and by their incorporation into DNA. This agent is of primary value in the treatment of pancreatic carcinoma and other gastrointestinal tumors.

OTHER ANTIMETABOLITES

Hydroxyurea[3] (H$_2$N-CO-NH-OH) is a close analogue of urea. It is a specific inhibitor of ribonucleotide reductase, interfering with DNA synthesis. It is used in myeloproliferative disorders including chronic myelocytic leukemia, thrombocythemia and polycythemia vera.

ALKYLATING AGENTS

Alkylating agents form covalent bonds with cellular targets. The cytotoxic effects result from their ability to bind to functional groups (OH, NH, SH) and to cross-link adjacent groups in DNA, RNA, and protein. Their principal effects are the production of DNA adducts, crosslinks, strand-breaks and disruption of replication, leading to the induction of apoptosis.

NITROGEN MUSTARDS [7] [8] [9] [12] (Figure 23-6)

The nitrogen mustards are so named because they are structurally related to the oily yellow blistering agent sulfur mustard – the mustard gas of World War I. The substitution of nitrogen for sulfur spawned the nitrogen mustard (HN2) series of alkylating agents.

The prototype HN2, mechlorethamine (Figure 23-6), is a simple bifunctional alkylating agent; following the release of Cl$^-$, it can covalently bind nucleophilic groups. The two active "arms" can form either intrastrand or interstrand bridging of DNA; this results in DNA dysfunction, strand-breaks, loss of replication, mutagenesis, or cell death. Its primary DNA target is the 7-amino group of guanine. HN2 and some of its clinically useful analogues are:

Mechlorethamine (HN2) is used in Hodgkin's disease and non-Hodgkin's lymphomas.

Chlorambucil (phenylbutyric acid mustard) is an oral agent used in low grade non-Hodgkin's lymphomas and in chronic lymphocytic leukemia.

Melphalan (L-phenylalanine mustard) has a particular role in the treatment of multiple myeloma and in a conditioning regimen for bone marrow transplantation.

Cyclophosphamide is activated *in vivo* by the p-450 mixed function oxidase system in hepatic microsomes. It is used in combination chemotherapy in lymphomas and solid tumours.

Ifosfamide is an analogue of cyclophosphamide. It also is activated by hepatic microsomal P-450. It is used in non-Hodgkin's lymphomas and in some solid tumours.

ALKANE SULFONATES [7] [8] [9] [12] (Figure 23-6)

Busulfan – a bifunctional alkylsulfonate that, like the mustards, can form DNA crosslinks. In contrast to the other alkylating agents, it is more myelotoxic than lymphotoxic. It is used in myeloproliferative diseases: chronic myelocytic leukemia, thrombocythemia. Because it is a potent carcinogen, its use in these diseases largely has been replaced by other agents.

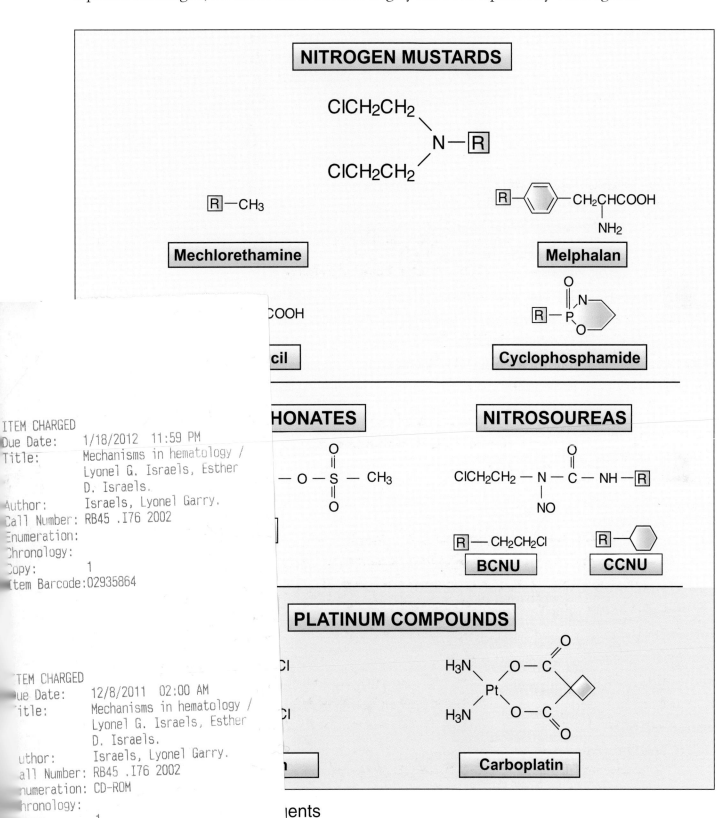

NITROSOUREAS [7] [8] [12] (Figure 23-6)

The primary action of these alkylating agents is the interstrand crosslinking of DNA. The preferred initial target is the 6-oxygen position of guanine. As the nitrosoureas are lipophilic, there is good penetration of the central nervous system.

BCNU (carmustine) and **CCNU** (lomustine) are used in combination therapy in lymphomas and in some solid tumour regimens.

PLATINUM COMPOUNDS [7] [8] [12] (Figure 23-6)

The platinum compounds **cisplatin** and **carboplatin** produce intrastrand and interstrand crosslinking of DNA, and interfere with the function of DNA as an RNA template. Their primary therapeutic role is in the treatment of solid tumours.

Other Alkylating Agents

Non-classical or atypical alkylating agents include **procarbazine and dacarbazine (DTIC)**. These agents undergo *in vivo* metabolic transformation to active intermediates with alkylating activity capable of forming DNA monoadducts and inhibition of DNA synthesis. Procarbazine is important in combination therapy for Hodgkin's and non-Hodgkin's lymphoma. Dacarbazine is used in Hodgkin's disease and in malignant melanoma.

NON-COVALENT DNA BINDING AGENTS

Anthracyclines [6] [7] [8] [9] [12] (Figure 23-7)

The **anthracyclines, daunorubicin, doxorubicin, and idarubacin,** belong to a large group of rhodomycins produced by various Streptomyces. These three molecules are identical but for minor substitutions on the four-ring structure. Their antitumour activity and their toxicity relate to multiple mechanisms: DNA binding stabilizes the *topoisomerase II-DNA complex,* inhibiting DNA synthesis and resulting in DNA single and double strand breaks (based on this mechanism of action, these agents also could be classified as topoisomerase inhibitors); interference with RNA synthesis; generation of free radicals by the quinone and hydroquinone groups of the parent molecule (this may be the mechanism of mitochondrial lipid peroxidation and cardiac toxicity); chelation of Ca^{2+}, Mg^{2+} and other metal ions.

They are used in combination with other agents in the treatment of lymphomas, the acute leukemias, and some solid tumours.

Mitoxantrone is a synthetic analogue of the anthracyclines; its mechanism of action closely parallels that of the anthracyclines. As mitoxantrone does not produce free radicals, it is less cardiotoxic than the anthracyclines. It is used primarily in the treatment of leukemias, lymphomas, and breast cancer.

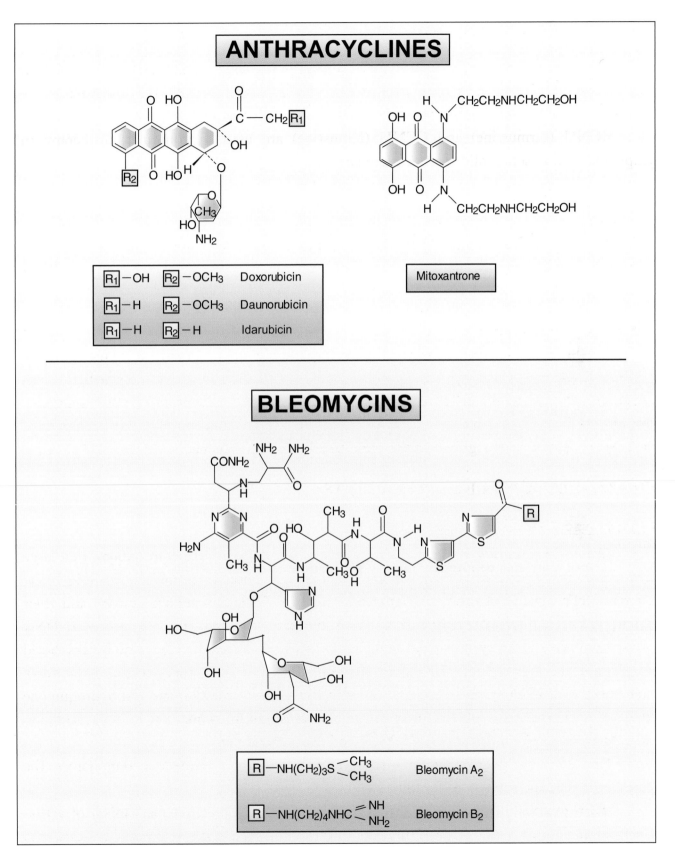

Figure 23-7 Noncovalent DNA Binding Agents

BLEOMYCIN [7] [12] (Figure 23-7)

Bleomycin consists of a mixture of glycopeptides which, in a complex with iron, binds to DNA. Redox cycling of the metal generates free radicals that produce DNA single and double strand breaks. It is used in combination chemotherapy of both Hodgkin's and non-Hodgkin's lymphoma, testicular tumors, and head and neck squamous cell carcinoma.

TOPOISOMERASE INHIBITORS [6] (Figure 23-8)

Topoisomerase enzymes form complexes with DNA and catalyze the unwinding and transient resealable breaks in DNA that facilitate structural changes in the molecule. This allows the relaxation and untangling of selected regions of the normally tightly packed DNA and permits the unwinding of the DNA strands for transcription and DNA synthesis. The enzymes are classified as **topoisomerase II** enzymes that break both DNA strands, or **topoisomerase I** enzymes that break only one DNA strand. Topoisomerase inhibitors stablize the DNA-enzyme complex preventing the normal function of the enzymes.

Epipodophyllotoxins [6] [12] (Figure 23-8)

Etoposide (VP-16) and **teniposide (VM-26)** are derived from mandrake root. They bind to tubulin at sites other than those bound by the vinca alkaloids. At therapeutic concentrations they do not block mitosis but inhibit **topoisomerase II** by stabilizing the enzyme-DNA complex – resulting in unrepairable double-strand breaks. Cells are arrested in G_2. These agents are used in the treatment of lymphomas and some solid tumours.

Camptothecins [6] [12] (Figure 23-8)

Irinotecan and **topotecan** inhibit **topoisomerase I**, resulting in DNA damage and cytotoxicity. These agents are of primary use in the treatment of solid tumors.

MICROTUBULE INHIBITORS

Vinca Alkaloids [11] [12] (Figure 23-9)

Vinblastine, vincristine and **vindesine** were derived originally from the periwinkle plant. They bind to tubulin, inhibiting microtubule production and formation of the mitotic spindle; the result is metaphase arrest. These are useful agents in the combination chemotherapy of Hodgkin's disease and non-Hodgkin's lymphomas.

Taxols [11] [12] (Figure 23-9)

Paclitaxel (originally extracted from the yew tree: Taxus brevifolia) and its semisynthetic analogue, **docetaxel (taxotere),** bind and stabilize tubulin. As a result, microtubule disassembly is prevented and cells are arrested at the G_2/M interface. These agents are used primarily in breast and ovarian carcinoma.

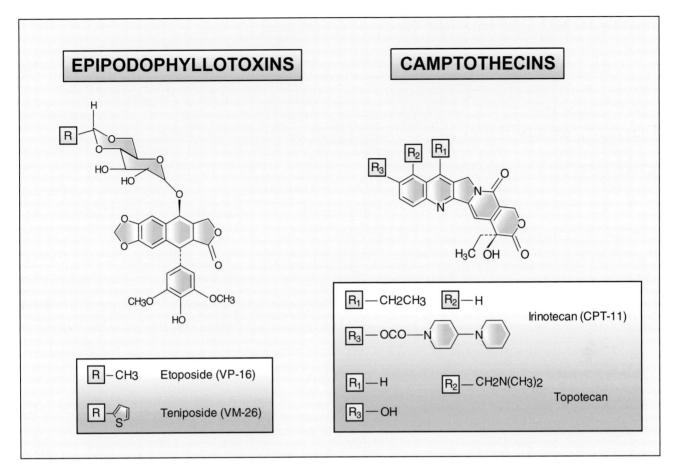

Figure 23-8   Topoisomerase Inhibitors

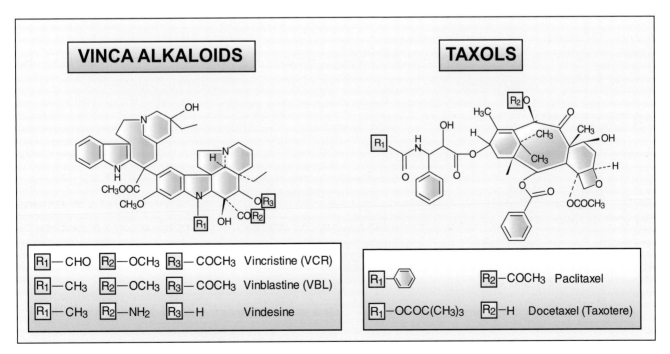

Figure 23-9   Microtubule Inhibitors

MONOCLONAL ANTIBODIES

Monoclonal antibodies targeted to specific antigenic sites expressed on the malignant cell offer the possibility of site-directed toxicity with little collateral damage. Cell kill may result from direct antibody-induced cell damage, induction of apoptosis, activation of complement-mediated cytotoxicity, or inhibition of cell-derived cytokines or growth factors. To reduce the immunogenicity of monoclonal antibodies, human sequences can be incorporated into the murine immunoglobulin, resulting in the formation of chimeric or humanized antibodies (Section 17). These antibodies also can be conjugated with direct cytotoxins (eg, ricin) or radionuclides (eg, iodine[131], yttrium[90]).

Monoclonal Antibodies for B-Cell Tumors

Rituximab is a chimeric murine/human monoclonal antibody specific for the CD20 antigen present on both normal and malignant B cells. The CD20 transmembrane protein is found on late pre-B and mature B lymphocytes. It is not expressed on early pre-B cells, plasma cells, or hematopoietic stem cells. CD20 probably regulates the cell cycle and is active during G_1. CD20 is not shed from the cell surface and is not present in plasma, therefore access of the antibody to the CD20 expressed on the cell is not impaired. CD20 is present on more than 90% of B-cell lymphomas. The variable CD20 binding site of the antibody is murine, the constant (C) regions are human. The C region both efficiently binds complement and interacts with human cytotoxic effector cells. Its primary therapeutic role is in non-Hodgkin's lymphomas, either alone or combined with cytotoxic chemotherapy.

Campath-1 is a humanized monoclonal chimeric antibody directed against the CD52 antigen. CD52 is expressed on all lymphocytes (both T and B cells) and monocytes. Its physiological role is unclear but it may mediate cell-cell interaction. Campath-1 probably induces direct cellular cytotoxicity, mediates complement cytoxicity, and induces apoptosis. It has been used for *in vitro* purging of donor lymphocytes in allogeneic bone marrow transplant, in graft versus host disease, in T-cell prolymphocytic leukemia, and in chronic lymphocytic leukemia.

Trastuzumab (Herceptin) is a monoclonal chimeric mouse/human antibody that targets the extracellular domain of Her-2, a cell membrane-associated tyrosine kinase. Her-2 is a member of the EGF receptor family. It has no known ligand but its expression is upregulated in 25-30% of breast cancers. The high concentration of Her-2 receptors probably results in homodimerization or heterodimerization with other EGF-like receptors, resulting in the activation of tyrosine kinases. Trastuzumab may trigger immune-mediated cell kill, downregulate the activated protein kinases, or induce inhibitors of the cyclin-dependent kinases. It is used in combination with paclitaxel or doxorubicin in the treatment of breast tumors.

OTHER AGENTS

L-Asparaginase [10] – an enzyme derived from E.coli. It hydrolyzes L-asparagine to aspartic acid and ammonia, thus interfering with protein synthesis. It is used in combination with other agents in the treatment of acute lymphoblastic leukemia.

STI571 – Chronic myelocytic leukemia (CML) is characterized by the 9q/22q translocation, presenting the Ph chromosome karyotype and the Bcr/Abl fusion protein. The new fusion protein is associated with increased tyrosine kinase activity and enhanced growth potential of the malignant clone (Section 22). STI571 (signal transduction inhibitor 571) is an inhibitor of the Bcr/Abl tyrosine kinase: it is a phenylamino-pyridine that blocks ATP access to the tyrosine kinase-binding pocket within Bcr/Abl. This precisely targeted inhibitor of the Bcr/Abl tyrosine kinase induces clinical remission accompanied by the disappearance of the Ph chromosome and the Bcr/Abl protein transcript. Clinical response occurs in most patients in chronic phase CML as well as in some patients in blast phase and in Bcr/Abl-positive patients with ALL. It also blocks the receptors for PDGF and stem cell factor – STI571 or its derivatives may be of value in tumors that overexpress these receptors.

Corticosteroids [12] – the glucocorticoids are strong inducers of apoptosis in lymphoid cells. They are useful adjuncts in the treatment of lymphomas, myeloma and acute lymphoblastic leukemia.

All-Trans Retinoic Acid – this agent is capable of producing cell maturation in acute promyelocytic leukemia (M3) associated with the t(15:17) chromosomal translocation. The site of the translocation on chromosome 17 includes the gene for the nuclear retinoic acid receptor (Section 22).

Interferons – these are a group of glycoproteins that are produced by normal cells in response to pathogens. They possess antiproliferative as well as antiviral activity. They are of use in hairy cell leukemia and as an adjunct in the treatment of chronic myelocytic leukemia and myeloma.

Inhibitors of Angiogenesis – Tumor growth and metastasis are dependent on new vessel formation. Inhibition of tumor associated angiogenesis produces tumor regression in mice. Antiangiogenic proteins include **angiostatin**, a 34 kD fragment of human plasminogen, and **endostatin**, a 20 kD fragment of collagen XVIII. The advantage of these agents is their low toxicity because the cycling fraction of tumor endothelial cells is some 2-3 logs higher than their normal counterparts.

DRUG RESISTANCE

Cellular drug resistance may be present at the start of therapy (intrinsic) or may be induced after an initial period of responsiveness (acquired). Malignant cells become resistant to chemotherapy through a number of mechanisms. A single drug may encounter or induce

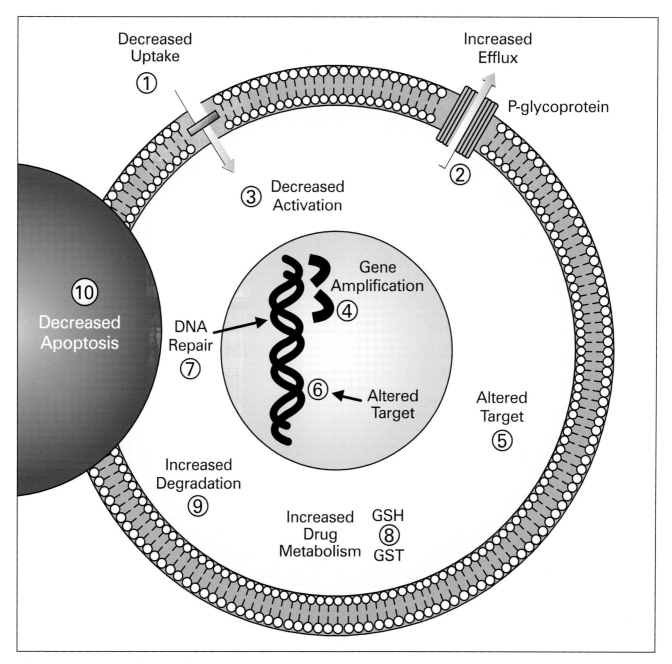

Figure 23-10 Drug Resistance

multiple modes of resistance. The numbers below refer to the site and mechanism of drug resistance diagrammed in Figure 23-10.

Decreased Drug Uptake [1]

This is due to changes in the cell membrane that result in decreased carrier-mediated uptake into the tumor cell. This mechanism may be responsible for resistance to the nucleoside analogues, nitrogen mustard, melphalan, and methotrexate.

Increased Drug Efflux [2]

A glycoprotein energy-dependent trans-membrane efflux pump is expressed normally in some cells for removal of potentially toxic xenobiotics that gain access to the organism. Malignant cells may exhibit intrinsic or acquired resistance by exploiting or amplifying this mechanism. The MDR1 (multiple drug resistance) phenotype is characterized by the presence of this trans-membrane multi-drug transporter (P-glycoprotein) for such drugs as the anthracyclines, vinca alkaloids, etoposide and taxol. The overexpression of P-glycoprotein results in the simultaneous resistance to a number of structurally unrelated drugs that share only the feature of being natural products isolated from plants or microorganisms. This resistance does not extend to synthetic agents such as antimetabolites, alkylating agents or platinum compounds. P-glycoprotein plays a normal protective role in xenobiotic excretion or exclusion in absorptive or excretory organs such as gut, liver and kidney; consequently, tumours arising from these tissues frequently are resistant to these natural products. Acquired resistance is associated with increased translation or amplification of the *mdr-1* gene sequences on chromosome 7 or on small extra-chromosomal pieces of DNA, termed double minutes, that code for P-glycoprotein. A variety of drugs, of unrelated structure, may partially reverse MDR1 multidrug resistance by directly interacting with P-glycoprotein; these include the calcium channel blockers, cyclosporin A, phenothiazines, and quinidine.

A second and distinct family of multiple drug resistance proteins (MRP) that confers inherent or acquired resistance to natural chemotherapeutic products has been identified. Overexpression of this MRP membrane transport protein also is associated with increased drug efflux. MRP is an ATP-dependent plasma membrane efflux pump that transports both physiological products (eg, bilirubin, leukotrienes) and natural chemotherapeutic products (eg, anthracyclines, vinca alkaloids, epipodophyllotoxins) out of the cell. This efflux is enhanced by prior conjugation of the substrate with glucuronic acid or glutathione.

Increased drug efflux also may be triggered by intracellular events. MTX is retained within the cell by polyglutamation as are its closely related folic acid congeners (Section 14). Decreased MTX polyglutamation or rapid degradation of the polyglutamate by increased hydrolase activity results in rapid loss of MTX from the cell and MTX resistance.

Decreased Drug Activation [3]

Reduced intracellular metabolism prevents conversion of a drug to its active form. Decreased kinase activity prevents the conversion of ara-C to its active form ara-CTP. Similarly, low kinase activity inhibits the phosphorylation of the nucleoside analogues DCF, 2-CdA and fludarabine to their active triphosphate forms. Drugs activated by the mixed function oxidase system (eg, cyclophosphamide) are vulnerable to reduced levels of cytochrome p450.

Gene Amplification [4]

In cells exhibiting the MDR1 phenotype, the *mdr-1* gene is amplified with increased P-glycoprotein expression and increased drug efflux. MTX resistance is associated with amplification of the gene for dihydrofolate reductase (DHFR), which may be increased several hundred-fold in resistant cells. Double minute chromosomes that are sites of gene reduplication are often present in these cells. Other examples of gene amplification are the genes for ribonucleotide reductase (the target enzyme of hydroxyurea), and adenosine deaminase (the target enzyme of deoxycoformycin).

Altered Target Enzymes [5] [6]

Induced changes in the normal target enzyme may result in decreased binding of drug. Some MTX-resistant cells have an altered dihydrofolate reductase incapable of binding MTX. Similarly, there is decreased binding of the 5-FU metabolite FdUMP to an altered thymidylate synthase that evolves in resistant cells. In some anthracycline-resistant cells, topoisomerase II, which mediates DNA cleavage by the anthracyclines, may undergo a structural change that is unreceptive to binding by these agents.

Increased DNA Repair [7]

The excision of the defective strand, its replacement by normal nucleotides and ligation of the repaired site is a principal mechanism of acquired resistance to alkylating and other DNA interacting agents. This mechanism is found in cells resistant to the alkylating agents and the anthracyclines.

Increased Drug Metabolism [8]

In normal cells, glutathione (GSH) plays a major role in the detoxification and excretion of physiological metabolites and xenobiotics by MRP transporters. These reactions are mediated by a family of glutathione S-transferases (GSTs). The emergence of resistance to a number of antitumour agents is associated with an increase in GST activity and GSH levels. This type of resistance may be induced by alkylating agents and anthracyclines.

Increased Degradation [9]

This may be due to up-regulation of metabolic or enzymatic activity. Deaminases, such as deoxycytidine deaminase, convert Ara-C to its inactive metabolite Ara-U. BCNU is metabolized by the mixed function oxidase system to a compound with little or no antitumour activity. Bleomycin is degraded by the enzyme bleomycin hydrolase. Activated cyclophosphamide is degraded by aldehyde dehydrogenase.

Table 23-1   Chemotherapeutic Antineoplastics

AGENTS	SITE OF ACTION	MECHANISMS OF RESISTANCE

Folate Antagonists
MTX
	Inhibits dihydrofolate reductase
	Blocks one-carbon transport
	Blocks purine and pyrimidine ring
	  synthesis
	Blocks thymidylate synthesis
		Decreased membrane transport
		Increased dihydrofolate reductase
		  (DHFR)
		Altered target enzyme (DHFR)
		Decreased cell retention

Purine Analogues 6MP, 6TG	Block purine synthesis Incorporation into DNA & RNA interferes with synthesis and funtion	Decreased conversion to nucleotides
Pyrimidine Analogues 5FU	Blocks thymidylate synthase (TS) Inhibits DNA synthesis Incorporated into dysfunctional RNA	Decreased activation Altered target enzyme (TS)

Purine Nucleoside
Analogues
DCF, F-Ara-A, 2-CdA
	Inhibit ribonucleotide reductase
	Inhibit DNA synthesis and repair
	Promote apoptosis
		Decreased activation - low kinase
		  activity prevents conversion to
		  triphosphates

Pyrimidine Nucleoside Analogues Ara-C, Gemcitabine	Incorporated into DNA Inhibit DNA synthesis and repair	Decreased activation - low kinase activity Decreased intracellular retention

Hydroxyurea	Inhibits ribonucleotide reductase	Increased levels or decreased
		  sensitivity of ribonucleotide
		  reductase

L-Asparaginase	Hydrolysis of L-asparagine Inhibits protein synthesis	Increased L-asparagine synthase
Alkylating Agents Nitrogen Mustards Busulfan Nitrosoureas Platinum Compounds	Crosslinking DNA, RNA, protein DNA strand breaks - disruption of replication Inhibit RNA synthesis Promote apoptosis	Decreased uptake Increased DNA repair Increased metabolism Increased degradation
Anthracyclines Doxorubicin, Daunorubicin, Idarubicin, Mitoxantrone	Inhibit topoisomerase II DNA strand breaks DNA intercalation - inhibit DNA & RNA synthesis	Increased drug efflux (MDR, MRP) Altered topoisomerase activity
Bleomycin	Induces DNA strand breaks	Increased DNA repair Increased degradation
Epipodophyllotoxins Etoposide, Teniposide	Inhibit topoisomerase II	Altered topoisomerase activity Increased drug efflux (MDR, MRP)
Camptothecins Irinotecan, Topotecan	Inhibit topoisomerase I	Altered topoisomerase activity
Vinca Alkaloids VP-16, VP-26	Prevent microtubule assembly Produce metaphase arrest	Increased drug efflux (MDR, MRP) Altered binding to tubulin
Taxols Paclitaxel, Docetaxel	Stabilize microtubules Produce metaphase arrest	Increased drug efflux (MDR) Altered binding to tubulin

Decreased Apoptosis [10]

In lymphomas, drug resistance may be due to mutated p53, up-regulation of Bcl-2 or alterations in the levels of caspases and other effectors of apoptosis, resulting in a delay or block in the apoptotic pathway to cell removal (Sections 2 and 4).

•••••●•••••

SUGGESTED READING

Arceci RJ. Clinical significance of P-glycoprotein in multidrug resistance malignancies. Blood 81:2215- 2222, 1993.

Chabner BA, Collins JA. Cancer Chemotherapy: Principles and Practice. J.B. Lippincott, 1990.

Druker BJ, Talpaz M, Resta DJ, et al. Efficacy and safety of a specific inhibitor of the Bcr/Abl tyrosine kinase in chronic myeloid leukemia. N Engl J Med 344:1031-1037, 2001.

Flynn JM, Byrd JC. Campath-1H monoclonal antibody therapy. Cur Opin Oncol 12:574-581, 2000.

Gibbs JB. Anticancer drug targets: growth factors and growth factor signaling. J Clin Invest 105:9-13, 2000.

Gorlick R, Goker E, Trippett T, Waltham M, Banerjee D, Bertino JR. Intrinsic and acquired resistance to methotrexate in acute leukemia. N Engl J Med 335:1041-1048, 1996.

Hannun YA. Apoptosis and the dilemma of cancer chemotherapy. Blood 89:1845-1853, 1997.

Hayes AJ, Li LY, Lippman ME. Antivascular therapy: a new approach to cancer treatment. BMJ 318:853-856, 1999.

Keshet E, Ben-Sasson SA. Anticancer drug targets: approaching angiogenesis. J Clin Invest 104:1497-1501, 1999.

Leget GA, Czuczman MS. Use of rituximab, the new FDA-approved antibody. Cur Opin Oncol 10:548-551, 1998.

Lowe SW, Ruley HE, Jacks T, Housman DE. p53 dependent apoptosis modulates the cytotoxicity of anticancer agents. Cell 74:957-967, 1993.

Lum BL, Gosland, MP. MDR expression in normal tissues: pharmacologic implications for the clinical use of P-glycoprotein inhibitors. Hematol Oncol Clin North Am 9:319-336, 1995.

O'Dwyer PJ, Yao K, Tew KD, Ozols RF. Modulation of glutathione and related enzymes in reversal of resistance to anticancer drugs. Hematol Oncol Clin North Am 9:383-396, 1995.

Pastan I, Gottesman MM. Multidrug resistance. Annu Rev Med 42:277-286, 1991.

Pratt WB, Ruddon RW, Ensminger WD, Maybaum J. The Anticancer Drugs. Oxford University Press, Second Edition,1994.

Preisler HD. Multidrug resistance is more than mdr1 activity. Leuk Res 19:429-431, 1995.

Reuter CWM, Morgan MA, Bergman L. Targeting the Ras signaling pathway: a rational, mechanism-based treatment for hematologic malignancies? Blood 96:1655-1669, 2000.

Spears CP. Clinical resistance to antimetabolites. Hematol Oncol Clin North Am 9:397-413, 1995.

Tannock IF, Hill RP. The Basic Science of Oncology. McGraw Hill, Third Ed, 1998.

COAGULATION CASCADE

*"After years of confusion, it seems that a relatively simple pattern
is emerging from present theories of blood coagulation"*
R.G. Macfarlane – Nature 1964

The maintenance of an intact vasculature is dependent upon a hemostatic mechanism requiring the participation of both cellular and plasma components. The coagulation system responds to vascular damage by the sequential conversion of precursor zymogens to their active serine proteases. Serial activation of these zymogens is achieved through enzymatic cleavage as the participating proteins are brought into close proximity on negatively-charged phospholipid membranes provided by activated platelets and endothelial cells. These linked reactions constitute an amplification cascade in which micromolar amounts of the initial reactants culminate in the conversion of fibrinogen to fibrin.

In Figure 24-1 the inactive factor is designated by a circle, the activated form by an ellipse. A number of these zymogens (shown in blue) are vitamin K-dependent proteins – factors II, VII, IX, and X. Factors V and VIII (in yellow) and tissue factor are not proteases but act as accelerating cofactors. The subscript "a" designates activated factors; "T" designates thrombin (factor IIa). Phospholipid membranes are represented by the red bars. Coagulation proceeds through the formation of three procoagulant enzyme complexes assembled on negatively-charged cell membranes: tissue factor complex, tenase and prothrombinase. Each of these complexes involves a vitamin K-dependent protein and a membrane-bound cofactor; limited proteolysis converts the vitamin K-dependent factors to serine proteases. The active site of the serine protease, located in the carboxyl terminal region of the molecule, consists of a catalytic triad: serine, aspartic acid and histidine.

The surface membranes of quiescent cells express non-thrombogenic neutral phospholipids that do not bind coagulation factors. Upon activation, platelets, monocytes, and endothelial cells display a procoagulant surface as the anionic phosphatidylserine (PS) from the inner leaflet is translocated to the outer leaflet of the cell membrane. The assembly of the enzyme-cofactor complexes on this phospholipid membrane increases the catalytic efficiency by three to five orders of magnitude. Coagulation is initiated, amplified, and propagated by the interaction of coagulation proteins on cell surfaces. The original concept of coagulation as an activation cascade has been modified by the recognition of the key role played by cell membranes in the process.

TISSUE FACTOR PATHWAY (EXTRINSIC PATHWAY)

Historically referred to as the *"extrinsic pathway,"* the tissue factor pathway is the primary initiator of *in vivo* hemostasis. The coagulation process is set in motion by tissue injury with exposure of cell membrane **tissue factor (TF)** – a glycoprotein that, normally, does not come into direct contact with circulating blood. TF is expressed constitutively on the surface of subendothelial cells (eg, fibroblasts) but is not present on healthy unstimulated endothelial cells. Endothelial cells and circulating monocytes express TF on their membranes only following direct injury or stimulation by cytokines, immune complexes, or bacterial products. (Platelets do not express TF). The membrane-anchored TF functions as a cofactor (allosteric regulator) for factor VIIa, markedly enhancing its enzymatic activity. In the circulating plasma, about one percent of factor VII is present as VIIa. TF binds both the factor VII zymogen and activated VIIa. Unbound VIIa does not induce cleavage/activation of other coagulation factors; the active site only becomes fully expressed when bound to TF. With formation of the VIIa/TF complex, referred to as **Tissue Factor Complex (TFC)**, VIIa rapidly activates factor VII, factor X and factor IX, as they assemble on the membrane surface with TFC. Feedback amplification occurs as VIIa, IXa and Xa activate additional factor VII bound to TF. With the formation of factor Xa, sufficient thrombin is generated from prothrombin to trigger the intrinsic pathway.

INTRINSIC PATHWAY

The coagulation process has been discussed, historically, in terms of the extrinsic and intrinsic pathways. Although this description is not an accurate reflection of physiological events, it has provided the framework for the evolution of current concepts, i.e. the important role of the membrane-bound enzyme complexes. The generation of thrombin through the tissue factor pathway is insufficient to support normal hemostasis; continuation of the process depends upon thrombin activation of coagulation factors in the intrinsic pathway. Thrombin formed by TF/VIIa activity is sufficient to activate platelets, exposing an anionic surface and receptors for factor XI; on the platelet surface, thrombin cleavage converts factor XI to XIa. In turn XIa activates factor IX to IXa. Thrombin also activates factors V and VIII to factors Va and VIIIa that function as cofactors to accelerate the reactions in which they participate. The complex of VIIIa and IXa in association with Ca^{2+} on the phospholipid surface, referred to as **tenase,** activates factor X. The association of factors Xa and Va on the cell surface membrane with Ca^{2+} constitutes **prothrombinase**, the active complex that converts prothrombin (factor II) to thrombin (Figure 24-2). Thrombin cleavage of fibrinopeptides A and B from fibrinogen to yield fibrin monomer is followed by self-assembly of the monomers and polymerization. Thrombin cleavage converts factor XIII to XIIIa which stabilizes the fibrin polymer to insoluble crosslinked fibrin (Section 29).

Although *in vivo* coagulation is initiated by the VIIa/TF complex, the amount of Xa that can be generated is relatively limited due to rapid inhibition of the complex by **tissue factor pathway inhibitor (TFPI)** (Figure 25-1). Sustained coagulation depends upon major

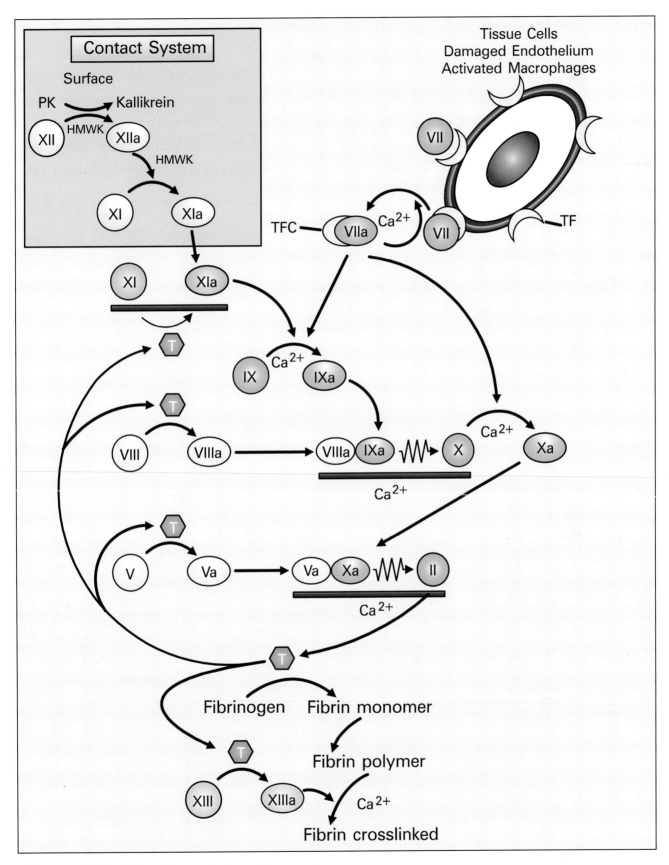

Figure 24-1 The Coagulation Cascade

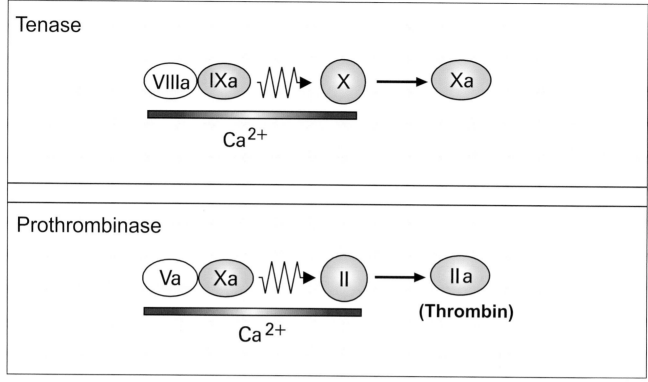

Figure 24-2 Tenase and Prothombinase

amplification of factor X activation by the intrinsic pathway. The importance of this augmenting pathway is emphasized by the profound bleeding manifestations of Hemophilia A and Hemophilia B (congenital deficiencies of factors VIII and IX, respectively) when insufficient Xa is produced to continue the coagulation process. Note: (1) the generation of thrombin, initially through the extrinsic pathway, feeds back to activate factors XI, VIII, V, XIII and platelets; (2) inactive factor VIII circulates bound to von Willebrand factor; cleavage by thrombin first dissociates the two molecules and then activates VIII to VIIIa; (3) the vitamin K-dependent factors interact with the phospholipid membrane via calcium-binding γ-carboxyglutamic acid residues; (4) specific cell membrane receptors and the negatively-charged phospholipids on activated cells profoundly enhance the rate at which the zymogens are converted to active serine proteases; (5) platelets have a primary role in sustaining and amplifying the coagulation process.

    Contact System – diagrammed in the upper left corner of Figure 24-1. The contact factors probably play a relatively minor role in hemostasis *in vivo*, although they are strongly reflected in *in vitro* laboratory tests of coagulation. *In vitro*, as demonstrated in the APTT test, autoactivation of factor XII to XIIa takes place on a negatively-charged surface in the presence of prekallikrein (PK) and high molecular weight kininogen (HMWK). Factor XIIa activates PK to kallikrein and factor XI to XIa. Kallikrein feeds back to activate additional factor XII, and cleaves HMWK to release bradykinin. Factor XIIa activation of factor XI initiates the "intrinsic pathway" *in vitro*.

In vivo, activation of these factors takes place on the surface of activated endothelial cells where they participate in fibrinolysis. Cell-surface receptors bind HMWK. PK and factor XI assemble on HMWK and are activated by cell-surface proteases; factor XII does not initiate these *in vivo* reactions but may increase the rate of activation.

Factor XI is activated *in vitro* by factor XIIa; *in vivo* activation is primarily the result of thrombin cleavage. Factor XI binds to high-affinity receptors on activated platelets where thrombin converts it to XIa. Surface-bound XIa, protected from circulating inhibitors, activates factor IX. *In vivo* activation of factor XI is not dependent on the contact proteins, thus explaining the absence of abnormal bleeding in patients with deficiencies of factor XII, PK, or HMWK.

Cofactors. Factors V and VIII and tissue factor are not enzymes but are essential for the assembly of coagulation factors on phospholipid membranes. Factors V and VIII are structurally and functionally homologous; they circulate in the plasma as inactive precursors that are activated by thrombin and by factor Xa. Factors Va and VIIIa are inactivated by activated protein C (Section 25). Factor VIII probably is synthesized in hepatocytes and reticuloendothelial cells. Factor V is synthesized in hepatocytes and in megakaryocytes; it is present in the α-granules of both megakaryocytes and platelets. Factor V released from activated platelets binds to the platelet surface; upon thrombin activation, the surface-bound factor Va assembles with the other components in the prothrombinase complex. Tissue factor, the receptor for factors VII and VIIa, is an integral membrane protein; it does not require proteolytic activation. TF is a member of the cytokine receptor family; with binding of its ligand VIIa, TF functions as a signaling receptor.

LABORATORY TESTS

In vitro, the coagulation process has been historically (and conveniently) described as a cascade – denoting the sequential activation of these factors; diagnostic tests based on this description of the interaction of the factors allows for their identification and measurement. The tests mimic *in vivo* events, although the use of high non-physiological concentrations of reagents alters the kinetics of the *in vitro* interactions. With results obtained from three screening tests (prothrombin time, activated partial thromboplastin time and thrombin time), it is possible to isolate an abnormality to a specific segment of the "cascade".

Prothrombin Time (PT) is determined by adding TF (thromboplastin) and $CaCl_2$ to plasma and timing the development of the clot. This reaction flows through the extrinsic pathway (on the right side of Figure 24-1); the test is a measure of factors VII, X, V. and II and fibrinogen. Note that, in this test, factor X is activated to Xa without intervention of factors VIII or IX; the PT is insensitive to reduced levels of factors VIII and IX and, therefore, is normal in patients with deficiencies of these factors (Hemophilia A and B). The PT is sensitive to decreased levels of the vitamin K-dependent factors (with the exception of factor IX); it is particularly useful for monitoring the clinical response to oral anticoagulants. The test results, expressed in seconds, are compared to a normal control (usually 10-12 sec.). However, for monitoring patients on oral anticoagulants, the PT is reported as the INR (**International Normalized Ratio**). This ratio, devised to correct for variations in instrumentation and reagents, compares or "normalizes" the results to an international standard thromboplastin; the standard is defined as equivalent to an INR of 1.0. The therapeutic INR range for warfarin-induced anticoagulation is between 2.0 and 3.5 – and as high as 4 to 4.5 in some therapeutic protocols.

Activated Partial Thromboplastin Time (APTT) depends on activation of the contact factors (XII and XI) by a negatively-charged surface such as kaolin or celite. In the presence of phospholipid and calcium, the sequential activation of the factors (illustrated on the left side of Figure 24-1) results in the conversion of fibrinogen to fibrin – usually in about 30-35 seconds. Note: the APTT is prolonged by low levels of all factors except VII and XIII. It also is prolonged in the presence of heparin, low or abnormal fibrinogen, and acquired inhibitors – most frequently lupus anticoagulants or anti-VIII antibodies.

Thrombin Time (TT) measures the rate of conversion of fibrinogen to fibrin upon the addition of thrombin to plasma. It is prolonged in the presence of heparin, low or abnormal fibrinogen, and fibrinogen/ fibrin degradation products.

Factor Assays - Each of the factors is individually assayed using modifications of the PT or the APTT. Fibrinogen is measured either by direct biochemical assay or by its rate of interaction with thrombin. The activity of factor XIII is determined by stability of a clot incubated in 5M urea which rapidly degrades fibrin that has not been crosslinked.

CLINICAL CORRELATES

Congenital Coagulation Disorders

Hemophilia A and B and von Willebrand disease are discussed in Sections 26 and 27, defects in fibrinogen and factor XIII in Section 29.

Factor XII, HMWK and Prekallikrein Deficiencies are inherited as autosomal recessive traits. Factor XII deficiency is present in up to 3% of normal blood donors; deficiencies of HMWK and prekallikrein are rare. A deficiency of one of these proteins is usually recognized when a prolonged APTT is discovered in an individual with no history of bleeding. The APTT is markedly prolonged with defects of factor XII and HMWK, less prolonged in prekallikrein deficiency. Factor XII (Hageman factor) deficiency may be a risk factor for thrombosis: the eponymous Mr. Hageman succumbed to a myocardial infarction.

Factor XI Deficiency is an autosomal recessive bleeding disorder. It occurs with high frequency in Ashkenazi Jews – approximately 5% of that population carry the gene and about 0.3% are homozygous for factor XI deficiency. Clinical manifestations are variable – usually mild, although severe bleeding can occur, and some patients are free of bleeding episodes. Platelet factor XI levels offer a possible explanation for this variable phenotype: in some factor XI deficient patients, the presence of a normal level of platelet factor XI probably is sufficient to support normal hemostasis.

Factor X Deficiency is an autosomal recessive defect; a number of dysfunctional factor X variants have been identified. Hemarthrosis, soft tissue hemorrhage and menorrhagia may occur when factor X levels approximate 1%; with factor X levels above 15%, bleeding episodes are infrequent and usually mild. An acquired factor X deficiency may be associated with light-chain **amyloidosis**. Factor X is adsorbed onto extracellular amyloid fibrils – as a result, the circulating factor X level may be low and bleeding severe. Replacement with factor X products may not be effective as the infused factor X is continuously removed by adsorption to the amyloid.

Factor VII Deficiency, inherited as an autosomal recessive trait, has an incidence of about 1 in 500,000. Homozygosity usually is associated with a significant bleeding tendency; hemarthrosis may occur at levels below one percent.

Factor V Deficiency, an autosomal recessive defect, may be due to decreased synthesis of the normal protein or synthesis of a non-functional variant. Platelet factor V is decreased in the rare autosomal dominant trait initially designated Factor V Quebec, and more recently referred to as Quebec Platelet Disorder (Section 30).

Prothrombin Deficiency, a rare autosomal recessive trait, may be present as hypoprothrombinemia or as dysprothrombinemia. A variety of mutations that result in substitution, deletion, or insertion of a single nucleotide have been identified. The severity of bleeding is variable.

Combined Deficiency of Factor V and Factor VIII. This is an autosomal recessive disorder associated with a moderate bleeding tendency; plasma levels of factors V and VIII range from 5% to 30% of normal. Factors V and VIII have both a structural and functional homology, and follow a similar post-translational pathway from the endoplasmic reticulum (ER) through the Golgi apparatus before exiting the cell. Efficient export of these factors requires the participation of ERGIC-53. This protein resides in the ER-Golgi intermediate compartment (ERGIC), a vesicular organelle essential to the secretory pathway. A defect in the *ERGIC-53* gene has been found in over 70% of patients with the combined V/VIII deficiency.

Combined Congenital Deficiency of the Vitamin K-dependent Proteins is very rare. There is reduced γ-carboxylation of factors II, VII, IX, X, and proteins C and S due to interruption of the oxidation-reduction cycle of vitamin K (Section 28). Two mutations have been identified: one in the gene for vitamin K_1-carboxylase and the second in the gene for K_1 epoxide reductase.

Disseminated Intravascular Coagulation (DIC)

Acute DIC usually presents as a catastrophic event with both arterial and venous thrombosis and bleeding into skin and mucous membranes. DIC is initiated by multiple mechanisms including: overwhelming bacterial sepsis, severe traumatic tissue injury, acute hemolytic transfusion reactions, acute promyelocytic leukemia, and obstetrical accidents (abruptio placentae and amniotic-fluid embolism). The process is the result of tissue factor release into the circulation with widespread activation of coagulation proteins; the production of thrombin results in intravascular deposition of fibrin and thrombotic occlusion of small vessels. Circulating micro-particles contribute to the process. These particles are derived from the cell membrane of activated platelets during the process of membrane remodeling as the anionic phospholipids are exposed on the plasma membrane; the micro-particles provide additional catalytic surfaces for the assembly of procoagulant enzyme complexes. Thrombocytopenia develops as platelets are activated and consumed in intravascular thrombi. Fibrin strands, that intersect the lumen of small vessels, shear off pieces of erythrocytes causing hemolysis and leaving tell-tales schistocytes as evidence of the process. This microangiopathic hemolytic anemia is amplified by complement-induced hemolysis.

Secondary activation of the lytic system with release of plasmin into the general circulation results in proteolysis of factors V and VIII and fibrinogen; fibrinogen degradation products (FDPs) appear in the plasma and urine. As thrombin is released into the circulation, there is depletion of its inhibitor ATIII. Unopposed thrombin induces activation of leukocytes, vascular smooth muscle cells and endothelial cells, with increased expression of inflammatory cytokines; the enhanced inflammatory process results in further tissue damage. Activation of the kinin system leads to increased vascular permeability with development of hypotension and shock. Laboratory findings include: prolonged PT and APTT, decreased levels of factors V and VIII, low fibrinogen, presence of soluble fibrin monomers and FDPs; D-dimers denote lysis of crosslinked fibrin. Plasma ATIII levels are markedly reduced.

Chronic (compensated) DIC may be associated with malignant tumours, aortic aneurysms and other vascular anomalies such as giant hemangiomas (Kasabach-Merritt syndrome). In these situations, there is local activation of coagulation with depletion of coagulation factors and platelets. As the process develops more slowly, the continuing synthesis of coagulation factors and inhibitors maintains the circulating level of these elements at near normal levels, although FDPs are elevated and D-dimers are present (Section 29). These patients may present with thrombotic events.

SUGGESTED READING

Bick R. Disseminated intravascular coagulation: pathophysiological mechanisms and manifesttions. Sem Thromb Haemost 24:3-18, 1998.

Broze GJ. Tissue factor pathway inhibitor and the revised theory of coagulation. Annu Rev Med 46:103-112, 1995.

Butenas S, van't Veer C, Mann KG. "Normal" Thrombin Generation. Blood 7:2169-2178, 1999.

Davie EW. Biochemical and molecular aspects of the coagulation cascade. Thromb Hemost 74:1-6, 1995.

Hoffman M, Monroe DM, Oliver JA, Roberts HR. Factors IXa and Xa play distinct roles in tissue factor-dependent initiation of coagulation. Blood 86:1794-1801, 1995.

Hoffman M, Monroe DM. A cell-based model of hemostasis. Thromb Haemost 85:958-965, 2001.

Levi M, tenCate H. Disseminated intravascular coagulation. N Engl J Med 341:586-592, 1999.

Mann KG. Biochemistry and physiology of blood coagulation. Thromb Haemost 82:165-174, 1999.

Nichols WC, Ginsburg D. From the ER to the Golgi: insights from the study of combined factors V and VIII deficiency. Am J Hum Genet 64:1493-1498, 1999.

Nichols WC, Terry VH, Wheatley MA, Yhang A, Zivelin A, et al. ERGIC-53 gene structure and mutation analysis in 19 combined factors V and VIII deficiency families. Blood 7:2261-2266, 1999.

Prydz H, Camerer E, Rottingen J, et al. Cellular consequences of the initiation of blood coagulation. Thromb Haemost 82:183-192, 1999.

Rapaport SI, Rao LVM. The tissue factor pathway: how it has become a "prima ballerina." Thromb Hemost 74:7-17, 1995.

Schmaier AH, Rajkjaer R. Shariat-Madar Z. Activation of the plasma kallikrein/kinin system on cells: a revised hypothesis. Thromb Haemost 82:226-233, 1999.

Zwaal RFA, Comfurius P, Bevers EM. Lipid-protein interactions in blood coagulation. Biochem Biophys Acta 1376:433-453, 1998.

REGULATORS OF COAGULATION

For every action there is an equal and opposite reaction –
Newton's Third Law of Motion.

Because the initiation of blood coagulation in response to injury is immediate, the amplification great, and the time from activation to fibrin production rapid, it is essential that the activity be confined and limited. Prevention of generalized systemic propagation depends upon a series of circulating inhibitors and membrane-bound molecules expressed on the surface of intact endothelial cells. The physiological regulators include tissue factor pathway inhibitor, antithrombin III, thrombomodulin, and proteins C and S.

Tissue Factor Pathway Inhibitor (TFPI) (Figure 25-1)

The targets for this physiological inhibitor are factor Xa and the factor VIIa/tissue factor complex. TFPI is a 42kD glycoprotein, synthesized and secreted primarily by vascular endothelial cells; about 8% is present in platelets. TFPI circulates in plasma associated with lipoprotein; it is increased after heparin infusion possibly by release from endothelial cells and released from platelets on stimulation with thrombin. It directly inhibits factor Xa by binding at or near the active site of the enzyme. The Xa-TFPI complex then interacts with and inhibits the VIIa/tissue factor proteolytic activity. Note: inhibition of the VIIa/TF complex is dependent upon the prior activation of factor X.

Antithrombin III (ATIII)

The terms antithrombin III and antithrombin (AT) are used interchangeably. (ATIII was the original designation for this protein, assigned when antithrombin activity had been attributed to six separate thrombin-protein interactions). ATIII is a glycoprotein homologous to other members of the family of serine protease inhibitors (**serpins**) that includes α_2-antiplasmin and α_1-antitrypsin. It is synthesized in liver parenchymal cells. ATIII circulates in a quiescent form that slowly reacts with and irreversibly inhibits most of the activated zymogens in the coagulation pathway. The primary targets are thrombin and factor Xa, but ATIII also inhibits IXa, XIa, XIIa, and VIIa (within the VIIa/tissue factor complex). Inhibition of these serine proteases occurs through formation of tight equimolar (1:1) covalent complexes between the active serine site of the coagulation factor and the exposed reactive site of ATIII; these complexes are removed rapidly from the circulation. Although the plasma ATIII level far exceeds the levels of the target factors, there is little interference with coagulation because the rate of ATIII inhibition is relatively slow – the reactive site of ATIII is incompletely exposed in the circulation. In contrast, when ATIII is bound to heparin (H) or heparan sulfate (HS), the reactive site is

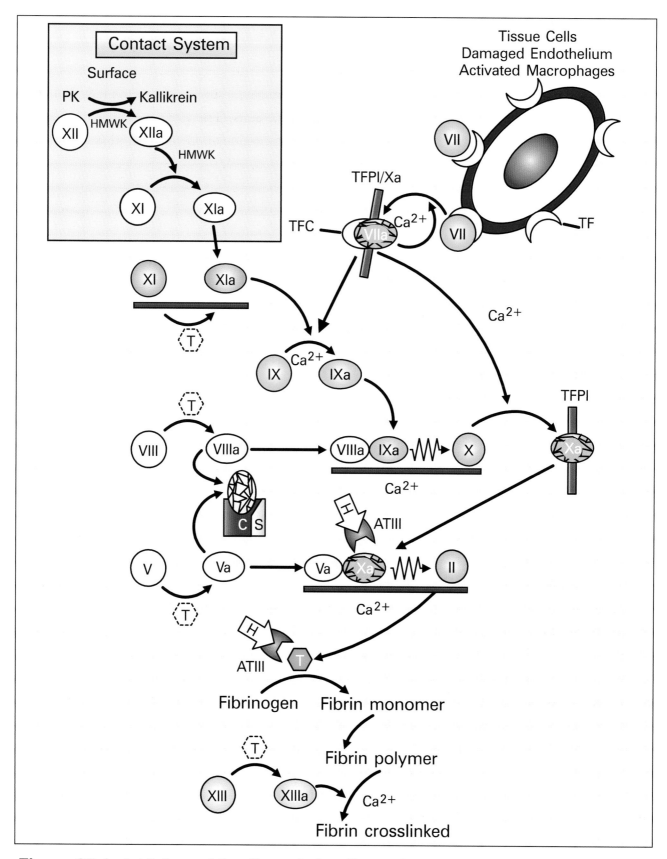

Figure 25-1　Inhibitors of the Coagulation Cascade

exposed and the rate of ATIII inhibition of the activated coagulation factors is accelerated over a thousand fold.

Heparin and heparan sulfate (proteoglycans) augment the activity of ATIII. Proteoglycans consist of glycosaminoglycans (long unbranched sugar polymers) attached to a core protein. **Heparin** is synthesized and stored in mast cells. The physiological function of heparin appears to be the regulation of mediators of inflammation and immunity (histamine and proteases) present in the cytoplasmic granules of the mast cell. Heparin is not present in blood and therefore may not be a physiological regulator of blood coagulation, although it is used therapeutically for this purpose. Specific sulfated pentasaccharide units in heparin glycosaminoglycans can bind ATIII, inducing a conformational change in the reactive site of ATIII that markedly increases ATIII-protease interactions; thrombin and factor Xa are the primary targets. Heparin/ATIII effectively inhibits thrombin activity – preventing thrombin conversion of fibrinogen to fibrin and also thrombin activation of factors V, VIII, XI and XIII.

The **heparans,** heparin-like proteoglycans, are components of the extracellular matrix and are abundant on cell surfaces. Heparan sulfate is present on endothelial cell membranes; specific pentasaccharide sequences on heparan sulfate bind ATIII, enhancing its physiological inactivation of coagulation proteases.

The Protein C Anticoagulant Pathway (Figure 25-2)

This pathway has a primary role in the regulation of thrombin formation and the prevention of microvascular thrombosis. The antithrombotic mechanism is complex, involving interaction of multiple proteins on cell surfaces. The major players are thrombin, thrombomodulin, proteins C and S. The targets are the cofactors Va and VIIIa – factors that are critical to the generation of thrombin.

Protein C is activated by the intravascular generation of thrombin (T). Excess thrombin, formed at sites of vessel injury, is washed downstream and binds to the endothelial transmembrane protein **thrombomodulin (TM)**. This high-affinity binding inhibits thrombin procoagulant activity and its ability to activate platelets; as TM binds thrombin through its fibrinogen-binding site, thrombin cleavage of fibrinogen is inhibited. TM now promotes stereochemical association of the active thrombin site with the cleavage site on protein C. Thus, TM acts as a molecular switch as it diverts thrombin from a procoagulant to an anticoagulant pathway.

Protein C is a vitamin K-dependent plasma protein with a half-life of eight to ten hours – significantly shorter than the other vitamin K-dependent coagulation factors with the exception of factor VII. Both protein C and its activated form (APC) bind reversibly to anionic phospholipid membranes in the presence of Ca^{2+}. Thrombin, bound to TM, cleaves a 12 residue peptide from the heavy chain of protein C converting it to the serine protease **activated protein C (APC)**. The affinity of the thrombin-TM complex for protein C is amplified when

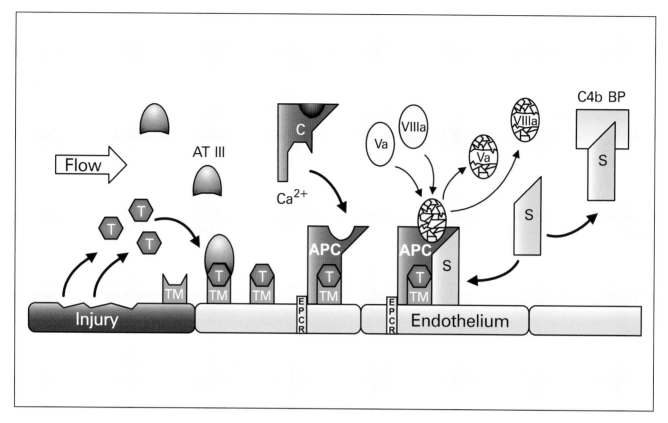

Figure 25-2 Protein C - Anticoagulant Pathway

protein C is bound to the **endothelial cell protein C receptor (EPCR)** – a transmembrane protein expressed at high levels on endothelial cells of large vessels and at lower levels in the capillaries of the microcirculation. Protein C is activated on the endothelial cell surface by the thrombin/TM/EPCR complex.

Protein S is homologous to the other vitamin K-dependent plasma proteins but is not a serine protease precursor. It functions as a cofactor to protein C – APC activity is increased ten-fold in the presence of protein S. In the circulation, sixty percent of protein S is associated with a regulatory protein of the complement system, **C4b-binding protein (C4bBP)**. Only free unbound protein S binds to and functions as a cofactor for APC; C4bBP appears to have a significant regulatory role in protein S cofactor activity. Protein S probably functions by positioning the active site of APC for optimal cleavage of substrate.

Proteins C and S assemble on the phospholipid surfaces of endothelium and platelets via their vitamin K-dependent γ-carboxyglutamic acid (Gla) binding sites (Section 28). Once APC is generated, it binds in a complex with its cofactor protein S; this complex now inactivates factors Va and VIIIa by cleavage at arginine sites. **Factor Va** is cleaved rapidly at Arg506, followed by slower cleavage at Arg306. Cleavage at Arg506 reduces factor Va activity; cleavage at Arg306 completely inactivates Va. Protein S enhances the rate of APC cleavage at Arg306. Proteolysis of **factor VIIIa** by APC occurs at two sites: cleavage at Arg336 in the A1 domain of VIIIa and/or cleavage at Arg562 in the A2 subunit result in loss of VIIIa cofactor activity (Figure 26-1). The cleavage at Arg562 is accelerated by protein S.

Other interactions have an impact on this pathway: (1) both factor V and protein S function synergistically as cofactors in the inactivation of factor VIIIa by APC; (2) protein S has anticoagulant activity independent of its cofactor role with APC – by binding to factors Va and Xa, protein S inhibits the prothrombinase activity of the factor Va-Xa complex assembled on endothelial cells and platelet membranes; (3) factor Va bound to prothrombin on membrane surfaces is resistant to inactivation by APC – thus, prothrombin appears to modulate the anticoagulant activity of APC (for clinical relevance, see Prothrombin 20210A in Clinical Correlates).

ATIII neutralization of thrombin is enhanced when thrombin is bound to TM on the endothelial surface – the activity of ATIII accelerated through interaction with cell surface heparans. The inactive thrombin/ATIII complex dissociates from TM and is cleared rapidly in the liver. The removal of thrombin prevents further protein C activation. Thus, when generation of thrombin at the site of injury ceases, activation of protein C also is terminated. Three plasma proteases are responsible for inactivation of APC: the protein C inhibitor, α_1-antitrypsin and α_2-macroglobulin. **Protein C inhibitor** is a serpin that inhibits a number of serine proteases, although it was originally identified as an inhibitor of APC. It is a major inhibitor of thrombin bound to TM; its inhibition of free thrombin is significantly slower. Note the multiple interactions that contribute to TM anticoagulant activity: (1) TM blocks thrombin coagulant activity, (2) it accelerates thrombin activation of protein C, (3) it enhances ATIII clearance of thrombin from the circulation, and (4) it augments the inhibition of thrombin by the protein C inhibitor. (TM also has a role in limiting fibrinolysis as thrombin bound to TM activates the fibrinolytic inhibitor TAFI – Section 29).

Table 25-1   Regulators of Coagulation

Regulator	Site of Synthesis	Primary Target
TFPI	Endothelium	Xa, VIIa/TF
ATIII	Liver	Thrombin, Xa
TM	Endothelium	Thrombin, Protein C
EPCR	Endothelium	Protein C
Protein C	Liver	Va, VIIIa
Protein S	Liver	Protein C Cofactor

CLINICAL CORRELATES

THROMBOPHILIA

Thrombophilia is defined as a tendency to thrombosis. Clinical disease most frequently is precipitated by the interaction of two or more predisposing risk factors, genetic and acquired. Acquired or environmental factors that influence the thrombotic risk include immobilization, infection, pregnancy, the use of oral contraceptives, surgery and malignant disease. A variety of genetic defects or polymorphisms are associated with the development of thrombotic disease:

ATIII Deficiency. Congenital deficiency of ATIII is due to either point mutations or gene deletions; inheritance is autosomal dominant with an incidence of 1/2000 - 1/5000. Patients with this defect are usually heterozygous; they have a 50% lifetime risk of venous thrombosis. The defect may be quantitative with a reduction in both ATIII antigen (protein) and activity, or qualitative with reduced ATIII functional activity although the antigen level is within the normal range. The dysfunctional variants are due to mutations that produce either a defective heparin (or heparan) binding site or interfere with ATIII binding to its target enzymes. The diagnosis of ATIII deficiency depends on the laboratory demonstration of reduced ATIII function/antigen levels. Because anticoagulants affect the plasma ATIII level, the assay should be delayed until anticoagulant therapy has been discontinued: heparin increases the rate of plasma ATIII clearance; oral anticoagulant therapy results in reduced ATIII consumption and, therefore, in a higher plasma concentration.

Conformationally unstable variants of ATIII have been identified in families with severe episodic thrombotic disease. Normal ATIII exists in a metastable form that undergoes a conformational change to a stable form as it reacts with thrombin. ATIII variants that undergo spontaneous inappropriate transition to a stable inactive conformation (referred to as a "latent" form) result in loss of ATIII activity. A slight increase in body temperature may trigger this transition – explaining the infection-related thrombotic events that occur in some of these patients.

Acquired ATIII deficiency occurs in: 1) disseminated intravascular coagulation – as clotting factors become activated (thrombin and Xa), ATIII is consumed; 2) cirrhosis with decreased protein synthesis; and 3) nephrotic syndrome with loss of ATIII in the urine.

Protein C and Protein S Deficiencies. These are autosomally inherited disorders that result in deficient or functionally abnormal variants associated with a high risk for venous thromboembolic disease; the clinical presentation is similar. Thrombotic events tend to increase with age although serious coagulation problems occasionally do appear in childhood. Infants with homozygous deficiency of either protein C or S have an increased risk for purpura fulminans. (Mutations in other proteins of the protein C pathway, TM and EPCR, are associated with venous thrombosis).

The levels of protein C and protein S (vitamin K-dependent factors) are reduced further when deficient patients are placed on oral anticoagulants. Protein C deficient patients may develop skin necrosis during the initial phase of warfarin anticoagulation; because of its short plasma half-life, protein C levels fall more rapidly than the other vitamin K-dependent factors (except factor VII), resulting in a severely depleted protein C pool before anticoagulation is achieved. To prevent this complication, protein C deficient patients should be heparinized prior to the initiation of warfarin anticoagulant therapy.

The risk of thrombotic disease in these patients is increased in gram-negative sepsis. This is related in part to the endotoxin-induced depression of thrombomodulin expression by endothelial cells, resulting in decreased protein C activation. In addition, with a rise in the level of circulating C4bBP (an acute phase reactant) there is increased protein S binding and a decrease in available free protein S. Post-infectious purpura fulminans has been documented in children with an acquired protein S deficiency due to autoantibodies directed against protein S; most reported cases have been associated with varicella.

Activated Protein C (APC) Resistance: Factor V Leiden. Congenital APC resistance is associated with an increased risk of venous thrombotic disease. The most common cause is a point mutation in the factor V gene that results in a single amino acid substitution (arginine 506 to glutamine) at the APC cleavage site. Because thrombin activation of factor V Leiden to Va is normal, the inability of activated protein C to cleave Va Leiden results in a hypercoagulable state. Inheritance is autosomal dominant. This genetic polymorphism has a high frequency of approximately 5 percent in Caucasians. Congenital deficiencies of ATIII, protein C, and protein S together account for about 5 percent of cases of deep vein thrombosis (DVTs); in Caucasians, APC resistance is estimated to account for 20 percent of DVTs.

In addition to factor V Leiden, APC resistance with an increased risk of thromboembolic disease is associated with the rare factor V mutation (arginine 306 to threonine), designated factor V Cambridge. APC resistance has been demonstrated in some patients in the absence of either mutation – other causes of APC resistance await identification.

Prothrombin 20210A is a risk factor for venous thrombosis. This common genetic variant is characterized by a single G to A nucleotide substitution at position 20210 in the $3'$-untranslated region of the prothrombin gene. An associated increase in plasma prothrombin concentration may be responsible for the increased thrombotic risk: because factor Va bound in the prothrombin-Va complex is resistant to APC inactivation, the higher prothrombin levels may increase the $t_{1/2}$ of Va by protecting it from APC cleavage. (The reason for the elevated plasma prothrombin levels has not been determined). The prevalence of this mutation in Caucasians is approximately 2%. The risk of venous thrombosis is compounded in patients heterozygous for both prothrombin 20210A and factor V Leiden.

Table 25-2   Antiphospholipid Syndrome

Clinical Manifestations	Primary	Secondary	Primary Antigenic Targets
Venous thrombotic disease Arterial thrombotic disease Recurrent fetal loss	No antecedent disease	Autoimmune disease Lymphomas Drugs	β_2-glycoprotein 1 Prothrombin Annexin V

Antiphospholipid Antibodies (aPL). These are a heterogeneous group of antibodies found in patients with autoimmune disorders such as collagen-vascular disease and lupus erythematosis, as well as in some apparently normal individuals. Two distinct groups of aPL antibodies are recognized. Type I antibodies are associated predominantly with infections (they may appear transiently after acute infections, and persist in chronic infections such as hepatitis C and HIV). They bind to phospholipid *in vitro* but appear to have no clinical significance. Type II antibodies are implicated in the development of thrombotic events, and frequently are associated with autoimmune disease. These antibodies do not recognize phospholipids but rather are directed against plasma proteins that bind to anionic phospholipids; the most common antigenic targets are the phospholipid-binding proteins β_2-glycoprotein 1 (β_2GP1) and prothrombin. Other possible targets are factor XI, proteins C and S, and annexin-V. The **antiphospholipid syndrome (APS)** is defined as the association of arterial or venous thrombosis, or recurrent fetal loss, with persistent aPL. In primary APS, there is no evidence of an underlying disease. APS is considered to be secondary when it occurs in association with other disorders, such as lupus or rheumatoid arthritis.

Some of these antibodies interfere with *in vitro* clotting assays and, therefore, are referred to as lupus anticoagulants although, clinically, they are associated with thrombotic events. (These "anticoagulant" antibodies were recognized originally in patients with lupus erythematosus). In the laboratory, the **lupus anticoagulant (LA)** is identified by a prolonged APTT that is corrected by additional phospholipid (provided by adding normal platelets or a phospholipid reagent to the test system). *In vitro*, prolongation of coagulation is due to the formation of high-affinity antigen-antibody complexes as LA binds to phospholipid – LA and coagulation factors compete for the same phospholipid catalytic surface. Many antiphospholipid antibodies do not interfere with clotting assays; some bind *in vitro* to cardiolipin and are known as **anticardiolipin antibodies (aCL).** They may be identified and quantitated in the laboratory using ELISA plates coated with cardiolipin. LA and aCL may be present singly or together in the same patient. LA appears to be a stronger risk factor for thrombosis than aCL.

Thrombotic disease may be due to interference with the activity of protein C, protein S,

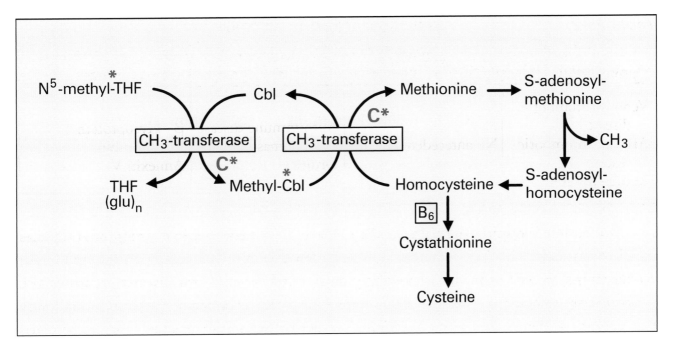

Figure 25-3   Homocysteine Metabolism

β_2GP1 or annexin-V. With the targeting of these proteins by aPL antibodies, a number of physiological processes may be compromised: proteins C and S anticoagulant activity, β_2GP1 clearance of anionic phospholipids from the circulation, and the antithrombotic function of annexin-V (it normally blocks the assembly of coagulation factor complexes on anionic phospholipid membranes). Annexin-V also is found on trophoblasts; if indeed annexin-V is the target of aPL antibodies, it may explain the placental changes that lead to fetal loss.

Hyperhomocysteinemia has been identified as an independent risk factor for atherosclerosis, cerebrovascular disease, deep vein thrombosis, and venous thromboembolism. Homocysteine is a sulfur-containing amino acid derived from the metabolism of methionine. The mechanism by which hyperhomocysteinemia acts as a thrombogenic risk factor appears to be related to its effect on the vessel wall – by inducing endothelial injury and dysfunction, thrombomodulin activity may be decreased and the vasoprotective functions of nitric oxide impaired (Section 31).

There are two homocysteine metabolic pathways: (1) Remethylation of homocysteine to methionine requires the cofactor activity of vitamin B_{12} and folate and is catalyzed by methionine synthase (a methyl transferase) – the methyl group donated by methyltetrahydrofolate via cobalamin (Section 14); methionine is converted to S-adenosylmethionine (a universal methyl donor); demethylation then regenerates homocysteine. (2) Irreversible degradation of homocysteine: transulfuration to cystathionine is catalyzed by cystathionine β-synthase (CBS) with pyridoxal $5'$ phosphate (vitamin B_6) as cofactor (Figure 25-3).

Severe congenital hyperhomocysteinemia (plasma levels above 100 μmol/L) is the result of defects in the metabolic pathways: 90% of cases are due to a homozygous deficiency of CBS, some 10% to defects in methylenetetrahydrofolate reductase (MTHFR). Patients present with venous thromboembolism, mental retardation and skeletal abnormalities.

Mild or moderate disease (plasma levels 16-100 μmol/L) is associated with genetic defects that cause a 50 percent reduction in one of the metabolic pathways: heterozygosity for CBS or MTHFR deficiency, or homozygosity for the C677T (alanine 677 → valine) MTHFR mutation. The latter is a thermolabile variant of MTHFR, present in up to 10% of healthy individuals; it has half the catalytic activity of the normal MTHFR enzyme. In mild disease, when folic acid levels are adequate, plasma homocysteine levels may remain normal. If random plasma levels are within the normal range (5-15 μmol/L), the abnormality may become apparent only by stressing the homocysteine/methionine pathway with oral methionine loading. Mild or moderate hyperhomocysteinemia is considered a risk factor for myocardial infarction, stroke, and other arterial thrombotic disease. Venous thrombosis may occur in the presence of additional risk factors.

Acquired hyperhomocysteinemia occurs with deficiencies of the vitamin cofactors, B_{12}, B_6 and folate, and with renal insufficiency. Vitamin deficiencies probably are responsible for the increased homocysteine levels in most subjects – the elderly are particularly vulnerable. Drugs, such as methotrexate, theophylline, and anticonvulsants that interfere in the metabolic pathway, may induce hyperhomocysteinemia.

Other genetic disorders that may be associated with thrombophilia include: dysfibrinogenemia, plasminogen deficiency or dysplasminogenemia, and factor XII deficiency (Sections 24 and 29). Dysfibrinogenemia, inherited in either a recessive or dominant manner, most commonly is associated with thrombotic events, rarely with bleeding. Mutations in thrombomodulin have been associated with myocardial infarction and venous thrombosis. Endothelial cell protein C receptor (EPCR) mutations carry a risk of venous and arterial thrombosis. Elevated plasma levels of normal coagulation factors (prothrombin, factors VIII, VII, and fibrinogen) and the fibrinolytic inhibitor PAI-1 confer a predisposition to thromboembolic events.

THERAPEUTIC (PHARMACOLOGICAL) INHIBITORS

The Antithrombins

Unfractionated Heparin. Heparin is a proteoglycan present in mast cell secretory granules. Pharmaceutical preparations, isolated from bovine lung or porcine gut, consist of a heterogeneous mixture of glycosaminoglycans ranging in size from 3 kD to 30 kD. Heparin anticoagulant activity is mediated through its interaction with plasma ATIII. This interaction induces a conformational change in ATIII that accelerates its binding to factor Xa and thrombin

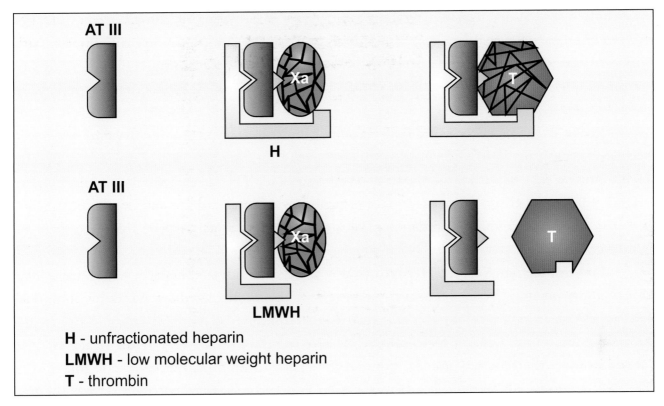

H - unfractionated heparin
LMWH - low molecular weight heparin
T - thrombin

Figure 25-4   Antithrombin III

(as well as other activated coagulation factors). Inactivation of Xa depends only on its binding to heparin-activated ATIII. In contrast, inhibition of thrombin requires the formation of a ternary complex: activated ATIII, a segment of the heparin molecule and thrombin. Heparin chains must be of sufficient length (present in unfractionated heparin) to bind simultaneously to both ATIII and thrombin. Because the reaction of heparin with ATIII is rapid, anticoagulation is achieved immediately upon intravenous injection. The half-life ($t_{1/2}$) of plasma heparin ranges from 1 to 2 hours – dependent upon the size of the intravenous bolus. Because of the short $t_{1/2}$, therapy usually is initiated by administration of a bolus injection followed by continuous intravenous infusion. Low dose prophylactic heparin may be administered subcutaneously. The APTT is useful for clinical monitoring; the specific heparin anti-Xa assay is preferred when there is prolongation of the APTT for other reasons (eg, the presence of a lupus anticoagulant).

   Heparin-induced thrombocytopenia (HIT), a complication of heparin therapy, is an immune disorder that may be accompanied by thrombosis. Heparin induces mild platelet activation with release of platelet factor 4 (PF4) molecules from platelet α-granules. PF4 binds to heparin forming immunogenic complexes that may stimulate production of IgG antibodies – these antibodies recognize conformational epitopes present on PF4 after it has bound to heparin. When the antibody binds to the heparin/PF4 complex, the Fc domain of the antibody reacts with the platelet surface Fcγ receptor. Clustering of the receptors results in platelet activation, aggregation, release of granule contents, and formation of thrombogenic platelet-derived microparticles that accelerate thrombin generation. In addition, the antibody may react with PF4 bound to heparan sulfate on the surface of endothelial cells: immunoinjury results in activation of the endothelial cells and upregulation of tissue factor expression, further enhancing thrombin generation.

In the event of heparin-induced thrombocytopenia (HIT), prompt discontinuation of heparin therapy is indicated. Anticoagulation may be maintained using other agents: antithrombins such as hirudin derivatives or a heparinoid. The latter, a low molecular weight glycosaminoglycan tissue extract (containing primarily heparan sulfate and dermatan sulfate), however, may exhibit minor immunological cross-reactivity with heparin. Synthetic heparin pentasaccharide derivatives appear promising.

Low Molecular Weight Heparin (LMWH) is a fractionated heparin with a molecular size of approximately 5 kD. Its anticoagulant effect also is mediated by ATIII binding. The LMWH/ATIII complex exhibits a relatively higher binding affinity for factor Xa than for thrombin: the shorter heparin molecules, while able to bind avidly to ATIII, are of insufficient length to form the ternary complex required for major thrombin inactivation (Figure 25-4). Therefore the anti-Xa assay, rather than the APTT, is recommended for monitoring LMWH levels. Because LMWH binds less avidly to plasma proteins and endothelium, it has a longer plasma half-life – approximately two to four times longer than unfractionated heparin. As a result, LMWH plasma levels can be maintained by administration of one or two daily doses. The incidence of thrombocytopenia is lower with LMWH therapy than with unfractionated heparin.

Hirudin, a polypeptide obtained from leech salivary gland, is a direct inhibitor of thrombin. It binds bivalently to the active proteolytic site and to the substrate recognition site of the enzyme, thus inhibiting thrombin participation in the coagulation cascade. ATIII does not participate in this reaction. Recombinant hirudin is available for clinical use.

Defibrinogenating Agents

A number of snake venoms are capable of depleting circulating fibrinogen. These venom proteases, in contrast to thrombin, cleave fibrinopeptide A but not fibrinopeptide B. The residual fibrinogen molecule is removed from the circulation without conversion to fibrin. Malayan Pit Viper venom (**ancrod or arvin**) depletes circulating fibrinogen directly without involvement of other coagulation factors. Therapy is monitored by assaying plasma fibrinogen levels.

Vitamin K Antagonists

The anticoagulants in this group are oral agents with structures related to bishydroxycoumarin; dicoumarol and warfarin are the preparations in common clinical use. These agents interrupt the vitamin K cycle by inhibition of vitamin K epoxide reductase, thus producing a functional vitamin K deficit. As a result, γ-carboxylation of the glutamic acid residues on the vitamin K-dependent proteins is blocked and their functional activity reduced; synthesis of the non-carboxylated inactive precursors continues (Section 28). Anticoagulation can be reversed within 4-6 hours by intravenous vitamin K_1.

The rate of response to warfarin is variable. There is evidence that genetic variation in the cytochrome p450 system influences the individual dose requirements and explains the need for careful monitoring of patients during the induction of anticoagulant therapy.

———————— •••●●●●●●• ————————

SUGGESTED READING

Aithal GP, Day CP, Kesteven PJ, et al. Association of polymorphisms in the cytochrome p450 CYP2C9 with warfarin dose requirement and risk of bleeding complications. Lancet 353: 717-719, 1999.

Brandt JT, Barna LK, Triplett DA. Laboratory identification of lupus anticoagulants: results of the second international workshop for identification of lupus anticoagulants. Thromb Haemost 74:1597-1603, 1995.

Carrell RW, Huntington JA, Mushunje A, Zhou A. The conformational basis of thrombosis. Thromb Haemost 86:14-22, 2001.

Clark, P, Greer IA, Walker ID. Interaction of the protein C/protein S anticoagulant system, the endothelium and pregnancy. Blood Rev 13: 127-146, 1999.

D'Angelo A, Selhub J. Homocysteine and thrombotic disease. Blood 90:1-11, 1997.

Esmon CT. Regulation of blood coagulation. Biochim Biophys Acta 1477:349-360, 2000.

Fuentes-Prior P, Iwanaga Y, Huber R, Pagila R, Rumennik G, et al. Structural basis for the anticoagulant activity of the thrombin-thrombomodulin complex. Nature 404:518-525, 2000.

Greaves M, Cohen H, Machin SJ, Mackie I. Guidelines on the investigation and management of the antiphospholipid syndrome. Br J Haematol 109:704-715, 2000.

Hillarp A, Dahlback B, Zoller B. Activated protein C resistance: from phenotype to genotype and clinical practice. Blood Rev 9:201-212, 1995.

Lane DA, Mannucci PM, Bauer KA, et al. Inherited Thrombophilia. Thromb Haemost 76:651-662 and 824-834, 1996.

Lane DA, Grant PJ. Role of hemostatic gene polymorphisms in venous and arterial thrombotic disease. Blood 95:1517-1532, 2000.

Mammen EF. Antithrombin: its physiological importance and role in DIC. Semin Thromb Haemost 24:19-25, 1998.

O'Brien LM, Mastri M, Fay PJ. Regulation of factor VIIIa by human activated protein C and protein S: inactivation of cofactor in the intrinsic factor Xase. Blood 95:1714-1720, 2000.

Rand JH, Wu X. Antibody-mediated disruption of the annexin-V antithrombotic shield: a new mechanism for thrombosis in the antiphospholipid syndrome. Thromb Haemost 82:649-655, 1999.

Rosendaal FR. Venous thrombosis: a multicausal disease. Lancet 353:1167-1173, 1999.

Taylor FB, Peer GT, Lockhart MS, Ferrell G, Esmon CT. Endothelial cell protein C receptor plays an important role in protein C activation in vivo. Blood 97:1685-1688, 2001.

Warkentin TE. Heparin-induced thrombocytopenia: a ten-year retrospective. Annu Rev Med 50:129-147, 1999.

FACTOR VIII AND FACTOR IX

"It is a surprising circumstance that males only are subject to this affliction (hemorrhagic disposition)."
"Although females are exempt, they are still capable of transmitting it to their male children."

J.C. Otto – 1803

Hemophilia, the most common of the severe congenital bleeding disorders, is due to the decrease or absence of functional factor VIII or factor IX. As early as the fifth century, it was recognized as a sex-linked defect. The risk of fatal bleeding at the time of infant circumcision in some families was acknowledged in the Talmud and rules pertaining to circumcision in these families were formulated. That the clinical disease is due to abnormalities in two distinct proteins was recognized in 1953 with the identification of factor IX by Biggs and McFarlane.

Factor VIII

Factor VIII has no intrinsic enzymatic activity – it functions as a cofactor to accelerate the activation of factor X by factor IXa. The liver appears to be the primary site of synthesis and the hepatocyte the major factor VIII-producing cell. The level of factor VIII in the circulation is very low (100ng/mL); as it is an acute phase reactant, levels increase with metabolic stress, vigorous exercise and pregnancy.

The factor VIII gene is one of the largest, spanning 186,000 base pairs on the X chromosome in proximity to the locus of the factor IX gene. It has major sequence homology with the gene for factor V. The primary molecular organization of factor VIII involves three structural units assembled in six discrete domains: A1-A2-B-A3-C1-C2 (Figure 26-1). Factor VIII is synthesized as a single-chain protein. In the endoplasmic reticulum, it undergoes post-translational modification that includes protein glycosylation and sulfation. Transport from the ER to the Golgi apparatus involves an intracellular membrane lectin, endoplasmic reticulum-Golgi intermediate compartment-53: ERGIC-53. (A mutation in the *ERGIC-53* gene is responsible for congenital combined factor V/factor VIII deficiency: Section 24). Limited proteolysis in the Golgi apparatus generates the two-chain heterodimer: the heavy chain (A1-A2-B) and the light chain (A3-C1-C2). These chains remain noncovalently associated through the A1 and A3 domains. When this heterodimer is secreted into the circulation, it immediately associates with von Willebrand factor (vWF) in a tight noncovalent complex; factor VIII binds to the vWF amino-terminal region (Figure 27-1). Two regions on the light chain of factor VIII (one at the amino-terminal of A3, the other in the carboxy-terminus of C2) are binding sites for vWF. In the three-dimensional configuration of the functional VIII molecule, close proximity of these two sites may provide a high-affinity binding site for vWF. The A and C domains are required for factor VIII procoagulant function; the role of the B domain is not known.

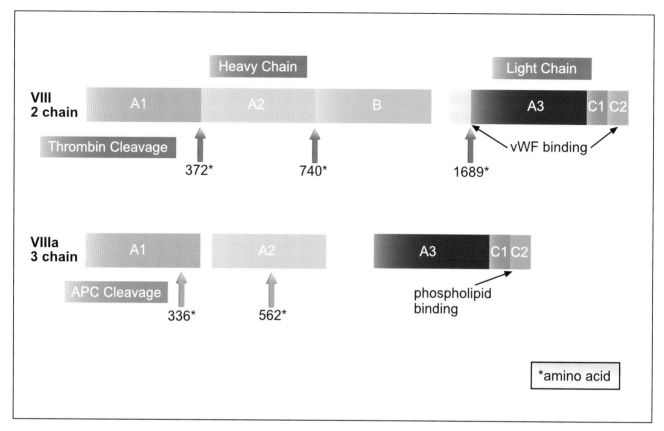

Figure 26-1   Factor VIII Molecule

In vitro, each subunit of the multimeric vWF molecule has the potential to bind one molecule of factor VIII. *In vivo*, changes in the plasma vWF level are accompanied by similar changes in the level of factor VIII: patients deficient in vWF also have low levels of factor VIII. Factor VIII bound to vWF has a half-life of 12 hours; free unbound factor VIII is rapidly degraded ($t_{1/2}$ of 0.5 hours). vWF-bound factor VIII is resistant to all proteolytic enzymes with the exception of thrombin. Proteolytic cleavage of the factor VIII light chain by thrombin frees VIII from vWF; subsequent cleavage of the heavy chain releases the B domain with conversion of the molecule to the three chain active factor VIIIa; the three chains are: A1, A2, and A3-C1-C2. The cofactor activity of factor VIIIa is the result of this cleavage-dependent configurational change.

When factor VIII is complexed with vWF, it cannot bind to phospholipid membranes; factor VIIIa binds readily. Phospholipid-bound factor VIIIa functions as a cofactor in the tenase complex (factors VIIIa, IXa, and X), inducing a conformational change in the factor IXa protease domain that markedly enhances the rate of factor IXa activation of factor X. Factor VIIIa is labile – spontaneous dissociation with loss of the A2 domain results in rapid loss of tenase activity. Selective proteolytic cleavage of factors Va and VIIIa by activated protein C (APC), in the presence of protein S, limits and regulates hemostasis (Section 25). The APC cleavage sites are indicated in Figure 26-1.

Factor IX

Factor IX is a vitamin K-dependent protein that circulates in plasma as the inactive zymogen. The zymogen has a molecular weight of 56 kD; its half-life in plasma is approximately 24 hours. The molecule is described and compared to other vitamin K-dependent proteins in Section 28. Activation of factor IX takes place on phospholipid membranes, initially by the tissue factor complex (TF/VIIa) and, subsequently, by factor Xa and factor XIa. Its role in hemostasis is described in Section 24.

CLINICAL CORRELATES

HEMOPHILIA

Hemophilia is a congenital sex-linked recessive hemorrhagic diathesis that gained notoriety as the scourge of European royal families. Genetic defects resulting in deficiencies of factor VIII or factor IX give rise to hemophilia A or hemophilia B, respectively. Approximately 30% of cases are the result of *de novo* (spontaneous) mutations. The incidence of the disease approximates 20 to 25 per 100,000 males; factor VIII deficiency accounts for about 85% of cases. The clinical picture in hemophilia A and B is similar: easy bruising, excessive bleeding following trauma or surgical procedures, and spontaneous joint and muscle hemorrhage. As platelet-vascular function is not compromised, the bleeding time and bleeding from minor cuts or abrasions are usually not abnormal.

With initiation of coagulation, factor IX is activated by the VIIa/tissue factor complex, and subsequently by thrombin-activated factor XI. Factor VIII is activated by thrombin. Factor IXa in conjunction with VIIIa activates factor X (Figure 24-1). The participation of factors IXa and VIIIa is critical for normal hemostasis – witnessed by the severe hemorrhagic diathesis associated with deficiencies of either protein.

Hemophilia A

The defects in the factor VIII gene on the X chromosome include: large deletions, small deletions and point mutations; intrachromosomal inversion of intron 22 is present in almost 50% of patients with severe hemophilia. More than 250 missense mutations in the factor VIII molecule have been identified. The severity of clinical manifestations depends upon the level of normally functioning factor VIII: severe bleeders have less than 1% functional factor VIII in circulating plasma, moderate bleeders 1-5%, and mild bleeders 5-30%. Major deletions of the VIII gene may result in complete absence of the factor VIII protein; these patients are antigen-negative. In antigen-positive patients, a functionally abnormal protein is present in the plasma. Patients lacking antigen are designated as CRM negative, and those expressing antigen as CRM positive (CRM: cross-reactive material).

Defects in the factor VIII gene in males is manifest by hemophilia A, in females by the carrier state. In carrier females, the defective X chromosome is present in approximately half the factor VIII-synthesizing cells, resulting in a 50% reduction of functional VIII levels. Most carriers do not have bleeding problems. The demonstration of a reduced factor VIII level is useful in carrier identification; however, as some carriers have factor VIII levels within the broad normal range, accurate carrier detection depends upon molecular genetic analysis. In the majority of families, DNA polymorphisms in linkage analysis provides accurate identification. In families with severe hemophilia A, the presence of the inversion mutation in intron 22 is diagnostic. Chorionic villus sampling in the first trimester permits prenatal diagnosis.

Hemophilia B

Hemophilia B is due to a deficiency of factor IX activity. The genetic abnormalities of the factor IX gene on the X chromosome include: large deletions, small deletions, point mutations, and missense mutations. Hemophilia B may be characterized immunologically as either antigen-negative or antigen-positive. The large deletions responsible for severe disease are associated with absence of detectable antigen. Antigen-positive hemophilia B occurs in about one-third of patients – the plasma level of the antigen may be normal but the protein is dysfunctional. The clinical presentation is heterogenous: severe disease is associated with less than 1% functional factor IX, moderate disease with 1-5% and mild disease with 5-25%. The level of factor IX in female carriers is usually about 50%; occasional carriers with levels under 20% present with a bleeding disorder.

Laboratory findings

APTT and PT are the standard laboratory screening tests: the PT is normal in hemophilia; the APTT is markedly prolonged in severe hemophilia and usually moderately prolonged in milder disease. In mild disease, the APTT may be within the normal range – in these patients, the clinical and family history of hemorrhage is a more reliable indicator of a bleeding disorder. Specific assays that measure factor VIII or factor IX functional activity provide a more definitive diagnosis.

Inhibitors

Inhibitors of factor VIII develop in up to 20% of hemophilia A patients, usually as an immune response to factor VIII replacement therapy. Inhibitor development is now the most serious treatment complication. Factor VIII inhibitors are polyclonal IgG molecules, predominantly of the IgG4 subclass. Because activated $CD4^+$ cells are required for antibody synthesis, existing inhibitors have disappeared in some patients with therapeutically-acquired HIV infection.

Inhibitors are significantly more frequent (up to 40%) in patients with severe hemophilia compared to those with mild disease. Severe hemophilia is more often the result of mutations, such as large deletions or inversions, that result in the absence of structurally normal circulating factor VIII antigen. Nonsense mutations causing premature translation stops which prevent factor VIII synthesis also are associated with a high incidence of inhibitors. The inhibitors are directed most frequently at epitopes in the A2 and C2 domains. Anti-A2 inhibitors block factor VIIIa function. Anti-C2 inhibitors block the binding of factor VIIIa to phospholipid, and also may interfere with vWF binding as both phospholipid and vWF bind to the carboxyl-terminus of the C2 domain. Not all patients with severe hemophilia develop clinically significant inhibitors; antibodies that do not interfere with factor VIII function usually escape detection.

Small deletions or point mutations are associated less frequently with inhibitor development; the VIII molecule, although functionally abnormal, may retain sufficient structural similarity to normal factor VIII to maintain immunological tolerance. When inhibitors do develop in these patients, they most commonly occur with mutations clustered in the same epitopes that are associated with inhibitor development in severe hemophilia. Some of these non-random mutations, such as $\text{Arg}^{593} \rightarrow \text{Cys}$ in the A2 domain, are responsible for conformational changes in the VIII molecule that make it antigenically distinct from normal VIII; inhibitors develop following exposure to exogenous factor VIII. When inhibitors develop in mild hemophilia, the patients' baseline factor VIII level is usually reduced to <1% — spontaneous bleeding in these patients may be the first indication of an inhibitor.

The risk of inhibitor development is not only related to the factor VIII genotype, it is also influenced by inherited differences such as the HLA class-II haplotype; this may account for the long recognized familial predisposition for inhibitor development. Inhibitors also develop more frequently with exposure to certain types of highly purified factor VIII concentrates; some processing methods induce antigenic changes in the molecule that render it immunogenic even in low risk patients.

Similarly, inhibitors of factor IX may develop in response to replacement therapy, and they occur most frequently in patients with gross deletions in the factor IX gene. The incidence is about 2-4% in severely affected hemophilia B patients — considerably lower than in hemophilia A. In some young children with major deletions, inhibitor development has been accompanied by anaphylactic reactions to factor IX concentrate. Inhibitors rarely develop in patients with mild disease.

Therapy

Treatment for most patients with hemophilia A and B requires replacement of factor VIII or IX with highly purified plasma-derived or recombinant factor concentrates. These agents can be used both prophylactically and therapeutically; the dose and choice of product is determined by the severity of the disease and the clinical situation. With use of recombinant preparations, the decreased exposure to human plasma reduces the risk of transfusion-transmitted disease. In the first generation recombinant factor VIII products, human albumin was added to stabilize factor VIII. In second generation recombinant factor VIII products, human albumin has been replaced by a high sucrose concentration, or by a modified recombinant factor VIII molecule – factor VIII lacking the large B domain is less sensitive to proteolytic degradation and does not require the addition of albumin. The recombinant factor IX preparations are formulated without addition of human plasma proteins. However, the recovery of factor IX (in the circulation) is lower than with plasma-derived factor IX – probably related to subtle structural differences in the recombinant product.

Patients with mild hemophilia A also can be treated with a synthetic analogue of vasopressin (DDAVP) – it induces a transient increase of factor VIII two to three times above baseline levels. As responses vary, preliminary DDAVP testing is recommended prior to selecting this agent for therapeutic use.

Treatment of hemophilia A patients with high titre inhibitors not responsive to factor VIII replacement requires the use of alternative agents. Low cross-reactivity of the inhibitor to porcine factor VIII makes this a valuable therapeutic agent. Products that bypass factor VIII (prothrombin complex concentrates or recombinant factor VIIa) are therapeutic alternatives. The induction of immune tolerance in patients with high titre inhibitors is achieved by exposure to high doses of factor VIII for prolonged periods of time, often in concert with immunosuppression; the reduction in anti-factor VIII inhibitors correlates with the production of anti-idiotypic antibodies (i.e. anti-antibodies). Low titre inhibitors may resolve spontaneously.

Future management of severe hemophilia is likely to include gene therapy. Technical problems, including choice of viral vectors, poor expression levels, and immune response to foreign protein are being addressed. Interim results from Phase I trials support continued development of gene transfer.

ACQUIRED HEMOPHILIA

Antibodies to factor VIII also arise *de novo* in non-hemophiliacs. They may develop in patients with autoimmune disease, with malignancies, in the postpartum period, but most frequently in apparently normal, often elderly individuals. The result is an acquired bleeding disorder, frequently life-threatening in its severity. In an adult with a low factor VIII level, the absence of previous bleeding or a family history is the clue to search for a factor VIII inhibitor. Successful treatment may require large amounts of factor VIII concentrate or products that bypass factor VIII, supplemented with plasmapheresis and immunosuppressive therapy. Antibody-induced factor IX deficiency is relatively rare.

SUGGESTED READING

Hay CRM. Why do inhibitors arise in patients with Haemophilia A? Br J Haematol 105:584-590, 1999.

Kaufman RJ, Pipe SW. Regulation of factor VIII expression and activity by von Willebrand factor. Thromb Haemost 82:201-208, 1999.

Lenting PJ, van Mourik, Martens K. The life cycle of coagulation factor VIII in view of its structure and function. Blood 92:3983-3996, 1998.

Lillicrap D. The molecular basis of haemophilia B. Haemophilia 4:350-357, 1998.

Peake I. The molecular basis of haemophilia A. Haemophilia 4:346-349, 1998.

Pruthi RK, Nichols WL. Autoimmune factor VIII inhibitors. Curr Opin Haematol 6:314-322, 1999.

von WILLEBRAND FACTOR

"Hereditär pseudohemofili"
Eric von Willebrand – 1926

Factor VIII and von Willebrand factor (vWF) are synthesized in different cells, have different functions, but circulate together in plasma in a noncovalently linked complex. vWF increases factor VIII survival, thereby playing a critical role in regulating factor VIII activity. Pathological processes that disturb the physiological interactions of these two proteins emphasize their importance in normal hemostasis.

vWF is a large multimeric glycoprotein synthesized in endothelial cells and megakaryocytes. It has two essential hemostatic functions: it stabilizes and prolongs the half-life of circulating factor VIII and it promotes platelet adhesion to subendothelial tissues at sites of vascular damage. The normal plasma level of vWF is broad, ranging from 50% to 240% (i.e. 50-240 U/dL). ABO blood group antigens are a major determinant of plasma vWF levels; plasma vWF antigen levels are 25-35% lower in blood group O individuals compared to the other ABO types. (ABO blood group antigens are covalently linked to oligosaccharide side chains of the vWF molecule – it has been suggested that the different carbohydrate structures exert subtle effects on plasma clearance of vWF). vWF behaves as an acute-phase reactant – levels increase transiently in response to a variety of events that involve adrenergic stimulation: exercise, trauma, and surgery. Levels increase during pregnancy, reaching a maximum late in the third trimester.

The vWF gene is located on chromosome 12 and spans 178 kilobases. vWF is synthesized as a precursor protein consisting of a large propeptide bound to a mature subunit. The propeptide is required for intracellular post-translational assembly of vWF multimers in the endoplasmic reticulum and Golgi apparatus; dimerization of the subunit, then multimerization, is followed by cleavage of the propeptide. The mature vWF and the propeptide are large polypeptides that are co-secreted on an equimolar basis. Plasma vWF and plasma propeptide are derived predominantly from endothelial cells rather than from platelet stores. Secreted propeptide has a very short half-life in plasma; in extracellular tissues, it may have a role in modulating cellular adhesion processes as it is cross-linked by factor XIIIa to the extracellular matrix. Because the plasma propeptide was detected initially by immunological methods, it also is referred to as vWF antigen II. Circulating vWF has a half-life of approximately 12 hours. The smallest secreted form of vWF is a 540 kD disulfide-linked homodimer; the multimers range in molecular size up to 20,000 kD – the largest are the most adhesive. The vWF molecule has specific binding sites for collagen, factor VIII, platelet GPIb and GPIIb/IIIa (Figure 27-1).

vWF synthesized in endothelial cells follows two secretory routes. 95% of newly synthesized vWF is secreted constitutively into both the circulation and the subendothelial

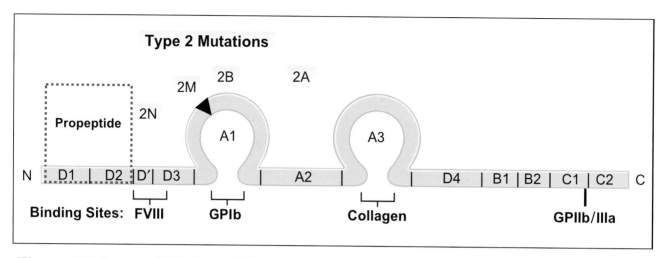

Figure 27-1   von Willebrand Factor

tissues, independent of stimulation by secretagogues. Proteolytic cleavage of the large multimers by a plasma metalloprotease leaves the smaller, less adhesive multimers in the circulation. This cation-dependent metalloprotease cleaves a site within the A2 domain of the vWF molecule – it is activated under conditions of high shear stress. (This vWF-cleaving protease is encoded by the gene *ADAMTS13* that maps to chromosome 9q34).

The regulated secretory pathway involves endothelial cell storage of the largest multimers in unique cytoplasmic vesicles, the Weibel-Palade bodies. The vWF propeptide is stored along with the multimers; they are released rapidly and in equimolar amounts in response to such agonists as thrombin, histamine, epinephrine, vasopressin, and the terminal complement complex 5b-9. These very large highly adhesive multimers, sequestered in Weibel-Palade bodies and released at sites of vascular injury, are critical to normal hemostasis.

Platelet vWF is not released constitutively. Large highly adhesive multimers synthesized by megakaryocytes are stored in platelet α-granules and released upon platelet activation at sites of vascular damage. The secreted vWF augments platelet adhesion to subendothelial tissues and platelet aggregation in the developing clot. Platelets contribute about 15% of the total blood vWF.

In the circulation, vWF does not interact with unstimulated platelets – vWF-platelet interactions are initiated at sites of vascular injury. With exposure of the subendothelial tissues, vWF binds to collagen and undergoes a conformational change that provides high-affinity binding sites for the platelet receptor GPIbα. Adhesion of platelets to vWF must counter the force of fluid shear stress; in areas of highest shear, GPIbα-vWF interaction is the primary initiator of hemostasis. This initial interaction, between GPIbα and the A1 domain of vWF, results in reversible tethering that slows the platelet and sets the stage for integrin-dependent platelet immobilization. vWF binding to GPIbα generates an intracellular platelet signal that produces a conformational change in the extracellular region of the integrin GPIIb/IIIa ($\alpha_{IIb}\beta_3$), resulting in irreversible binding; GPIIb/IIIa binds to RGD (Arg-Gly-Asp) sequences in the vWF subunit (and to RGD sequences in other adhesive molecules such as fibrinogen). vWF functions as a bridge to connect platelets to the subendothelial matrix (platelet adhesion) and to each other (platelet aggregation: Figure 30-3).

Tissue factor activity in areas of vessel injury initiates coagulation with the generation of thrombin. Thrombin activation of nearby platelets and endothelial cells results in release of large multimeric vWF. The binding of these multimers to the GPIIb/IIIa integrin on activated platelets enhances platelet adhesion and aggregation. Thrombin also activates the factor VIII carried into the area on vWF, augmenting coagulation and local fibrin deposition.

High shear stress at sites of vascular pathology may promote changes in circulating vWF that result in exposure of GPIb-binding sites. Under these circumstances, vWF binds to GPIbα on unactivated platelets; the subsequent binding of vWF to activated GPIIb/IIIa results in platelet aggregation. These events occur in areas of high turbulence associated with cardiac valve abnormalities and sites of vascular stenosis, and may result in platelet aggregation and deposition of platelet aggregates on endothelial surfaces – as a consequence, there is local consumption of vWF and the level of circulating vWF may be reduced.

CLINICAL CORRELATES

VON WILLEBRAND DISEASE (vWD)

In 1926, Erik von Willebrand described a bleeding disorder in a family living on the island of Föglö in the Åland Archipelago (Finland). Repeat studies in 1957 established this family as the prototype for von Willebrand disease. vWD is the most common hereditary bleeding disorder, with a prevalence of 1-2% of the population. It is characterized by mucous membrane bleeding, excessive bleeding following invasive surgical or dental procedures, and easy bruising. Administration of the vasopressin analogue DDAVP (1-desamino-8-D-arginine vasopressin) induces vWF release from endothelial cell Weibel-Palade bodies, resulting in increased levels in the circulation. Recent studies suggest factor VIII may be stored in ECs with vWF as the plasma level of both proteins increase simultaneously in response to DDAVP.

Laboratory studies include both screening tests and definitive assays. The bleeding time (or the *in vitro* closure time) is usually prolonged. The *in vitro* closure time appears to be more reproducible than the bleeding time and equally sensitive to reduced platelet and vWF function – the test determines the ability of platelets to occlude a small membrane aperture. The APTT reflects the level of factor VIII; it is often normal in mild vWD. Plasma levels and the multimeric composition of the vWF antigen are determined by immunological assays.

Table 27-1   Classification of Congenital von Willebrand Disease

	Platelet Count	Bleeding Time	VIII Coagulant	vWF Antigen	vWF: RCo*	RIPA**	Plasma Multimers	Platelet Multimers
Type 1	N	N / ↑	↓	↓	↓	N / ↓	↓	N / ↓
Type 2A	N	↑	N / ↓	N / ↓	↓	↓	HMW↓	HMW↓
Type 2B	↓	↑	N / ↓	N / ↓	↓	↑	HMW↓	HMW present
Type 2M	N	↑	N	N	↓	↓	N/Abnormal	N/Abnormal
Type 2N	N	N	↓	N	N	N	N	N
Type 3	N	↑	–	–	–	–	–	–
Pseudo	↓	↑	N / ↓	N / ↓	N / ↓	↑	HMW↓	HMW present

*   vWF:RCo (ristocetin cofactor activity) measured by mixing the patient's plasma with formalin fixed normal platelets, adding ristocetin and assaying the aggregation response.

** RIPA (ristocetin-induced platelet aggregation) assayed by measuring platelet aggregation on addition of ristocetin to the patient's own platelet rich plasma.

N - Normal
↓ - Decreased
↑ - Increased
– - Absent
HMW - High Molecular weight multimers

Functional assays include: vWF ristocetin cofactor (vWF:RCo) activity, ristocetin-induced platelet aggregation (RIPA), and vWF collagen-binding activity (vWF:CBA). vWF binding to GPIb is reproduced *in vitro* in the presence of the antibiotic ristocetin. In the vWF:RCo assay, vWF adhesion to GPIb is assessed by the aggregation of formalinized donor platelets in the presence of ristocetin. RIPA measures plasma vWF function in a similar assay but the patient's own platelets provide the GPIb-binding site. (Ristocetin was withdrawn from clinical use due to the high incidence of thrombocytopenia). vWF:CBA evaluates the capability of plasma vWF to bind to collagen – the test is sensitive to reduced levels of the large multimers.

Low levels of vWF antigen II (vWF propeptide) reflect decreased vWF synthesis. It may be useful in distinguishing congenital vWD from acquired vWF deficiency; as vWF synthesis is unimpaired in acquired vWD, the level of vWF antigen II is normal. It also may serve as a marker for endothelial cell (EC) perturbation, as both vWF and the propeptide are released from stimulated ECs.

Classification of von Willebrand Disease

vWD is divided into three groups: quantitative deficiencies, partial or complete (Types 1 and 3 respectively); and qualitative defects – Type 2. A rare pseudo-vWD is due to a platelet anomaly in vWF binding. This classification is summarized in Table 27-1.

Type 1 – the most common form (representing 70-80% of cases) has an autosomal dominant inheritance and is manifest by decreased production of normal vWF. Factor VIII levels in plasma are reduced proportionately to the vWF, reflecting the role of vWF in binding and stabilizing circulating VIII. Thus, there is an equivalent reduction of factor VIII, vWF antigen and vWF activity in plasma. These patients have a variably prolonged bleeding time (or *in vitro* closure time). Although the total vWF protein is decreased, the immunoelectrophoretic multimeric pattern of the protein is normal. A disproportionately large number of these patients are blood group O. Administration of the synthetic analogue of vasopressin, desmopressin (DDAVP), raises plasma vWF levels in the majority of these patients.

Type 2 is separated into four groups: 2A, 2B, 2M and 2N – each characterized by a different structural and functional defect. Patients with types 2A, 2B and 2M have a prolonged bleeding time (or *in vitro* closure time) and reduced vWF functional activity; the total vWF antigen may be within normal limits; factor VIII levels may be normal or decreased.

Type 2A is characterized by selective absence of large and mid-sized multimers, the result of missense mutations most frequently found within the A2 domain. The absence of large multimers is due to two mechanisms: defective intracellular transport with impaired storage and secretion of large multimers, or increased susceptibility of the molecule to proteolytic cleavage in plasma; the vWF-cleaving protease is probably responsible for this proteolysis. Inheritance is usually autosomal dominant, rarely autosomal recessive. Responses to DDAVP are variable and may be poor.

Type 2B – In this dominant phenotype, the large multimers of the mutant vWF have an increased affinity for GPIb – they bind spontaneously to the surface of non-activated platelets. The mutations that have been identified are all within the GPIb-binding region (the vWF A1 domain). Because these platelet/vWF complexes are cleared rapidly from the circulation, thrombocytopenia is frequently present. The bleeding diathesis is related to the poor adhesive activity of the remaining small multimers. Due to the attachment of the large vWF multimers to the platelet membrane, there is enhanced *in vitro* ristocetin-induced platelet aggregation (**RIPA**) and an absence of high molecular weight multimers in the plasma. Note: therapy with DDAVP may induce further endothelial cell release of the abnormal multimers – resulting in increased platelet aggregation and significant thrombocytopenia.

Type 2M is a heterogeneous group with defective vWF-dependent platelet adhesion. Although the multimeric pattern may appear normal, the large multimers are functionally defective. Missense and small frameshift mutations have been identified in the A1 domain that impair binding to platelet GPIb. *In vitro*, this is demonstrated by abnormal functional activity.

Type 2N is a rare autosomal recessive variant (vW Normandy) due to mutations in the vWF-binding site for factor VIII in the D' and D3 domains. The vWF multimeric pattern and platelet-dependent functions are normal. Because the abnormal vWF cannot bind factor VIII, plasma levels of factor VIII are decreased (usually to about 25% of normal). The clinical picture resembles mild hemophilia A but can affect females as well as males. The response to infusion of VIII concentrate is poor as unbound factor VIII is cleared rapidly from the circulation. In contrast, because factor VIII production and function are normal, plasma levels of VIII increase with the infusion of vWF concentrates.

Type 3 is an autosomal recessive defect with little or no vWF synthesis. There may be total or partial deletions of the vWF gene, nonsense or frameshift defects. These patients have a markedly prolonged bleeding time, absent ristocetin cofactor activity, and absent vWF antigen. Concomitantly, factor VIII also is decreased – plasma levels are usually less than 10%. Clinically, these patients may be confused with hemophilia A; however, in hemophilia A, vWF activity and antigen level are normal. Treatment requires replacement therapy with vWF/factor VIII concentrates. Alloantibodies to vWF develop in 5-10% of patients following replacement therapy.

Pseudo or Platelet-Type vWD is due to gain-of-function mutations of the platelet receptor GPIbα, involving amino acid substitutions within a restricted area of the vWF-binding domain. In vWD Type 2B, the mutant vWF has a high affinity for normal platelet GPIbα; it adheres to circulating platelets producing both thrombocytopenia and vWF depletion. Its mirror image is Pseudo-vWD in which the mutated platelet GPIbα has an increased affinity for normal vWF. The binding of normal high molecular weight multimers causes platelet aggregation, and the removal of the aggregates from the circulation results in thrombocytopenia. The clinical and laboratory presentation of Type 2B and Pseudo-vWD is similar – in both, the large multimers are missing from plasma but are present on platelet membranes. Pseudo vWD can be differentiated by molecular characterization of platelet GPIbα; the mutations are restricted to a seven amino acid span (residues 233-239) of the GPIbα chain, producing a molecular configuration with enhanced vWF binding.

ACQUIRED VON WILLEBRAND DISEASE

This syndrome presents with laboratory findings similar to congenital vWD, usually in patients with no personal or family history of a bleeding diathesis. Acquired vWD occurs most commonly in patients of advanced age in association with a variety of other diseases: neoplasia, autoimmune disorders, clonal diseases (eg, myeloma, Waldenström's macroglobulinemia, leukemia), and cardiac/vascular disorders. The mechanisms responsible for decreased levels of vWF include: (1) circulating autoantibodies that bind and remove vWF, and (2) more commonly, selective adsorption of the largest vWF multimers onto tumor cells or activated platelets; platelet activation occurs in areas of vascular turbulence or high shear stress – as in valvular heart disease and in areas of angiodysplasia.

Laboratory findings confirm the reduced level of circulating vWF due, primarily, to loss of the high molecular weight multimers. vWF propeptide levels, however, are normal or increased, reflecting normal synthesis of vWF. Abnormal functional assays (ristocetin cofactor activity and collagen-binding activity) reflect the loss of the large multimers from the circulation. Inhibitory antibodies can be demonstrated only in a minority of cases.

THROMBOTIC THROMBOCYTOPENIC PURPURA (TTP)

TTP, a disseminated thrombotic microangiopathy described by Moschowitz in 1924, is characterized by extensive platelet thrombi in the arterioles and capillaries in target organs, typically brain and kidneys. Patients may present with the classical pentad: thrombocytopenia, hemolytic anemia, fever, renal dysfunction, and neurologic abnormalities. In the early stages of the disease, microangiopathic hemolytic anemia may be the only finding.

The development of TTP may be immune-mediated, familial, or secondary to pre-existing conditions. Although the clinical presentations are similar, differences in the pathogenesis of the disease support this clinical classification. Impaired function of the vWF-cleaving protease has been identified in many of these patients; defective vWF-cleavage leads to formation of platelet thrombi as the superadhesive multimers bind and aggregate platelets.

Primary (acute) TTP characteristically develops in previously healthy individuals. Unusually large vWF multimers are present in the plasma. An IgG autoantibody directed against the vWF-cleaving protease is responsible for deficient protease activity in most of these patients. The plasma protease is reduced or completely absent during the acute illness but returns to normal after recovery. Therapeutic plasma exchange results in antibody removal with concomitant enzyme replacement. (The hemolytic uremic syndrome (HUS) is a microangiopathy of the kidney and other organs that usually occurs following infection with Shiga toxin-producing bacteria, such as E. coli 0157:H7. Although the clinical and histopathological manifestations are similar to TTP, the vWF-cleaving protease activity usually is normal – reduced protease levels have been reported in some cases of HUS).

Secondary TTP, which represents 25-50% of cases, has been associated with bone marrow transplantation, HIV infection, pregnancy, and drug therapy – particularly ticlopidine, quinine and chemotherapeutic agents. Endothelial damage is common. In marrow transplant-associated TTP, the protease is normal. Most cases of ticlopidine-associated TTP have autoantibodies to the vWF-cleaving protease – the course of the disease is similar to acute primary TTP and also responds to plasma exchange.

Familial chronic relapsing TTP is an autosomal recessive disease due to mutations in the *ADAMTS13* gene on chromosome 9 that codes for the vWF-cleaving protease. There are recurring episodes of thrombocytopenia and microangiopathy. Very large vWF multimers in the patient's plasma are detected most readily between acute episodes. The factors responsible for the recurrent acute episodes have not been identified. Therapeutic plasma infusions replace the absent protease.

SUGGESTED READING

Federici AB, Rand JH, Bucciarelli P, Budde U, van Genderen PJJ, Mohri H, Meyer D, et al. Acquired von Willebrand syndrome: data from an international registry. Thromb Haemost 84:345-349, 2000.

Levy GG, Nichols WC, Lian EC, et al. Mutations in a member of the *ADAMTS* gene family cause thrombotic thrombocytopenic purpura. Nature 413: 488-494, 2001.

Mannucci PM. Desmopressin (DDAVP) in the treatment of bleeding disorders: The first 20 years. Blood 90:2515-2521, 1997.

Mannucci PM. Thrombotic thrombocytopenic purpura: a simpler diagnosis at last? Thromb Haemost 82:1380-1381, 1999.

Miller JL. Platelet type von Willebrand disease. Thromb Haemost 75:865-869, 1996.

Ruggeri ZM. Structure and function of von Willebrand factor. Thromb Haemost 82:576-584, 1999.

Ruggeri AM. Developing basic and clinical research on von Willebrand factor and von Willbrand disease. Thromb Haemost 84:147-149, 2000.

Sadler JE. Biochemistry and genetics of von Willebrand factor. Annu Rev Biochem 67:395-424, 1998.

Sadler JE, Mannucci PM, Berntorp E, Bochkov N, Boulyjenkov V et al. Impact, diagnosis and treatment of von Willebrand disease. Thromb Haemost 84:160-174, 2000.

Veyradier A, Jenkins CSP, Fressinaud E, Meyer D. Acquired von Willebrand syndrome: from pathophysiology to management. Thromb Haemost 84: 175-182, 2000.

VITAMIN K

"It is proposed to term this factor vitamin K (Koagulations Vitamin)"
Henrik Dam – 1935

In 1929, Henrik Dam began a series of experiments in which he demonstrated that removal of a fat-soluble element from the diet of chicks resulted in hemorrhage and death. He subsequently isolated the "Koagulation Vitamin" – vitamin K.

The K vitamins are 2 methyl-1, 4 naphthoquinones with repeating 5 carbon prenyl units at position 3. Vitamin K_1 (phylloquinone), found primarily in leafy green vegetables and vegetable oils, supplies the daily dietary requirement of about 1 μg/kg. Additional K activity may be provided by vitamin K_2 (menoquinones) synthesized by intestinal gram-negative bacteria; however, the exact physiological role of K_2 remains unclear. Synthetic vitamin K_3 (menadione) has no side chain and no intrinsic activity until it undergoes *in vivo* conjugation at position R (Figure 28-1) to form an active menaquinone.

Vitamin K is an essential cofactor for the microsomal γ-carboxylation of the N-terminal glutamyl residues of the Ca^{2+}- binding coagulation factors II, VII, IX, X and proteins C and S, as well as osteocalcin and matrix Gla protein of bone, and other Ca^{2+}-binding proteins (including protein Z) whose functions remain less well defined. Quantitatively, the major site of K_1-mediated protein γ-carboxylation is the liver; however, γ-carboxylation is probably ubiquitous – it has been identified in most organs, as well as in a number of tumors. Its presence in these extrahepatic sites may relate to its role in cell signaling.

The hydroquinone form of vitamin K functions as a cofactor for a membrane-associated **K-dependent carboxylase**. In the presence of CO_2 and O_2, this enzyme generates additional carboxyl groups on glutamic acid sites on precursors of the K-dependent proteins. The result is a series of γ-carboxyglutamic acid (Gla) residues in juxtaposition to the N-terminus of these proteins. Depending upon the protein, the post-translational carboxylation takes place on from 9 to 12 N-terminal glutamic acid residues. It is this γ-carboxyglutamic acid "Gla" region that mediates the Ca^{2+}- binding of the protein to anionic phospholipid surfaces, thereby assuring close proximity and interaction with other components of the coagulation sequence and with cell receptors for vitamin K-dependent ligands. Excess Gla proteins are excreted in the urine. In the absence of vitamin K, the coagulation protein precursors continue to be synthesized but are not γ-carboxylated; the non-functional *descarboxy* forms, referred to as PIVKA (protein induced by vitamin K absence), appear in the plasma.

A microsomal oxidation-reduction system recycles vitamin K for continuing use in the γ-carboxylation reaction (Figure 28-1). The carboxylation of the precursor proteins results in

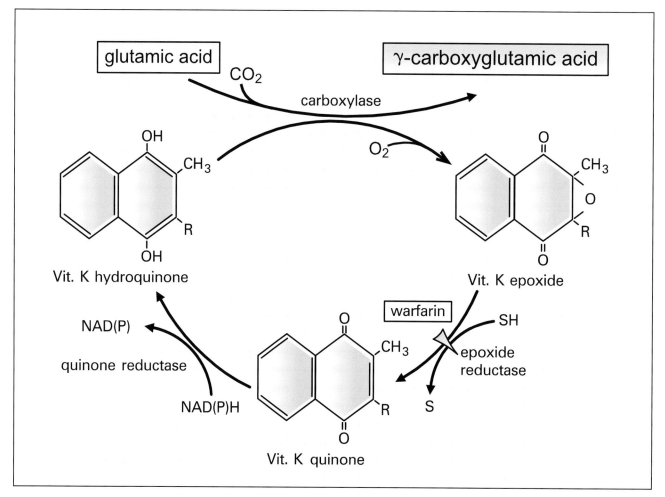

Figure 28-1 Vitamin K_1 Cycle

oxidation of the vitamin K *hydroquinone* to the *epoxide*. The epoxide, in the presence of **epoxide reductase** and dithiols as reductants, yields the *quinone* form of vitamin K. A subsequent, NADPH or NADH-dependent **quinone reductase** reaction, completes the cycle as the hydroquinone is resynthesized. The cycle can be inhibited by the coumarin anticoagulants (eg, warfarin); these agents block the reduction of the K epoxide to the quinone by epoxide reductase and, to a lesser degree, inhibit the quinone reductase.

The Vitamin K-Dependent Coagulation Proteins

There is major homology of the vitamin K-dependent coagulation proteins (Figure 28-2). Each molecule is synthesized with an amino-terminal start signal peptide, followed by a propeptide domain. The signal peptide directs the protein to the endoplasmic reticulum where the signal peptide is cleaved. The propeptide contains the recognition site for initiation of the γ-carboxylation reaction; the subsequent removal of the propeptide, that takes place within the Golgi complex, leaves the γ-carboxyglutamic acid rich (Gla) domain at the N-terminal portion

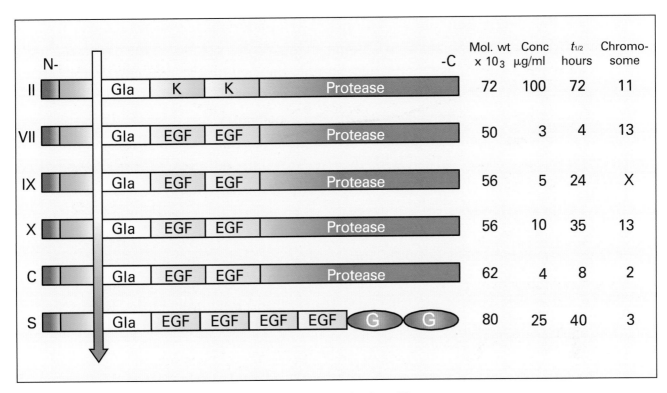

Figure 28-2 Vitamin K Dependent Coagulation Factors

of the secreted protein. The active catalytic C-terminal end of the molecule is a serine protease closely resembling the proteolytic enzymes trypsin and chymotrypsin. In factors VII, IX, X and protein C the C-terminal end is separated from the Gla region by two epidermal growth factor (EGF) sequences; in prothrombin (factor II) this intermediate region consists of two disulphide bonded triple loops (kringle domains). The coagulation factors II, VII, IX and X are zymogens that participate in a cascade of sequential activation; the activated precursor ignites the next one in the sequence (Section 24). Protein S, which functions as a cofactor for protein C (Section 25), has a Gla rich N-terminal domain separated from the C-terminal domain by four joining EGF segments. The C terminal end of protein S is not a protease but a duplex sex hormone binding globulin-like (SBHG) cassette known as the **G region**. The G region is the site of interaction with protein C, of binding to C4b-binding protein, and of interaction with the growth regulatory receptor tyrosine kinase (RTK) Sky.

Protein Z (PZ), a vitamin K-dependent protein, is a 60,000 MW glycoprotein with a plasma half-life of 2-3 days. The structure of the PZ molecule is similar to factors VII, IX, X, and protein C but the active catalytic site at the C-terminal is missing; like protein S, PZ does not function as a protease. PZ circulates in plasma in a complex with the protease inhibitor ZPI (PZ-dependent protease inhibitor), a recently identified member of the serpin family of protease inhibitors (Section 26). PZ acts as a cofactor for ZPI inhibition of factor Xa – the physiological significance of this PZ/ZPI activity is unclear.

The Growth Regulatory Function of Vitamin K$_1$-Dependent Ligands (Figure 28-3)

Recently, K-dependent proteins have been identified as ligands for cell membrane receptors that mediate tyrosine kinase phosphorylation, stimulating cell growth and cell transformation. Two K$_1$-dependent ligands, protein S and Gas6, have been identified as growth regulatory proteins. Gas6 is of similar size and major structural homology to protein S. It was isolated initially from cells undergoing artificially-induced growth arrest – overproduction of Gas6 in these cells apparently was associated with their re-entry into cell cycle. Three closely related receptor tyrosine kinases, Axl, Sky and Mer, are receptors for Gas6; Sky is also a receptor for protein S. All three receptors share similar extracytoplasmic regions: two fibronectin domains followed by two immunoglobulin-like N-terminal domains. These receptors are present on normal cells and in a number of tumor cells. The ligands attach initially through their G domain and, secondarily, through the Gla region as they fix Ca^{2+}. With ligand engagement, the activated receptors can stimulate growth and cell transformation, and inhibit apoptosis. Recent studies indicate that these receptors and their ligands, protein S and Gas6, have an important role in immune regulation.

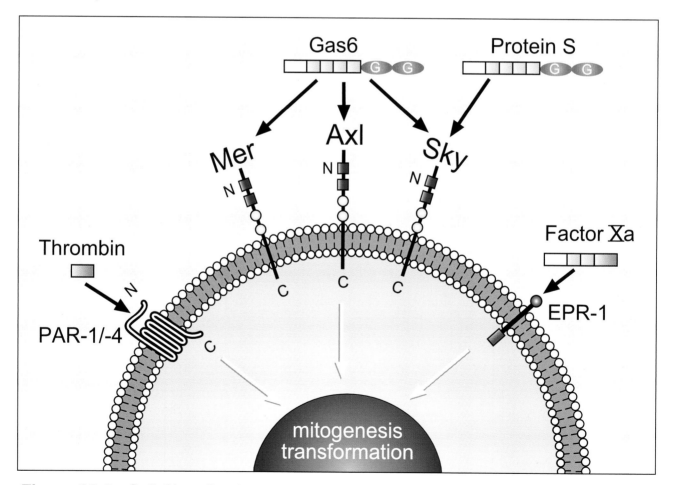

Figure 28-3 Cell Signaling by Vitamin K Dependent Proteins

The serine proteases thrombin and factor Xa derived from the vitamin K-dependent proteins prothrombin and factor X, respectively, are mitogenic, primarily for vascular smooth muscle. Thrombin binds to the cell membrane proteolytic activated receptors, PAR-1 and PAR-4 (Section 30); factor Xa binds to its specific receptor, EPR-1 (effector cell protease receptor-1). The fact that both thrombin and factor Xa are mitogenic for vascular smooth muscle suggests they have a potential role in atherogenesis.

CLINICAL CORRELATES

Decreased Vitamin K_1 Activity

This may result from deficiency of vitamin K or from the metabolic blockade of vitamin K re-cycling by warfarin or related drugs (coumarins). Vitamin K deficiency is associated with: (1) poor oral intake in the acutely ill and in those receiving antibiotics that alter bowel flora; (2) biliary obstruction – vitamin K is a fat soluble vitamin requiring bile salts for absorption; (3) the normal fetus and newborn. Functional vitamin K deficiency is seen most commonly in patients on oral anticoagulants. Because of the short $t_{1/2}$ and rapid turnover of the K-dependent coagulation factors, warfarin blockade of coagulation is achieved in 72 to 96 hours and is reversible by intravenous vitamin K_1 within 6-12 hours.

As the levels of the vitamin K-dependent coagulation factors are not sensitive indices of K_1 deficit, depletion of the normally small body storage pool and of K_1-dependent protein synthesis is compatible with a normal prothrombin time. More sensitive indicators of vitamin K_1 deficiency are: (1) increased levels of PIVKA in plasma and (2) decreased excretion of Gla proteins in urine. The liver is the primary storage pool for vitamin K_1. Because the pool is small, young healthy adults on a K_1-free diet begin to show increased PIVKA levels in plasma within one week. This calls into question the role of the K_2 series of menaquinones in the presence of a K_1 deficit.

The mammalian fetus is maintained in a "K deficient" state as evidenced by the low functional levels of the vitamin K-dependent coagulation factors during fetal development and at birth. The transplacental gradient between mother and fetus makes it virtually impossible to increase fetal levels by administration of K_1 to the mother. The teleological explanation for maintaining the K-dependent factors in their undercarboxylated state is unclear. Recent findings, that the K-dependent proteins, protein S and Gas6, are ligands for receptor tyrosine kinases and can function as growth promoters by upregulation of a tyrosine phosphorylation cascade, may explain the need for the tight control of vitamin K_1 levels in the rapidly proliferating cell systems of the fetus. The low levels of K-dependent coagulation factors at birth may result in hemorrhagic disease of the newborn in those babies not supplemented with vitamin K_1. Because K_1 is a fat soluble vitamin, this risk is greatest in neonates with liver disease or cholestasis.

Warfarin is known to cross the placenta – the adverse clinical effects have been well documented. Warfarin embryopathy results from administration of the drug during pregnancy. The growth and skeletal anomalies are similar to those of congenital K_1 epoxide reductase deficiency and congenital chondrodysplasia: short stature, phalangeal hypoplasia and radiological demonstration of stippled epiphysis. The embryopathy associated with warfarin or epoxide reductase deficiency may reflect the depletion of the K_1-dependent ligands essential to growth regulatory pathways. Congenital deficiency of the γ-carboxylated K-dependent proteins is associated with a mutation in the gene for vitamin K_1-carboxylase.

Vitamin K-dependent Gla proteins, osteocalcin and matrix Gla protein, are important to the structural integrity of bone; they are demonstrable also at sites of ectopic calcification. Vitamin K- deficiency, with reduced availability of these Gla proteins, is probably a factor in postmenopausal osteoporosis and hip fracture in the elderly.

———————— ••••●●•••• ————————

SUGGESTED READING

Booth SL, Suttie JW. Dietary intake and adequacy of vitamin K. J Nutr 130:1S Suppl:785-788, 2000.

Broze GJ. Protein Z-dependent regulation of coagulation. Thromb Haemost 86:8-13, 2001.

Furie B, Furie BC. The molecular basis of vitamin K-dependent gamma-carboxylation. Blood 75:1753-1762, 1990.

Israels LG, Israels ED. Observations on vitamin K deficiency in the fetus and newborn: Has nature made a mistake? Semin Thromb Hemost 21:357-363, 1995.

Israels, LG, Israels, ED. The riddle of vitamin K_1 deficit in the newborn. Semin in Perinatology 21: 90-96, 1997.

Lu Q, Lemke G. Homeostatic regulation of the immune system by receptor tyrosine kinases of the tyro 3 family. Science 293:306-311, 2001.

Price PA. Vitamin K nutrition and postmenopausal osteoporosis. J Clin Invest 91:1268, 1993.

Saxena S, Israels ED, Israels LG. Novel vitamin K-dependent pathways regulating cell survival. Apoptosis 6:57-68, 2001.

Shearer MJ, McCarthy PT, Crampton OE, Mattock MB. The assessment of vitamin K status from tissue measurements. In: Current Advances in Vitamin K Research. Suttie JW ed. New York: Elsevier Science 1988: 437-452.

Shearer MJ. Vitamin K. Lancet 345: 229-234, 1995.

Varnum BC, Young C, Elliott G, Garcia A, Bartley TD, et al. Axl receptor tyrosine kinase stimulated by the vitamin K-dependent protein encoded by growth-arrest-specific gene 6. Nature 373:623-626, 1995.

Uotila L. The metabolic functions and mechanisms of action of vitamin K. Scand J Clin Lab Invest Suppl 201:109-117, 1990.

FIBRINOGEN, FACTOR XIII AND FIBRINOLYSIS

"Oh what a tangled web we weave"
Marmion, Sir Walter Scott

FIBRINOGEN

The conversion of soluble fibrinogen to insoluble fibrin by the proteolytic action of thrombin is the final step in the coagulation cascade. Fibrinogen, a 340 kD glycoprotein synthesized in the liver, is present in plasma at the highest concentration of all the coagulation factors (2-4 g/L), with a half-life of approximately 4 days. Substantial amounts also are present in platelet α-granules. Fibrinogen is a dimer consisting of 3 paired chains, Aα, Bβ, and γ, held together by disulfide bonds. The three genes coding for the α, β, and γ chains are clustered on chromosome 4. The initial event in the conversion of fibrinogen to fibrin is the thrombin-catalyzed removal of the A and B peptides. Thrombin cleaves one peptide bond in the amino terminal of each Aα chain to release the two fibrinopeptide A segments then, at a slower rate, releases the two fibrinopeptide B segments from the β chains. The residual molecule is **fibrin monomer** – with three symmetrical paired chains: α, β and γ. On electron microscopy, fibrinogen and fibrin monomer molecules appear as tri-nodal structures resembling the diagram in Figure 29-1, the outer nodes larger than the central node. The central node is referred to as the E domain and the lateral nodes as D domains. The six amino terminals of the three paired polypeptide chains are gathered together at the centre of the molecule – in the E domain.

Fibrin monomer is a soluble protein that undergoes spontaneous polymerization to form insoluble fibrin. In the circulation, fibrin monomer forms soluble complexes with fibrinogen; polymerization occurs when the concentration of the monomer exceeds the binding capacity of plasma fibrinogen. The formation of the fibrin polymer takes place by self-assembly of the monomers – end to end association of the D domains, and the side to side association of one E domain with two D domains of adjacent chains. During the polymerization process with formation of the fibrin net, **factor XIIIa** introduces covalent cross-links, first between the juxtaposed γ chains and later between the α chains. Crosslinked fibrin is resistant to fibrinolysis; in the absence of factor XIIIa the clot remains weak, friable, and easily lysed.

FACTOR XIII (Figure 29-2)

Factor XIII converts the loose fibrin polymer into a firm, organized structure resistant to fibrinolysis. XIIIa is a transglutaminase that catalyzes the crosslinking of α and γ chains of fibrin through the formation of glutamine-lysine covalent bonds. Like all transglutaminases, factor

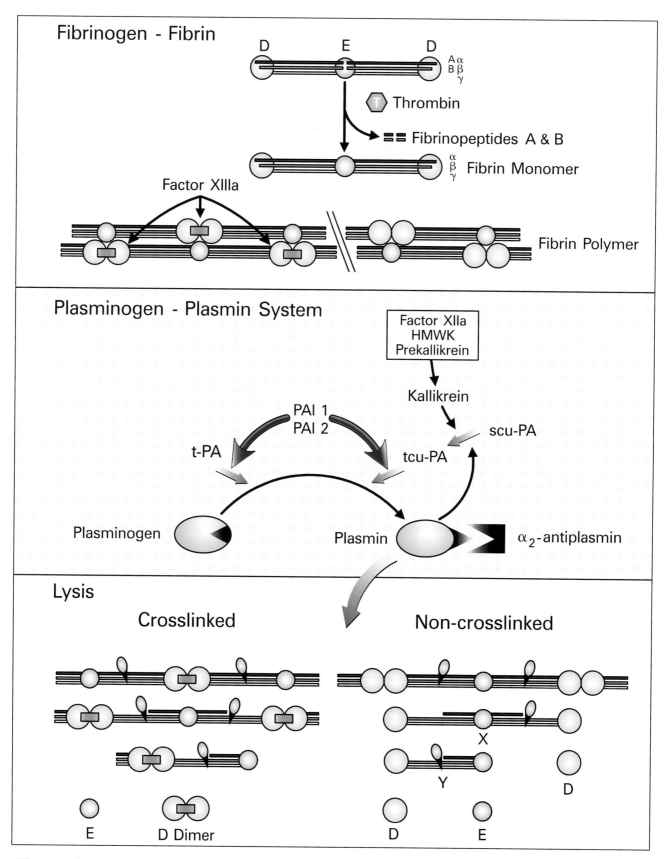

Figure 29-1   Fibrinogen / Fibrin / Fibrinolysis

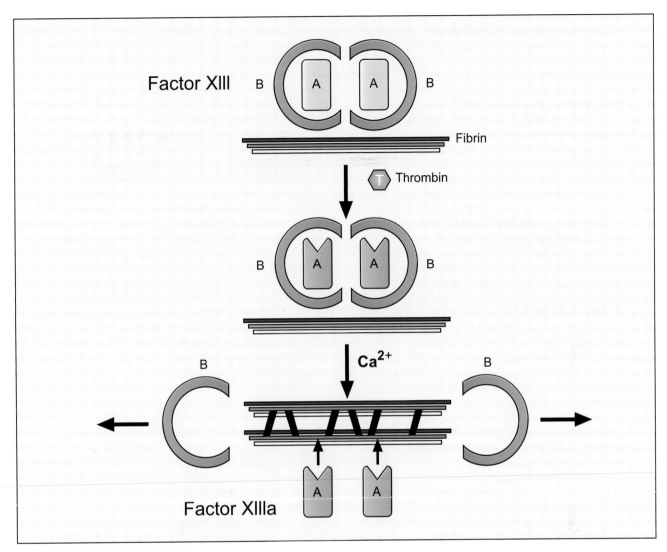

Figure 29-2 Activation of Factor XIII

XIIIa is a cysteine protease; the other coagulation enzymes are serine proteases. In addition to cross-linking fibrin chains, XIIIa induces covalent bonding of α_2-antiplasmin and fibronectin to fibrin, further enhancing the mechanical stability of the fibrin clot and its resistance to fibrinolysis.

The 330 kD factor XIII zymogen circulates in plasma as a heterotetramer, A_2B_2, consisting of two catalytic A subunits and two noncatalytic carrier B subunits. The tetramer is held together by noncovalent bonds. Dimers of subunit A (A_2) are present in platelets and in monocytes; the A_2 dimers in platelets account for 50 percent of the factor XIII in peripheral blood. The A subunit probably is synthesized in megakaryocytes and monocytes in the bone marrow and in hepatocytes, the B subunit in hepatocytes. Following their secretion into the plasma, the subunits come together as the tetramer. Activation of XIII requires both thrombin and calcium, and takes place in two steps: (1) limited proteolysis by thrombin cleaves an arginine-lysine bond in the A subunits, (2) dissociation of the B subunits, in the presence of Ca^{2+}, exposes the active site on the A subunits (XIIIa). The physiological concentration of calcium in plasma is sufficient to induce dissociation of the B subunits.

THE FIBRINOLYTIC SYSTEM (THE PLASMINOGEN SYSTEM)

The proteins in this system participate in two processes: (1) fibrinolysis and (2) degradation of extracellular matrix. The term, the plasminogen system, acknowledges this dual role.

Fibrin clots provide a temporary scaffold on which wound healing takes place; eventually they must be dismantled. The fibrinolytic dissolution of fibrin clots maintains and restores blood vessel patency and expedites wound healing. The major enzyme of the fibrinolytic pathway, plasmin, is derived from the precursor molecule plasminogen; activators of plasminogen convert it to the active enzyme. Plasmin degrades fibrin into soluble fibrin degradation products (FDPs). Inhibitors of plasminogen activation and of plasmin regulate this fibrinolytic activity. Fibrin also is degraded by proteases released by neutrophils and other cells in the area – the products are removed by phagocytosis.

The activity and regulation of the fibrinolytic system involves: (1) serine proteases – tissue-type plasminogen activator (t-PA), urokinase-type plasminogen activator (u-PA), and plasmin; (2) serine protease inhibitors (serpins) – plasminogen activator inhibitors 1 and 2 (PAI-1 and PAI-2) and α_2-antiplasmin (α_2-AP). The active site of the serine protease is located in the carboxyl terminal region of the molecule. Serine proteases are regulated by serpins; the amino acid sequence in the reactive centre of the serpin molecule determines selectivity for specific proteases. Upon interaction with its target, the serpin undergoes a conformational change that irreversibly locks the two molecules together, distorting and inactivating the catalytic site of the protease. The complex then is cleared by the liver.

The interaction of components of the fibrinolytic system involves the lysine-binding sites on t-PA, u-PA and plasminogen/plasmin and lysine residues on fibrin (Figure 29-4). Binding of these proteins to fibrin localizes their fibrinolytic activity and protects them from their inhibitors. The fibrinolytic inhibitor α_2-antiplasmin also binds via its lysine-binding sites to fibrin.

Plasminogen is a single chain zymogen synthesized in the liver; it has a molecular mass of 92 kD and circulates in plasma at a concentration of $1.5 - 2 \mu M$. The molecule is organized into seven structural domains: an NH_2-terminal activation peptide, five homologous folded structures called kringle domains, and the protease domain. Lysine-binding sites on the kringle domains anchor it to the lysine residues on fibrin and endothelial cell surface receptors, eg, annexin II. (Lysine analogues such as epsilon-aminocaproic acid (EACA) and tranexamic acid are used therapeutically to inhibit fibrinolysis: Figure 29-3).

Native plasminogen, **Glu plasminogen**, has an N-terminal glutamic acid that is cleaved

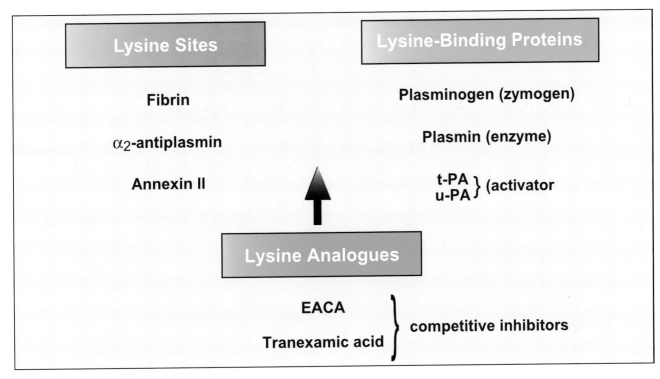

Figure 29-3 The Lysine Connection

by limited plasmin activity, resulting in a major conformational change to **Lys-plasminogen** with an N-terminal lysine. Lys-plasminogen is activated more readily by plasminogen activators and binds more avidly to fibrin. This positive feedback mechanism of plasminogen cleavage by plasmin amplifies lytic activity. In addition, the initial plasmin lytic attack on fibrin exposes new C-terminal lysines; the availability of additional lysine sites augments plasminogen binding to fibrin. Cleavage of a single peptide bond (Arg 560-Val 561) by t-PA or u-PA converts plasminogen to the active serine protease plasmin.

The plasminogen gene on chromosome 6 is linked closely to the structurally similar apolipoprotein (a) gene: this gene product associates with a low density lipoprotein to form **lipoprotein (a)**. By molecular mimicry, Lp(a) competes with plasminogen for the annexin II binding domain on the endothelial cell surface (Figure 29-5). Lp(a) is highly atherogenic – its competitive interference with the binding of plasminogen probably plays a role in development of the atherogenic plaque.

Plasmin. When plasminogen is cleaved, plasmin remains bound to fibrin, protected from its inhibitors and optimally positioned to degrade fibrin; circulating plasmin is neutralized rapidly by α_2-antiplasmin. (In pathological states such as disseminated intravascular coagulation (DIC), increased generation of circulating plasmin may exceed the capacity of the inhibitors α_2-antiplasmin and α_2-macroglobulin; under these circumstances, plasmin will target and degrade circulating fibrinogen and factors V and VIII). Plasmin activity is not confined to the vascular system – it has an important role in the cellular microenvironment. Cell-bound plasmin activates matrix metalloproteins (MMPs), thus mediating dissolution of the extracellular matrix (Figure 29-6).

Plasminogen is converted to the active enzyme by specific serine proteases – **tissue-type plasminogen activator (t-PA)** and **urokinase-type plasminogen activator (u-PA)** also referred to as **urokinase** (Figure 29-1). In the circulation, t-PA is the principal activator of plasminogen. t-PA is synthesized primarily by endothelial cells and released into the circulation in response to a variety of stimuli such as thrombin, vasopressin (and its analogue DDAVP), fibrin deposition and venous occlusion. Bradykinin, released by kallikrein proteolysis of HMWK (Section 17), is a potent stimulator of t-PA release. t-PA has a high affinity for fibrin; its lysine-binding sites interact with lysine residues on fibrin, in juxtaposition to fibrin-bound plasminogen. The co-assembly of t-PA and plasminogen on fibrin increases plasmin generation 500 fold. Until it is bound to fibrin, t-PA has little activity – making it a highly selective mediator of plasminogen activation and fibrin lysis. Unbound t-PA in the plasma forms a complex with **plasminogen activator inhibitor 1 (PAI-1)** and is cleared rapidly from the circulation; fibrin-bound t-PA is protected from PAI-1 inhibition. When fibrin is cross-linked by XIIIa, fewer lysine sites are available to t-PA and fibrinolysis is inhibited.

u-PA, originally isolated from urine, is of primary importance in a number of biological processes, including local fibrinolysis, angiogenesis, inflammation, and extracellular matrix remodelling during wound healing and development. Binding of urokinase to specific receptors provides cells with a localized proteolytic potential. The inactive single chain precursor, scu-PA (prourokinase) is synthesized and secreted by a number of cells, including renal parenchymal cells, monocytes/macrophages, fibroblasts, and epithelial cells. scu-PA has a high affinity for fibrin-bound plasminogen. As plasmin is generated, it cleaves scu-PA to its active two chain form (tcu-PA) which then activates additional plasminogen. Plasminogen and u-PA also associate with cell membranes – co-localization on the cell surface increases the efficiency of plasminogen activation and subsequent plasmin-dependent proteolysis. At sites of vascular injury, **kallikrein** generated from prekallikrein on the surface of endothelial cells activates scu-PA (Figure 29-1).

Inhibitors of Plasminogen Activation (Figure 29-1)

The physiological role of these inhibitors is to block lysis beyond the immediate area of injury – the fibrinolytic enzymes bound to fibrin are protected from inhibition. The **plasminogen activator inhibitors 1 and 2 (PAI-1 and PAI-2)** are serpins. PAI-1, the major inhibitor of both t-PA and u-PA, is the critical regulator of plasminogen activation. It is found primarily in endothelium and in platelet α-granules – its release from these cells produces a high concentration at the site of injury. Release of PAI-1 from endothelial cells is regulated by cytokines and growth factors – as an acute phase reactant its concentration is increased by inflammatory stimuli.

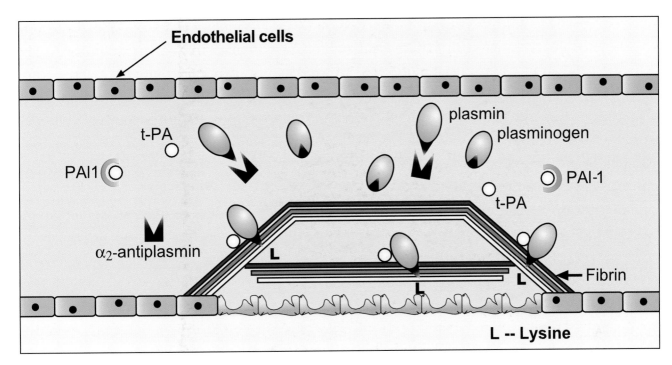

Figure 29-4 The Fibrinolytic System

PAI-1 forms tight 1:1 stable complexes with t-PA and u-PA that are cleared from the circulation by hepatic cells.

In the circulation and in the extra-cellular matrix (ECM), PAI-1 is present primarily in a complex with the glycoprotein vitronectin. Vitronectin-binding appears to be critical for the control and localization of PAI-1: the interaction stabilizes PAI-1 in its active conformation and enhances PAI-1 binding to fibrin. The association of vitronectin, plasminogen activators, and PAI-1 may regulate cell migration in areas of wound healing.

PAI-2 is found in most cells, notably in monocytes/macrophages; it also is present in the trophoblastic epithelium. PAI-2 is secreted into the ECM but is not detectable in plasma except during pregnancy. In tissues, it may contribute to the regulation of plasminogen activator activity on cell surfaces and in the pericellular space.

Thrombin-activatable fibrinolysis inhibitor (TAFI) is a procarboxypeptidase that is synthesized in the liver and circulates in the plasma as an inactive zymogen. TAFI provides an important link between coagulation and fibrinolysis: activation of TAFI by the coagulation system results in downregulation of fibrinolytic activity. TAFI is activated by high concentrations of thrombin; cleavage by thrombin produces the active carboxypeptidase. Thrombin-catalyzed activation of TAFI is increased many fold when thrombin is bound in a complex with thrombomodulin (Section 25).

Activated TAFI (TAFIa) attenuates fibrinolysis by removing carboxy-terminal lysines from fibrin. Because these lysine residues are binding sites for t-PA and plasminogen, their removal by TAFIa inhibits plasmin production and local fibrinolytic activity. Disturbances in the coagulation pathway with reduced production of thrombin results in decreased TAFI activation and an increased rate of clot lysis – this mechanism may contribute to the premature lysis of clots in hemophilia patients. TAFIa rapidly loses its activity through a conformational change and by plasmin proteolysis. (TAFIa also inactivates complement-derived C3a and C5a; in this capacity it is referred to as carboxypeptidase R: Section 20).

Inhibitors of Plasmin (Figure 29-4)

α_2-antiplasmin (α_2-AP) is synthesized in the liver and also is present in platelet α-granules. This serpin circulates at a concentration of 1mM, half the concentration of circulating plasminogen. α_2-AP is the primary inhibitor of plasmin; its inhibitory action is dependent on the availability of both free (i.e. unbound) lysine-binding sites and the free active catalytic site in the plasmin molecule. When plasmin is generated on fibrin strands, its lysine-binding sites are bound to lysine residues on fibrin and its active enzymatic site is engaged in fibrin degradation – thus bound plasmin is protected from inactivation by α_2-antiplasmin. Unbound, circulating free plasmin is a ready target for α_2-AP inhibition: α_2-AP interacts with the lysine-binding sites on plasmin to form an irreversible 1:1 stoichiometric complex that is cleared in the liver.

α_2-macroglobulin is a non-specific protease inhibitor (not a serpin) that inactivates a broad spectrum of substrates. It is synthesized by endothelial cells and macrophages, and is present in platelet α-granules. As a second-line inhibitor of plasmin and t-PA it becomes important only in the event of major systemic activation of the lytic system.

Cell Surface Receptors (Figure 29-5)

Cell surface receptors localize and regulate components of the fibrinolytic system. Plasminogen receptors are expressed on a variety of cells – the receptors that have been identified include: gangliosides, the glycolytic enzyme α enolase, and the integrin $\alpha_{IIb}\beta_3$ (GPIIb/IIIa) on activated platelets. The receptor **annexin II**, bound to phosphatidylserine expressed on the surface of activated endothelial cells, binds both plasminogen and t-PA. Because the plasminogen and t-PA lysine-binding sites interact with lysine residues on annexin II, the enzymes are protected from their inhibitors and, with their location on the endothelium, they are well-positioned to regulate fibrinolysis at adjacent sites of vessel injury and fibrin deposition. (Annexins are a class of phospholipid-binding proteins with a preference for negatively charged phospholipids like PS. Annexin V is discussed in Section 25).

The **u-PA receptor** (u-PAR) serves to localize u-PA activity, resulting in cell-surface activation of plasminogen. u-PAR is expressed on the surface of activated monocytes/macrophages, endothelial cells, platelets and fibroblasts. HMWK binds both to cell surfaces and

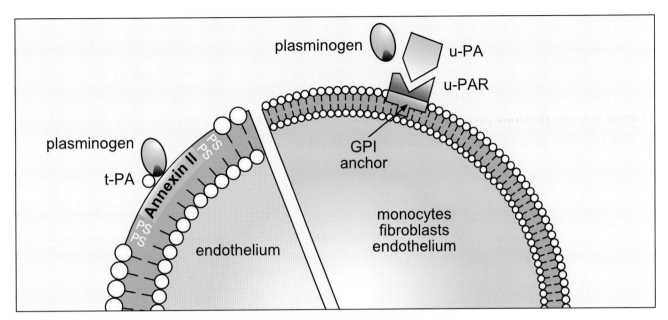

Figure 29-5   Cell Receptors for Plasminogen and Plasminogen Activators

to u-PAR, bringing the components of the kininogen/kinin system into close proximity with fibrinolytic proteins; kallikrein activates scu-PA (Figure 29-1).

u-PAR is linked to the cell membrane by a glycosylphosphatidylinositol (GPI) anchor (Figure 29-5). As with other GPI-anchored proteins, u-PAR is deficient in paroxysmal nocturnal hemoglobinuria (PNH) – whether the high incidence of venous thrombosis associated with PNH is related to the deficiency of u-PAR is uncertain (Section 10).

Fibrin-Fibrinogen Degradation Products (FDPs)

The process of lysis depends on the substrate; the end-products formed when fibrinogen and non-crosslinked fibrin are lysed differ from those formed on lysis of crosslinked fibrin (Figure 29-1). Plasmin cleavage of crosslinked fibrin first releases a series of large molecular weight products; further digestion yields the two terminal digestion products, E piece (50 kD) and a crosslinked D-D (D-dimer) piece (180 kD). Plasmin degradation of fibrinogen and non-crosslinked fibrin yields a different series of breakdown products: the earliest to appear is the large fragment X (240 kD); further lysis generates fragment Y (165 kD) and one D piece; Y is subsequently degraded to one D piece (90 kD) and one E piece.

When present in the circulation (eg, in DIC), these products are of functional significance as they interfere with coagulation: fragments X and Y are competitive inhibitors of thrombin and interfere with fibrin polymerization; D and E interfere with platelet function. FDPs can be identified in plasma; D and E also are found in urine. Identifying D-dimers in plasma provides evidence for the presence of crosslinked fibrin in the circulation and supports the diagnosis of on-going intravascular clotting.

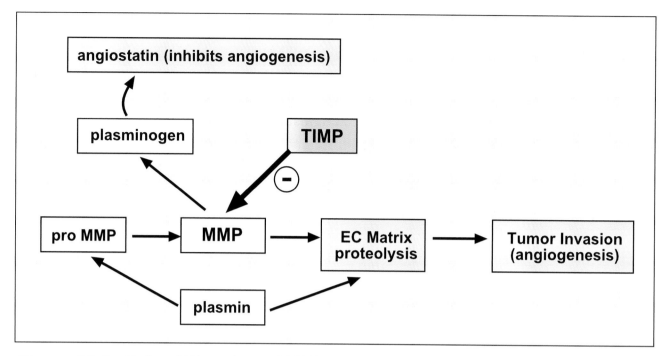

Figure 29-6   Role of Plasmin and MMP in Tumor Invasion

Matrix Metalloproteinases (MMPs) (Figure 29-6)

The extracellular matrix (ECM) is an intricate meshwork of proteinaceous fibres (eg, fibrillar collagen) and other macromolecules. Degradation of ECM takes place during cell migration and tissue remodeling and involves two proteolytic systems: the fibrinolytic and MMP systems. Plasmin can degrade only some of the components of ECM, such as laminin and fibronectin, but it plays a role in activation of proMMPs. MMPs degrade other components such as elastin and collagen.

MMPs are a family of zinc-dependent enzymes that can be divided into two structurally distinct groups: secreted MMPs and membrane-type MMPs. The secreted MMPs include collagenases, gelatinases, and stromelysins. The majority of MMPs are secreted as zymogens (proMMPs) and are activated extracellularly by a variety of proteases including plasmin. The membrane MMPs are expressed at the cell surface in activated form. MMP expression is regulated transcriptionally by growth factors, cytokines, cell-matrix and cell-cell interactions. MMP activity also is regulated by a family of proteins referred to as **tissue inhibitors of metalloproteinases (TIMPs)**. TIMPs can bind both proMMP and activated MMP to limit and regulate proteolysis.

Proteolysis of the ECM by MMPs is essential to normal physiological processes: tissue remodelling, wound healing, angiogenesis, and embryogenesis. MMPs also contribute to microbial and tumor cell invasion, to metastasis, and to degenerative diseases. Most tumors are supported by normal stroma; during tumor progression, the stromal cells are stimulated to produce proteases, inhibitors, and other regulatory factors. Interactions between tumor and stromal cells involve the two protease systems, uPA/uPAR/plasminogen and the MMPs, that are primarily responsible for extracellular proteolysis. Activation of these proteases on the surface of tumor cells promotes tumor invasion.

MMP cleavage of plasminogen releases **angiostatin**, a plasminogen fragment consisting of kringles 1-4. Angiostatin is a circulating inhibitor that binds to the endothelial surface ATP synthase responsible for angiogenesis. Angiostatin-binding may promote apoptosis, thus inhibiting endothelial cell proliferation and angiogenesis. Because angiostatin inhibits tumor vascularization, it may have a major role in the inhibition of tumor growth.

CLINICAL CORRELATES

Fibrinogen

Congenital deficiency of fibrinogen is inherited as an autosomal recessive disorder; hypofibrinogenemia is more common than afibrinogenemia. Congenital afibrinogenemia is due to mutations in the fibrinogen gene cluster on chromosome 4. In the majority of Caucasian patients, there are truncating mutations in the fibrinogen Aα gene. Bleeding usually appears at fibrinogen levels below 0.5 g/L and varies from moderate to severe; umbilical cord bleeding, mucosal bleeding, and menorrhagia are common. In afibrinogenemia, laboratory tests (PTT, PT and TT) are infinitely prolonged. Antibodies to fibrinogen may develop following fibrinogen replacement therapy.

Congenital dysfibrinogenemia is characterized by a structurally abnormal molecule with abnormal function. A number of functional abnormalities have been described: (1) impaired fibrinopeptide release, (2) defects in polymerization, and (3) defective cross-linking. Because fibrin formed from abnormal fibrinogens frequently is more resistant to lysis, these patients may present with thrombotic disease rather than with a bleeding diathesis.

Acquired disorders of fibrinogen include: (1) increased levels associated with inflammatory disease as fibrinogen is an acute phase reactant, (2) hypofibrinogenemia due to impaired synthesis in hepatocellular disease, or increased consumption in DIC and fibrinolytic states, (3) dysfibrinogenemia associated with acute or chronic liver disease or primary hepatic tumours; the abnormal fibrinogen is characterized by defective fibrin polymerization – the structural defect, the result of post-translational modification, is due to an increase in the amount of sialic acid attached to carbohydrate side chains.

Defibrinogenating agents derived from snake venom (eg, ancrod) are anticoagulants, not lytic agents. They catalyze the conversion of fibrinogen to fibrin by selectively removing fibrinopeptide A. Because ancrod does not activate factor XIII, this soluble fibrin, with residual intact fibrinopeptide B, is not crosslinked and is removed rapidly from the circulation by the reticuloendothelial system and by fibrinolysis. As a result, there is no intravascular deposition of fibrin associated with the rapid depletion of plasma fibrinogen.

Factor XIII

Deficiency of factor XIII is a rare autosomal recessive disorder, most frequently due to a primary defect in the catalytic A subunit. More than one-third of these patients have point mutations that cause amino-acid substitution. Rarely, there is a primary defect in the carrier B subunit that results in a secondary decrease in plasma subunit A; as the A_2 dimer in platelets is not affected, these patients have a mild bleeding disorder. Patients with homozygous factor XIII (A subunit) deficiency characteristically present with severe delayed bleeding 12-36 hours after trauma or surgery; although poor wound healing was described in the original patient, it is not common. Because there is bleeding at the time of umbilical cord separation, the deficiency usually is apparent in the neonatal period. Intracranial hemorrhage is the most serious complication in untreated patients.

Reduced levels of factor XIII are present in liver disease (decreased synthesis) or with increased consumption (in inflammatory bowel disease, septicemia, major surgery, and DIC). Acquired factor XIII inhibitors are rare but have been described in the elderly associated with autoimmune disease, and in patients receiving prolonged therapy with a number of drugs including isoniazid; hemorrhagic complications may be life threatening.

In factor XIII deficiency, routine coagulation screening tests are normal. Diagnosis depends on the demonstration of increased solubility of the fibrin clot in 1% monochloroacetic acid or 5M urea; confirmation is provided by immunoelectrophoresis or by specific assays that measure the enzymatic activity of factor XIII. The clot solubility test is positive only when the plasma factor XIII level approximates zero, therefore, the test is not reliable if the patient has received blood products within the preceding five to six weeks. Factor XIII concentrates are used to control severe bleeding; plasma may be used for milder episodes. Because the half-life of infused factor XIII is long (11 to 14 days), prophylactic infusions can be given at five to six week intervals.

Fibrinolysis

Acute promyelocytic leukemia (APL) patients (t[15;17]) frequently present with a hemorrhagic diathesis manifest by bleeding into skin and mucous membranes and at venipuncture sites; the incidence of intracranial hemorrhage is high. Increased fibrinolysis, critical to the pathological process, is the result of multiple interacting factors: (1) The high expression of the plaminogen/t-PA receptor annexin II on the surface of the leukemic cells results in increased plasminogen activation, formation of plasmin, and consumption of the inhibitors α_2-AP and PAI-1. (2) The release of plasminogen activators by the leukemic cells augments the fibrinolysis.

(3) TAFIa activity is limited due to its inactivation by plasmin. The life-threatening bleeding may be reversed by early treatment with all-trans-retinoic acid – ATRA (Section 22).

Therapeutic Clot Lysis.

Thrombolysis may be activated pharmacologically in the treatment of vascular and, particularly, coronary artery occlusion. The agents in clinical use are: recombinant t-PA, urokinase, prourokinase (scu-PA), and streptokinase. Streptokinase (SK), derived from β hemolytic streptococci, has no intrinsic enzymatic activity until complexed with plasmin or plasminogen to produce a potent activator of plasminogen; SK forms a complex with plasminogen on an equimolar basis – the SK-plasminogen complex converts plasminogen to plasmin.

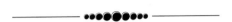

SUGGESTED READING

Anwar R, Miloszewski KJA. Factor XIII deficiency. Br J Haemat 107: 468-484, 1999.

Blomback B. Fibrinogen and fibrin - proteins with complex roles in hemostasis and thrombosis. Thromb Res 83:1-75, 1996.

Browder T. Folkman J, Pirie-Shepherd S. The hemostatic system as a regulator of angiogenesis. J Biol Chem 275:1521-1524, 2000.

Collen D. The plasminogen (fibrinolytic) system. Thromb Haemost 82:259-270, 1999.

Hajjar KA. Changing concepts in fibrinolysis. Curr Opin Hematol 2:345-350, 1995.

Ichinose A. Physiopathology and regulation of factor XIII. Thromb Haemost 86:57-65, 2001.

Kohler HP, Grant PJ. Plasminogen-activator inhibitor type 1 and coronary artery disease. N Engl J Med 342:1792-1801, 2000.

Marder VJ, Francis CW. Plasmin degradation of cross-linked fibrin. Ann N Y Acad Sci 408:397-406, 1983.

McDonagh J, Fukue H. Determinants of substrate specificity for factor XIII. Semin Thromb Hemost 22:369-376, 1996.

Meijers JCM, Oudijk EJD, Mosnier LO, et al. Reduced activity of TAFI (thrombin-activatable fibrinolysis inhibitor) in acute promyelocytic leukaemia. Br J Haematol 108:518-523, 2000.

Menell JS, Ceserman GM, Jacovina, McLaughlin MA, Lev EA, Hajjar KA. Annexin II and bleeding in acute promyelocytic leukemia. N Engl J Med 340: 994-1004, 1999.

Nelson AR, Fingleton B, Rothenberg ML, Matrissian LM. Matrix metalloproteinases: biologic activity and clinical implications. J Clin Oncol 18:1135-1149, 2000.

Pepper MS. Extracellular proteolysis and angiogenesis. Thromb Haemost 86:346-355, 2001.

Plow EF, Herren T, Redlitz A, Miles LA, Hoover-Plow JL. The cell biology of the plasminogen system. FASEB J 9:939-945, 1995.

Podor TJ, Peterson CB, Lawrence DA et al. Type 1 plasminogen activator inhibitor binds to fibrin via vitronectin. J Biol Chem 275:19788-19794, 2000.

Robbins KE. Dysplasminogenemias. Prog Cardiovasc Dis 34:295-308, 1992.

Roberts HR, Stinchcombe TE, Gabriel DA. The Dysfibrinogenemias. Br J Haemat 114:249-257, 2001.

PLATELET STRUCTURE AND FUNCTION

Sara Israels
Esther Israels

*"Il existe dans le sang trois espèces de particules: 1° les globules rouges
(the red globules); 2° les globules blancs (the white globules);
3° les globulines (the little globules – the platelets)"*
Alfred Donné - Paris Academy of Sciences – 1842

Donné's report to the Paris Academy of Sciences in 1842 is probably the first microscopic description of the platelet. These small anucleate cells, formed in the bone marrow by fragmentation of megakaryocyte cytoplasm, carry the intracellular components that will serve them in the peripheral circulation over their lifespan of seven to twelve days. The metabolic repertoire of this small anucleate cell is large and complex.

MEGAKARYOCYTES AND THROMBOPOIESIS

Megakaryocytes (MKs) are derived from pluripotent bone marrow stem cells that, under cytokine stimulation, become committed to the MK lineage. Development of MKs evolves through the proliferation of progenitor cells and generation of immature MKs, culminating in the appearance of mature post-mitotic cells.

Thrombopoietin (TPO) is the primary regulator of thrombopoiesis. The TPO gene has been mapped to chromosome 3. TPO has a molecular weight of 31-35 kD; it contains two domains – one of these, the amino-terminal domain, has significant homology with erythropoietin. (TPO also contributes to the proliferation of erythropoietic progenitors). It is produced primarily in the liver, but also in the kidney. Binding of TPO to the Mpl receptor on MK progenitors initiates signal transduction that results in the proliferative response.

The TPO receptor gene initially was recognized as the human homologue of the transforming viral gene *v-mpl* of the myeloproliferative leukemia virus (MPLV). The normal cellular proto-oncogene (*c-mpl*) encodes the TPO receptor (**Mpl**) expressed on the surface membrane of MK-lineage cells and platelets. Binding of TPO through its amino-terminal domain to Mpl results in receptor dimerization and intracellular signaling. Like other cytokine receptors, Mpl does not possess intrinsic tyrosine kinase activity; the cytoplasmic domains of the activated dimerized receptor induce activation of the tyrosine kinase JAK2 and tyrosine phosphorylation of a number of targets through the JAK/STAT signal transduction pathway (Section 1), triggering nuclear signaling and MK proliferation.

Following the proliferative phase, TPO induces maturation of the diploid (2N) MK precursors. An increase in ploidy is the result of the unique process of **endomitosis**: DNA replication is uncoupled from cell division, resulting in a cell that contains multiples (up to 64 times) of the normal chromosomal complement (2N) within a single nucleus. Once the polyploid nucleus is formed, there is a dramatic increase in the amount of cytoplasm and an increase in the number of platelet specific granules; the cell volume is correspondingly larger. Demarcation by invagination of the plasma membrane results in the cytoplasmic partitioning that is a precursor to the release of mature platelets.

The TPO level in the circulation is regulated by a feedback mechanism that involves TPO binding to Mpl on platelets and MKs; bound TPO is degraded. During normal hemostasis, the platelet count (mass) remains constant and circulating TPO is maintained at basal levels. In thrombocytopenia, the drop in platelet mass results in a reduced number of peripheral binding sites for TPO; with the increase in unbound TPO there is enhanced stimulation of MK precursors. The reverse process operates in thrombocytosis: TPO binding by the elevated platelet/MK mass reduces the level of circulating TPO, limiting thrombopoiesis.

PLATELET STRUCTURE

The circulating platelet is an irregular disc with an average diameter of 3.5 μm and a thickness of 0.9 μm. A number of morphological structures are unique to platelets (Figure 30-1). The **surface-connected canalicular system** weaves throughout the platelet – the membrane is continuous with the plasma membrane and during platelet activation it provides the additional membrane surface required for formation of pseudopodia and platelet spreading. Although the canalicular system opens to the external milieu, energy is required for the uptake of molecules into these channels. The **dense tubular system,** a closed channel consisting of narrow tubules, is considered analogous to the sarcoplasmic reticulum of smooth muscle. It is the site of calcium storage – platelet activation triggers Ca^{2+} release into the cytoplasm.

The platelet **cytoskeleton** supports the plasma membrane and is primarily responsible for maintaining the shape of both resting and activated platelets. It consists of three major structures: (1) a membrane-associated cytoskeleton composed of actin, actin-binding protein, spectrin, α-actinin, and a number of other proteins that contribute to maintaining the discoid shape; the cytoplasmic domains of the membrane glycoproteins GPIIb/IIIa and GPIb/IX/V are associated with the membrane cytoskeleton; (2) a microtubule coil at the periphery is a tightly wound polymer of tubulin that helps maintain the discoid shape of the platelet; when the platelet is activated, contraction of this coil may move the platelet granules to the centre of the cell; (3) a cytoplasmic network consisting of long interconnecting actin filaments.

There are three primary types of **platelet granules**: lysosomes, and two types of platelet specific granules (electron dense granules and alpha-granules). The soluble acid hydrolases present in **lysosomes** are involved in intracellular protein degradation. **Dense granules** (delta (δ) granules) contain non-protein agonists: serotonin, Ca^{2+}, and the non-metabolic pool of adenine nucleotides (ADP and ATP); CD63 (a tetraspanin) is present in the granule membrane. Release of the contents promotes platelet activation. There are 3 to 8 dense granules per platelet; because of their high calcium content, they appear as dense bodies in electron micrographs of whole platelets. The **alpha-granules** are the predominant granule – about 50 per platelet. They contain a broad range of proteins: (1) adhesive proteins (vWF, fibrinogen, fibronectin, vitronectin, thrombospondin, membrane P-selectin and GPIIb/IIIa), (2) procoagulants (factors V, XI, XIII), (3) anticoagulant factors (protein S), (4) anti-lytic factors (plasminogen activator inhibitor-1), (5) anti-heparins (platelet factor 4), (6) growth-promoting factors for angiogenesis and repair (platelet derived growth factor, transforming growth factor-β, thrombospondin). Some of these proteins are synthesized by MKs, eg, vWF, platelet factor 4 (PF4), β-thromboglobulin, and factor V. Other proteins are acquired from the plasma by endocytosis, eg, fibrinogen, albumin, and IgG.

THE PHOSPHOLIPID MEMBRANE

Intact platelets in the circulation normally present a non-thrombogenic surface. The anionic phospholipids, phosphatidylserine (PS) and phosphatidylethanolamine (PE), are sequestered in the inner leaflet of the plasma membrane; neutral phospholipids, phosphatidyl-choline (PC) and sphingomyelin (SM), predominate in the outer leaflet. This asymmetry is

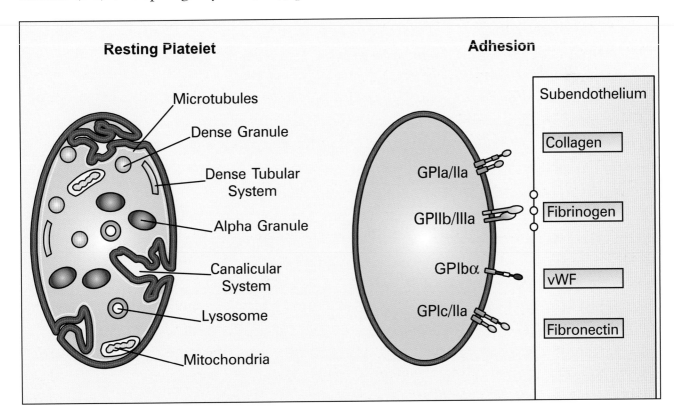

Figure 30-1 Platelet Structure and Adhesion Receptors

maintained by a dynamic process involving two ATP-dependent enzymes: **translocase** and **flopase**. Translocase (also referred to as flipase) rapidly transports PS and PE from the outer surface of the membrane to the inner surface; flopase slowly transfers PC and other phospholipids to the outer surface. With activation of platelets, there is extensive remodeling of the surface membrane: an increase in the level of intracellular calcium blocks translocase and flopase activity, while a third enzyme, the Ca^{2+}-dependent **scramblase** is activated. Scramblase induces rapid movement of phospholipids in both directions (referred to as "lipid scrambling") – the result is loss of asymmetry and exposure of PS and PE on the cell surface; this is associated with the appearance of small PS-rich membrane "microparticles" in the plasma. PS plays a critical role in platelet-mediated blood coagulation: when exposed on the outer leaflet, this anionic phospholipid provides a procoagulant surface for the assembly of the tenase and prothrombinase complexes leading to the generation of thrombin (Section 24). The membrane microparticles probably provide additional surface for the assembly of these coagulant proteins. (The procoagulant phospholipid surface previously was referred to as "platelet factor 3 activity").

RECEPTOR-MEDIATED ADHESION

Platelets support primary hemostasis at sites of vascular injury. A number of platelet membrane receptors are poised for immediate interaction with specific adhesive proteins when an area of vascular damage is encountered. These constitutively expressed receptors mediate adhesion to subendothelium; subsequent platelet activation and aggregation result in the formation of a firm platelet plug at the site of the vascular leak.

Deposition of platelets on exposed subendothelium is influenced by shear forces within the vessel. The velocity of blood in the vessel is highest in the centre of the stream and lowest near the vessel wall. There is a shearing effect between the layers of fluid moving in parallel at different rates – sheer stress is greatest near the vessel wall (Figure 30-2). Red cells predominate in the axial stream; platelets are marginated along the vessel wall by the shear forces and by collisions with red cells. As a result of these physical and kinetic factors, platelets are well-positioned to monitor the integrity of the vessel wall and respond immediately at sites of vessel damage. This is illustrated by the prolonged bleeding time associated with a decrease in red cell mass, such as in the anemia of renal failure: correction of the hematocrit by blood transfusion shortens the bleeding time in these patients.

When platelets encounter an area of denuded endothelium, they adhere to the subendothelial matrix, undergo a dramatic change in shape to an irregular sphere with multiple pseudopods, and spread to increase their area of surface contact. Agonists in the microenvironment interact with specific receptors on the platelet surface. A number of glycoproteins (GPs) on the

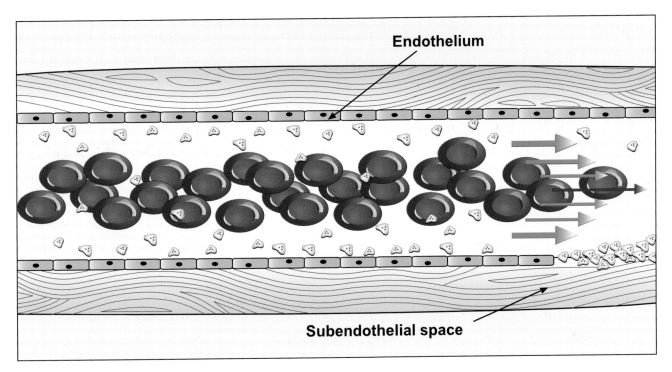

Figure 30-2 Sheer Stress

platelet membrane are receptors for adhesive proteins present in the vessel wall and in plasma. (The numbering of GPs from I to IX is based on separation patterns obtained on polyacrylamide gel electrophoresis; further subdivisions are designated a or b). Some of these glycoprotein receptors are integrins (Section 3); the integrin subunit composition is designated in parenthesis. GPVI and GPIb/IX/V are non-integrin receptors. The platelet adhesion receptors and their ligands include: GPIa/IIa ($\alpha_2\beta_1$) and GPVI for collagen, GPIc/IIa ($\alpha_5\beta_1$) for fibronectin, GPIb (located within the GPIb/IX/V complex) for vWF; $\alpha_V\beta_3$ for vitronectin, fibrinogen, vWF, and thrombospondin; and GPIIb/IIIa ($\alpha_{IIb}\beta_3$) for vWF, fibrinogen, fibronectin and vitronectin (Figure 30-1). The redundancy of receptors enhances platelet engagement with matrix proteins; a single ligand binding to different receptors may initiate several functional responses.

The capacity of platelets to adhere to the vessel wall is pivotal to normal hemostasis (and to formation of thrombi). At sites of exposed subendothelial matrix, platelet attachment must resist the force of blood flow – highest shear rates are present in the microcirculation and in areas of vessel narrowing. Platelet interaction with vWF is indispensible for adhesion in areas of high shear stress. At high shear rates, the initial adhesive event is platelet tethering mediated by subendothelial-bound vWF interacting with the platelet GPIb/IX/V complex. Subendothelial vWF is bound through its A3 domain to collagen; its A1 domain binds to platelet GPIbα (Section 27). This initial adhesion is rapid, enabling the capture of circulating platelets, but the bond is transient and is sufficient only to slow platelet passage (comparable to leukocyte rolling in areas of inflammation: Section 7). Firm adhesion requires interaction of other platelet receptors with the subendothelial matrix, notably collagen or immobilized fibrinogen. The interaction of platelet GPIb with vWF induces intracellular signaling that triggers activation of membrane GPIIb/IIIa; vWF in the extracellular matrix now binds irreversibly to the activated GPIIb/IIIa, producing firm adhesion of the platelet to the vessel wall (Figure 30-3).

The highest shear stress occurs in areas of vascular turbulence, eg, in the presence of prosthetic cardiac valves or pathological vessel narrowing. Under these circumstances, conformational changes are induced in circulating vWF that increase its binding affinity for platelet GPIb (Section 27).

In areas of low shear stress, adhesion is less dependent upon GPIb/IX/V. Platelet adhesion at these sites involves interaction with other subendothelial matrix adhesive proteins: fibronectin, collagen and fibrinogen. The platelets adhere through GPIc/IIa to fibronectin, through GPIa/IIa and GPVI to collagen, and through GPIIb/IIIa to the immobilized fibrinogen.

RECEPTOR-MEDIATED SIGNAL TRANSDUCTION

A variety of agonists are involved in transforming the circulating resting platelet into an adherent platelet. Interaction with surface receptors induces the intracellular signaling that results in platelet activation, secretion and aggregation.

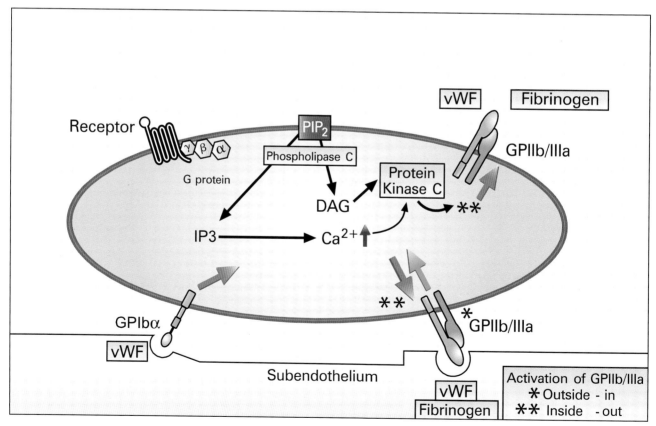

Figure 30-3 Platelet Signaling

Phospholipid Signaling Pathways (Figures 30-3, 30-4, 30-5)

Membrane phospholipids are substrates for two inter-related signaling pathways that mediate platelet activation: the phosphoinositide pathway and the arachidonic acid pathway. The primary membrane phospholipids are phosphatidylcholine (38%), phosphatidylethanolamine (27%), phosphatidylserine (10%), and phosphatidylinositol (5%). Two other inositol containing

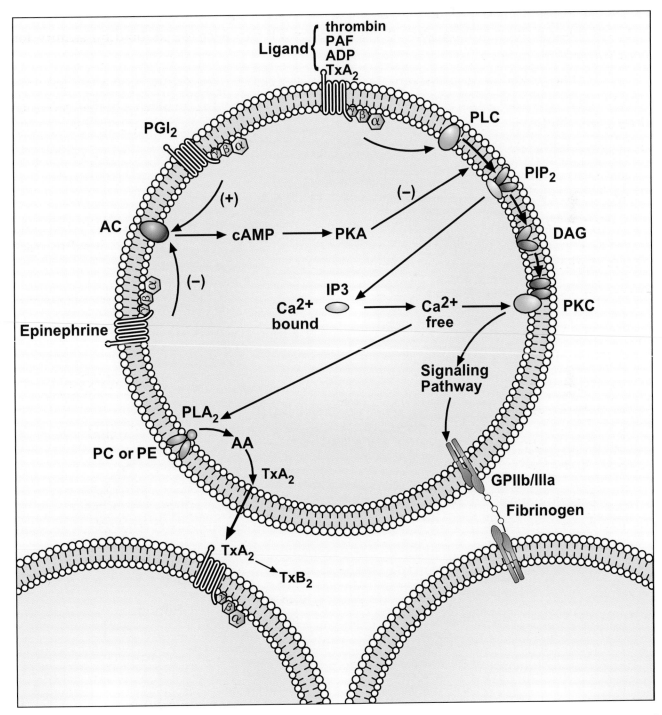

Figure 30-4 Platelet Activation - Inhibition

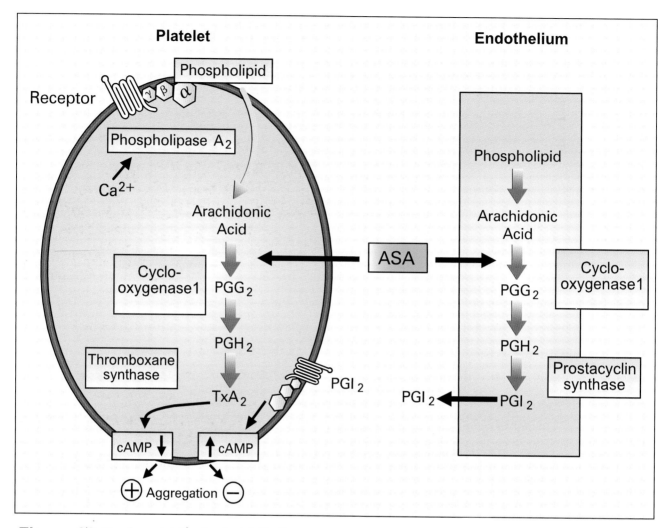

Figure 30-5   Arachidonic Acid Pathways

phospholipids are derived by phosphorylation of phosphatidylinositol (PI): phosphatidylinositol 4-phosphate (PIP) and phosphoinositol 4,5-bisphosphate (PIP_2).

    Phosphoinositide Pathway. Agonist binding to specific G protein-coupled receptors (GPCRs) results in the activation of plasma membrane **phospholipase C (PLC);** this enzyme hydrolyzes **PIP_2** in the plasma membrane to two potent second messengers: inositol triphosphate (**IP3**) and diacylglycerol (**DAG**). DAG activates **protein kinase C (PKC)**; PKC phosphorylation of target proteins induces granule secretion and up-regulation of the receptor GPIIb/IIIa. Soluble IP3 diffuses from the plasma membrane to the dense tubular system, where it binds to specific receptors that cause Ca^{2+} channels to open. Sequestered Ca^{2+} is released into the cytosol from the dense tubular system; there is also an increase in trans-membrane Ca^{2+} influx through opening of plasma membrane ligand-gated Ca^{2+} channels. The sharp rise in cytosolic Ca^{2+} triggers granule secretion and secondary activation of phospholipase A_2. Also, the increase of cytosolic Ca^{2+} causes cytosolic PKC to bind to the plasma membrane where it can be activated by the membrane-associated DAG – thus activation of PKC depends on both Ca^{2+} ions and DAG. (In the resting platelet, cytosolic Ca^{2+} is maintained at a low level by Ca^{2+} efflux from the cell and sequestration in the dense tubular system).

Arachidonic Acid (AA) Pathway. AA is the major polyunsaturated fatty acid in humans. Its oxygenated derivatives are the prostanoids (members of a large group of oxygenated fatty acids known collectively as **eicosanoids,** a family of potent signaling molecules that act within short range of the cells that produce them). The AA pathway is initiated by agonist binding to specific platelet receptors and stimulation of signaling pathways that lead to activation of cytosolic **phospholipase A_2 (PLA$_2$).** PLA$_2$ hydrolyzes membrane phospholipids, primarily phosphatidylethanolamine **(PE)** and phosphatidylcholine **(PC),** with release of arachidonic acid. The enzyme **cyclooxygenase-1** (COX-1) catalyzes oxidation of arachidonate to produce the eicosanoid prostaglandin PGG$_2$. A subsequent peroxidase reaction converts PGG$_2$ to PGH$_2$. In platelets, PGH$_2$ is converted by **thromboxane synthase** to thromboxane **(TxA$_2$),** a potent short-lived platelet excitatory agonist. TxA$_2$ exits the platelet and binds to a specific G protein-coupled receptor (GPCR) on the same platelet or on nearby platelets. Binding of TxA$_2$ results in the activation of phospholipase C, thereby activating the phosphoinositide pathway with formation of the second messengers, IP3 and DAG. TxA$_2$ is highly labile and degrades spontaneously to the inactive metabolite **TxB$_2$.**

In other cells eicosanoid synthesis follows the same initial sequence, but PGH$_2$ is converted via specific synthases to other biologically active end products. In endothelial cells, PGH$_2$ is converted by **prostacylin synthase** to prostacylin **(PGI$_2$),** an inhibitor of platelet aggregation. PGE$_2$ and PGD$_2$ also are inhibitors of platelet aggregation – inflammatory cells are one source of these prostanoids.

Cyclic AMP (Figure 30-6)

Cyclic AMP (cAMP) is a second messenger formed from ATP by the membrane enzyme **adenylyl cyclase (AC).** cAMP activity is terminated when it is hydrolyzed to AMP by **cAMP phosphodiesterase.** Adenylyl cyclase is stimulated by the binding of agonists such as PGI$_2$, PGE$_2$, and PGD$_2$ to platelet receptors. Increased levels of cAMP inhibit aggregation – this is the result of activation of the cAMP-dependent **protein kinase A (PKA).** Phosphorylation of target proteins by PKA decreases platelet activity, probably by reducing phosphoinositide hydrolysis and levels of IP3, DAG, and free cytosolic Ca^{2+}. In contrast, when cAMP levels fall, platelet aggregation is enhanced. Receptor-binding of agonists such as thrombin, ADP, TxA$_2$, and epinephrine initiate signaling pathways that lead to inhibition of adenylyl cyclase, thereby suppressing cAMP synthesis.

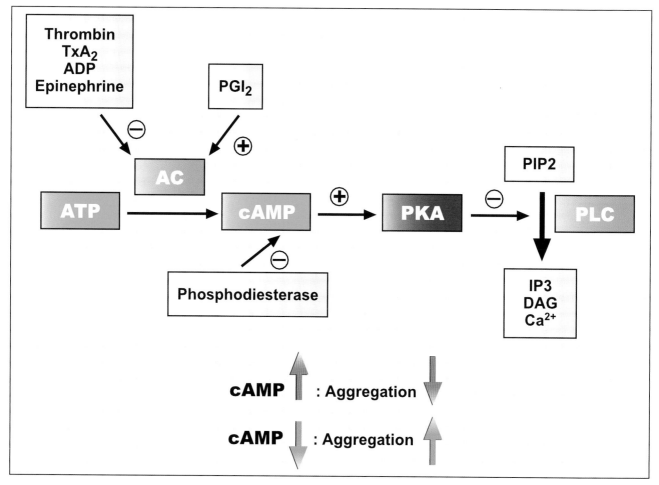

Figure 30-6 The Role of cAMP

Receptor Ligands

Agonist occupancy of specific receptors is coupled to cell signaling. vWF, thrombin, collagen, ADP, TxA$_2$, and PAF induce activation of phospholipase C; ADP and epinephrine inhibit adenylyl cyclase. Agonists that bind to platelet membrane GPCRs include thrombin, epinephrine, PAF, ADP, and TxA$_2$.

vWF adhesion to the GPIb/IX/V complex on platelets initiates the events that result in either hemostasis or thrombosis. The plasma membrane GPIb-IX-V complex consists of four transmembrane units: GPIbα, GPIbβ, GPIX and GPV. In the normal circulation, vWF does not adhere to platelets. Both immobilization of vWF (in the subendothelial matrix) and high shear stress alter the conformation of the A1 domain of vWF, making it a high-affinity ligand for the GPIb/IX/V complex. vWF binds to at least three regions in the N-terminal domain of GPIbα, inducing signaling that involves elevation of Ca^{2+} and activation of protein kinase C and, ultimately, results in 'inside-out' activation of GPIIb/IIIa (Section 3).

At sites of vascular injury, the exposure of **tissue factor**, expressed constitutively on the surface of cells in the subendothelium, results in formation of the tissue factor/factor VIIa complex that leads to the local generation of thrombin from prothrombin (Section 24). **Thrombin** binding to the platelet receptors **PAR-1** and **PAR-4** (protease activated receptor-1 and -4) triggers platelet secretion and aggregation. These GPCRs are activated by a novel mechanism: thrombin cleaves the receptor at a single peptide-bond in the amino-terminal extracellular domain to unmask a new amino-terminus that then functions as a tethered ligand; binding of the new NH_2-terminus to a site within the extracellular portion of the receptor induces receptor self-activation. (Like other G protein-coupled receptors, activated PAR-1 and PAR-4 are internalized and rapidly degraded – thus terminating signal transduction). The glycoprotein complex **GPIb/IX/V** also has been recognized as a thrombin receptor; thrombin first cleaves GPV from the complex and, subsequently, binds to GPIbα. Thrombin binding generates intracellular signals that lead to GPIIb/IIIa activation. Recent evidence indicates that **activated factor XII (XIIa)** is a ligand for GPIbα – this interaction has the capacity to regulate thrombin binding to GPIbα and thereby inhibit thrombin-induced platelet aggregation.

Collagen is the most thrombogenic matrix protein and a major platelet agonist. Platelet-collagen interaction involves the GPIa/IIa and GPVI receptors. With initial binding of collagen to GPVI, GPIa/IIa ($\alpha_2\beta_1$) undergoes a conformational change to a high-affinity state. Binding of both platelet receptors to collagen is required for optimum intracellular signaling that leads to phospholipase C activation.

The adhesive protein **thrombospondin** (TSP) is present in α-granules and is secreted during platelet activation; it binds to a specific five-transmembrane-spanning receptor, inducing an intracellular signal that converts GPIIb/IIIa from a resting to an active configuration.

ADP activates platelets by binding to three purine receptors ($P2Y_1$, $P2Y_{12}$, and $P2X_1$) on the platelet surface. $P2Y_1$ is a GPCR that, on ADP binding, activates phospholipase C with formation of IP3 and release of Ca^{2+} from intracellular stores. ADP binding to the GPCR $P2Y_{12}$ inhibits platelet adenylyl cyclase, reducing the level of cAMP. Simultaneous stimulation of these two receptors by ADP is required to induce platelet aggregation. The $P2X_1$ receptor is a ligand-gated ion channel that mediates rapid transient Ca^{2+} influx in response to ADP binding. ADP amplifies platelet aggregation, secretion, and procoagulant activity induced by other platelet agonists (eg, collagen).

Epinephrine stimulates platelets by binding to specific GPCRs, the α_2-adrenergic receptors that inhibit adenylyl cyclase activity. **PAF** is a lipid mediator produced by endothelial and other cells including activated neutrophils. PAF binds to a high-affinity GPCR on platelets, stimulating aggregation and secretion through PLC activation.

There are three **eicosanoid receptors**: two inhibitory and one stimulatory. The inhibitory eicosanoids interact with a PGI_2/PGE_2 receptor and a PGD_2 receptor; when activated by agonist binding, these receptors induce intracellular signals that stimulate adenylyl cyclase, thereby increasing cAMP and inhibiting platelet activation and aggregation. PGI_2 is the most important of these platelet inhibitors. Binding of the eicosanoid **thromboxane A_2** to its high affinity GPCR stimulates platelet activation via the PLC pathway.

Negative Regulators of Platelet Activation

Circulating platelets are maintained in a non-reactive state until they are recruited to sites of vascular damage. Inappropriate adherence to normal endothelium or to other platelets is prevented or terminated by a number of internal and external factors. Intrinsic platelet factors contribute to maintenance of this inactive state: (1) The negative surface charge on platelets prevents interaction with red cells, leukocytes, endothelial cells, or other platelets. (2) The active form of GPIIb/IIIa is not expressed constitutively on resting platelets; it must undergo a conformational change before it reacts with plasma fibrinogen. If minimal activation of the receptor occurs, internalization of GPIIb/IIIa bound to fibrinogen may clear the receptor/ligand complex from the platelet surface. (3) Tight regulation maintains cytosolic Ca^{2+} at a low level. (4) Platelet surface ADPases hydrolyze ADP secreted by platelets and other circulating cells. (5) The potent platelet agonist thromboxane (TxA_2) is converted rapidly to the inactive metabolite TxB_2. (6) Phosphatases limit kinase-dependent signaling. (7) Rapid desensitization of activated GPCRs is accomplished by phosphorylation of their serine and threonine residues.

Endothelial cells also prevent platelet activation: (1) Constitutively-expressed platelet receptors (eg, GPIb/IX/V and GPIa/IIa) are separated from their ligands (collagen, fibronectin) by the physical barrier provided by intact endothelium. (2) PGI_2 is produced and released by endothelial cells; binding of PGI_2 to a specific platelet surface GPCR activates adenylyl cyclase resulting in increased cAMP levels. (3) Nitric oxide produced in endothelial cells diffuses across the platelet plasma membrane, binding to guanylyl cyclase and enhancing cyclic GMP (cGMP) production; a cGMP-dependent protein kinase inhibits platelet activation. NO and PGI_2 may act synergistically. (4) The ecto-ADPase on the surface of endothelial cells augments ADP degradation (Section 31).

SECRETION (Figure 30-7)

Exocytosis of platelet contents at sites of vascular injury provides the high local concentration of effector molecules essential for hemostasis. This process amplifies platelet activation and consolidates thrombus formation. Ligand occupancy of platelet receptors induces platelet shape change and activation that precedes the release of granule contents. During shape change, the granules coalesce in the centre of the cell, fuse with the surface-connected canalicular system or with the plasma membrane and discharge their contents outside the cell. (SNARE proteins are a superfamily of proteins that are involved in vesicle trafficking and exocytosis in

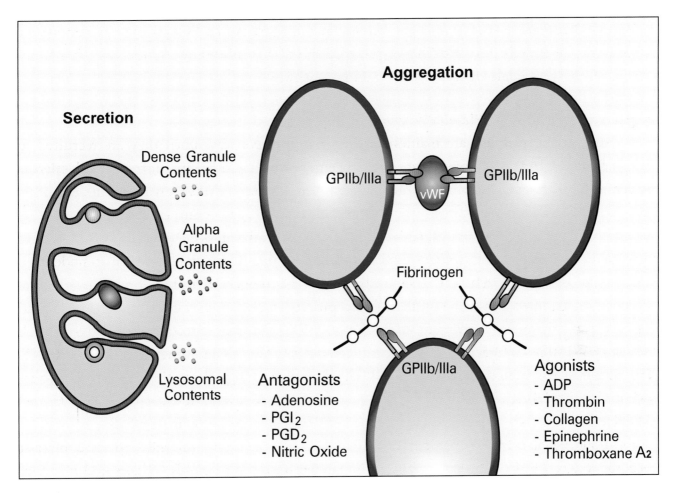

Figure 30-7 Platelet Secretion and Aggregation

nucleated cells – proteins of this family also appear to mediate the secretion of platelet granule contents). Secretion of dense granule contents induces a variety of reponses by neighbouring cells: vasoconstriction by serotonin, platelet activation by ADP, and the increased local concentration of calcium further augments activation, adhesion, and aggregation. Proteins released from alpha-granules augment platelet adhesion and activation. Upon platelet activation, P-selectin in the α-granule membrane is phosphorylated and moves to the surface of the plasma membrane, functioning as an adhesion receptor that interacts with other cells: it upregulates tissue factor expression on monocytes and recruits leukocytes to areas of vascular injury.

AGGREGATION (Figure 30-7)

When platelets adhere to exposed subendothelial tissue, additional platelets accumulate and adhere to one another in a process referred to as platelet aggregation. Aggregation is an active metabolic process: agonist binding initiates signaling pathways that convert GPIIb/IIIa from a latent to an activated state, enabling this receptor to bind soluble macromolecular ligands, such as plasma fibrinogen and vWF.

GPIIb/IIIa ($\alpha_{IIb}\beta_3$) is a member of the large family of cell surface adhesion receptors, the **integrins** (Section 3). It is a bi-directional conduit for information flow across the plasma membrane: (1) Reactions with an extracellular ligand (fibrinogen bound to exposed subendothelial matrix or to an activated platelet) induce conformational changes in the receptor, transducing a signal to the interior of the platelet followed by activation and secretion – this is referred to as outside-in signaling; (2) Inside-out signaling results when vWF attaches to GPIb, and also when excitatory agonists such as thrombin, ADP, or TxA_2 bind to their specific receptors – the transmission of a cytoplasmic signal activates GPIIb/IIIa, inducing the conformational change that promotes binding to fibrinogen and vWF. Fibrinogen and vWF are multivalent ligands that function as bridges between the GIIb/IIIa receptors on adjacent platelets, thus allowing platelet aggregation to proceed. The symmetrical fibrinogen molecule can bind to two platelets – there are approximately 50,000 copies of GPIIb/IIIa on the platelet surface. GPIIb/IIIa interaction with fibrinogen, vWF, and some other ligands is through recognition of a specific tripeptide, the RGD (arginyl-glycyl-aspartic acid) sequence on these proteins (Section 3). There are two RGD sequences in the Aα chain of fibrinogen.

Laboratory Assessment of Platelet Aggregation.

Platelets suspended in plasma *in vitro* do not aggregate until an agonist is introduced into the system. Platelet aggregation is assessed by the response to ADP, collagen, epinephrine, arachidonic acid, and thrombin. The addition of the agonist to platelet rich plasma, in the presence of calcium, initiates intracellular signaling, inducing shape change and alterations in GPIIb/IIIa that promote binding to plasma fibrinogen and platelet aggregation. The rate and degree of aggregation are assayed spectrophotometrically.

Clot Retraction

After formation of the platelet-fibrin hemostatic plug, the clot is reduced in volume and becomes more compact through the process of clot retraction. The forces responsible for clot retraction are generated by the platelet actin-myosin cytoskeleton. When platelets are activated, phosphorylation of the myosin light chain induces contractile forces that are transmitted through the myosin heavy chain to actin filaments. Actin filaments are anchored to membrane GPIIb/IIIa integrins which, in turn, are linked to fibrin strands outside the cell. As the clot retracts, serum is extruded from the interstices of the fibrin mesh with reduction in clot volume. Because of the failure of surface GPIIb/IIIa expression in Glanzmann thrombasthenia, clot retraction is absent. Poor clot retraction also is associated with thrombocytopenia, low fibrinogen levels and factor XIII deficiency.

CLINICAL CORRELATES

CONGENITAL DEFECTS IN PLATELET FUNCTION (Tables 30-1 and 30-2)

Platelet functional defects may be congenital or acquired. All are manifest by easy bruising, bleeding from mucous membranes and increased bleeding with trauma.

Defective Adhesion

The rare autosomal recessive disorder **Bernard-Soulier Syndrome (BSS)** is characterized by large platelets and thrombocytopenia; the bleeding time is long. BSS is due to a mutated GPIb-IX-V complex that results in deficiency or dysfunction with loss of binding to vWF. The principal hemostatic function of the complex is to initiate the arrest of platelets at sites of vascular injury; the GPIbα moiety binds to vWF in the exposed subendothelium. BSS most commonly is associated with mutations in the GPIbα gene; mutations also have been located on

Table 30-1   Molecular Basis of Platelet Dysfunction

Functional Defect	Molecular Defect
Adhesion Bernard Soulier Syndrome	GPIb/IX/V
Aggregation Glanzmann Thrombasthenia	GPIIb/IIIa

Secretion
    Dense Granules
        Hermansky-Pudlak Syndrome
        Chediak-Higashi Syndrome
        Empty Sack Syndrome
    Alpha Granules
        Gray Platelet Syndrome
        Quebec Platelet Disorder
	HPS protein; AP-3β3A
	Lysosomal trafficking factor
	?
	
	? α-granule membrane defect
	u-PA expression ↑

Cytoskeleton Wiskott-Aldrich Syndrome	WAS protein
Coagulant Surface Scott Syndrome	Scramblase function

Signaling
    Membrane Receptors
        Platelet-type vWD
        TxA$_2$ Receptor Defect
        Glanzmann Thrombasthenia
        Bernard Soulier Syndrome
    Signal Transduction
        Cyclooxygenase Deficiency
        Thromboxane Synthase Deficiency
	
	GPIbα
	TxA$_2$-GPCR
	GPIIb/IIIa
	GPIb/IX/V
	
	COX-1
	Thromboxane synthase

Table 30-2   Functional Defects in Platelet Disorders

CONGENITAL	SITE	DEFECT	FUNCTION
Bernard Soulier Syndrome	GPIb/IX/V ↓	vWF binding ↓	Adhesion ↓
Glanzmann Thrombasthenia	GPIIb/IIIa ↓	vWF binding ↓ Fibrinogen binding ↓	Aggregation ↓
Gray Platelet Syndrome	Alpha granules ↓	Secretion of Adhesive Proteins ↓	Aggregation ↓
δ-Storage Pool Syndromes	Dense granules ↓	Secretion of ADP ↓	Aggregation ↓
Platelet-type vWD	GPIbα mutation	Spontaneous vWF binding to abnormal GPIbα (plasma vWF↓)	Adhesion ↓
ACQUIRED	**SITE**	**DEFECT**	**FUNCTION**
Drug Induced (ASA, NSAIDs)	Cyclooxygenase ↓	TxA_2 ↓	Aggregation ↓
Uremia	Multiple	Uremic plasma factor(s) Anemia	Adhesion ↓ Aggregation ↓

GPIbβ and GPIX. BSS can be differentiated from other bleeding disorders by platelet aggregation studies: the *in vitro* platelet aggregation response to ADP, collagen and epinephrine is normal, however, platelets fail to aggregate in the presence of ristocetin. Ristocetin is a promoter of GPIb-vWF binding in normal platelets; although ristocetin induced aggregation is an *in vitro* phenomenon, it is an indicator of *in vivo* physiological interaction of platelets with exposed subendothelial tissues (Section 27). Flow cytometry is used to confirm the absence of the platelet GPIb/IX/V complex.

Defective Aggregation

Glanzmann thrombasthenia (GT) is an autosomal recessive disorder due to a dysfunctional or absent GPIIb/IIIa. The genes for GPIIb and GPIIIa are closely linked on chromosome 17. Mutations in either GPIIb or GPIIIa may be associated with failure of expression of the heterodimer on the plasma membrane as assembly in the endoplasmic reticulum requires the presence of both glycoproteins. Most GT phenotypes are associated with absence of GPIIb/IIIa. In some GT variants, there may be reduced surface expression or an impairment in functional activity. Dysfunction may be due to failure to bind ligand, or failure to induce signaling when the ligand is bound. The platelet antigen HPA1 (Pl[A1]) is a structural component of GPIIIa and, as such, usually is absent in Glanzmann thrombasthenia. *In vitro*, there is poor or absent platelet aggregation to ADP, epinephrine, and collagen; the response to ristocetin, mediated by GPIb, is normal. Clot retraction is absent.

Defective Storage Granules

Dense granule storage pool disease (SPD) is a heterogeneous group of disorders that may be divided into those associated with albinism (the Hermansky-Pudlak syndrome and the Chediak-Higashi syndrome) and those with normal pigmentation. Patients present with a mild to moderate bleeding diathesis; the number of dense granules is decreased. In some cases of non-albino SPD, the platelet content of CD63 (a tetraspanin protein present in dense granule and lysosomal membranes) is normal, indicating that the membrane is present although the contents of the dense granules are missing; this disorder has been termed the **empty sack syndrome**.

The **Hermansky-Pudlak Syndrome (HPS)** is a rare autosomal recessive disorder associated with a bleeding diathesis. All patients have some degree of oculocutaneous tyrosine-positive albinism and deficiency of platelet dense granules (storage pool deficiency); many have ceroid-lipofuscin deposits in cells of the reticuloendothelial system, although this is not considered essential for diagnosis of HPS. Patients may develop progressive pulmonary fibrosis or granulomatous colitis. There is defective biosynthesis of three related cytoplasmic organelles: melanosomes, platelet dense granules, and lysosomes. In the northwest region of Puerto Rico, where the incidence of HPS is high (with a gene frequency of 1 in 21), the affected individuals are homozygous for the specific *HPS1* mutation. The *HPS1* gene has been localized to chromosome 10q23. Most mutations result in a HPS1 protein with a truncated carboxy terminus.

In non-Puerto Rican patients, fewer than 50% have mutations in the HPS gene. In a subset of these patients (designated HPS type 2), there is a mutation in the *ADTB3A* gene that encodes a subunit (AP-3β3A) of the AP-3 adaptor complex. These adaptors are heterotetrameric complexes that effect inclusion of cargo proteins into transport vesicles for delivery to specific secretory granules. AP-3 is involved in sorting newly synthesized cargo proteins from the trans-Golgi network into transport vesicles destined for delivery to melanosomes, lysosomes, and platelet dense granules. As a result of the defective β3A subunit, protein delivery to these organelles is impaired. Because the clinical manifestations are similar in the Puerto Rican patients, it is probable that the HPS protein also has a role in the trafficking of vesicular proteins. HPS type 3, a recently recognized variant with mild symptoms, is due to mutations in a gene located on chromosome 3q24.

The autosomal recessive **Chediak-Higashi syndrome (CHS)** is characterized by partial albinism, dysfunctional neutrophils with giant lysosomal granules and recurrent pyogenic infections. Neutropenia is common. Mild bleeding is related to the decrease in platelet dense granules. Giant lysosomes in granulocytes and giant melanosomes are pathognomonic.

Mutations have been identified in the *LYST* gene on chromosome 1q42 that encodes the cytosolic LYST protein, the lysosomal trafficking regulator. The primary defect may be in endosomal sorting and/or vesicle budding with failure in the delivery of proteins to appropriate cellular sites.

Selective **deficiency of platelet α-granules** occurs in the rare autosomal disorder referred to as the **gray platelet syndrome**. The name is derived from the presence of large platelets that appear pale gray in a stained blood smear. The defect is probably the inability to form normal alpha-granule membranes – in some patients the membrane-specific P-selectin is reduced. Alpha-granule constituents are found in the cytoplasm, indicating that there is defective packaging with premature release. The patients manifest mild mucocutaneous bleeding; thrombocytopenia is variable. *In vitro*, the platelet aggregation response to thrombin is frequently abnormal; the aggregation response to other agonists is normal.

The **Quebec platelet disorder** is a rare autosomal dominant trait typically associated with delayed bleeding that appears 12-24 hours following trauma or surgery. There is proteolytic degradation of α-granule proteins, including fibrinogen, von Willebrand factor, and factor V. The α-granule protein multimerin appears to be quantitatively deficient. There is an unusually large amount of urokinase-type plasminogen activator (u-PA) in the α-granules (up to 100-fold more than in normal platelets), far in excess of the u-PA inhibitor, PAI-1. Proteolysis probably is due to u-PA activity. The bleeding can be controlled by fibrinolytic inhibitors (tranexamic acid and epsilon aminocaproic acid) but not by platelet transfusions (Section 29).

Defective Coagulant Surface

A rare autosomal recessive bleeding disorder, **Scott syndrome**, is due to a defect in the outward transmembrane migration of procoagulant phospholipids. There is decreased cell surface exposure of phosphatidylserine on activated platelets (and on other peripheral blood cells). In the absence of this procoagulant surface, the assembly of tenase and prothrombinase components is compromised. This defect probably is due to the absence of scramblase activity, although the protein is present.

Defective Cytoskeleton

The X-linked **Wiskott-Aldrich syndrome (WAS)** is characterized by actin cytoskeletal defects that lead to thrombocytopenia, eczema, and immunodeficiency. **X-linked thrombocytopenia (XLT)**, a milder form of the disease, is limited to platelet abnormalities. Small platelets are common to both phenotypes. The disorder is due to mutations in the Wiskott-Aldrich syndrome protein (WASP) family. WASP is expressed exclusively in hematopoietic cells. (A homologous protein, N-WASP, is widely distributed). WASP proteins regulate the assembly of actin monomers into filaments and, thus, are important regulators of the cytoskeletal organization and motility of cells. WASP signals to the cytoskeleton by binding to a̲ctin-r̲elated p̲roteins in the Arp2/3 complex, an assembly that promotes actin polymerization thereby regulating the structure and dynamics of actin filament networks. In platelets, this cytoskeletal reorganization is essential for the formation of actin-rich pseudopodia. In T cells, WASP-mediated cytoskeletal reorganization is critical for normal T cell activation (Section 19).

Defective Membrane Receptors

Platelet-type von Willebrand disease is due to mutations affecting the GPIb/IX/V complex on the platelet membrane that result in a dominant gain-of-function phenotype. Mutations produce an active configuration of GPIbα that binds circulating vWF with high affinity. Loss of the most active large vWF multimers from the plasma results in a bleeding diathesis resembling type 2B von Willebrand disease (Section 27).

Defects in the **thromboxane receptor,** in **ADP receptors,** and in **collagen receptors** have been described.

Defective Signal Transduction

Aspirin-like functional defects are present in the rare congenital **cycloxygenase deficiency,** characterized by a long bleeding time, easy bruising, and abnormal *in vitro* platelet aggregation. **Thromboxane synthase deficiency** has been reported in a small number of cases.

THROMBOCYTOPENIA (Table 30-3)

Thrombocytopenia is the most common cause of platelet-associated bleeding. It may be due to: (1) impaired production resulting from megakaryocyte depletion as a result of drug or chemical toxicity, immunological suppression, or as part of general bone marrow aplasia with stem cell failure, or (2) increased platelet destruction by immunological mechanisms.

Congenital amegakaryocytic thrombocytopenia is a rare disease characterized by severe thrombocytopenia in infancy that develops into pancytopenia in later childhood. The basis of the abnormality appears to be an intrinsic stem cell defect due to mutations in the c-mpl gene. Mpl is either absent from the surface of these cells or is present in a truncated form. Serum TPO is high due to the low number of binding sites associated with the absence of platelets and megakaryocytes.

Immune Thrombocytopenic Purpura (ITP) (Figure 30-8)

ITP may be acute or chronic. Children most commonly present with the acute form of the disease; the onset is sudden, developing usually in patients with a history of an antecedent infection. Spontaneous remission occurs in over 90% of cases. Chronic ITP develops more slowly and may be associated with other autoimmune disease; spontaneous remissions are less common.

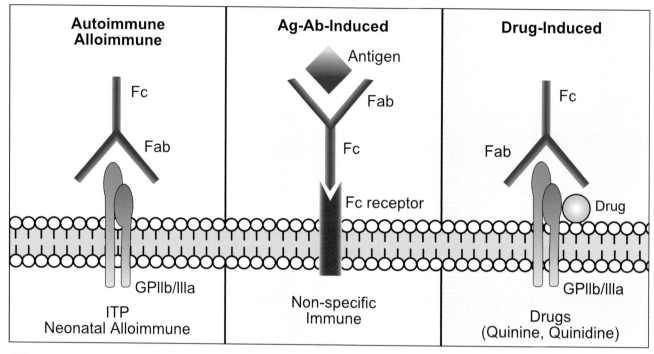

Figure 30-8 Immune Thrombocytopenia

ITP is a result of the development of IgG autoantibodies to a platelet protein; the most frequent targets are GPIIb/IIIa and GPIb/IX. The Fab portion of the antibody binds to the platelet antigen; interaction of the Fc portion of the bound antibody with Fc receptors on reticuloendothelial macrophages leads to phagocytic platelet removal. These antibodies may cross the placenta and react with the fetal platelets, resulting in **neonatal autoimmune thrombocytopenia** (Section 11).

Neonatal alloimmune thrombocytopenia is a more severe neonatal disorder. It is due to the presence of fetal platelet-specific antigens that are not expressed on maternal platelets. As a result of fetomaternal bleeds, with entry of fetal platelets into the maternal circulation, alloantibodies against fetal platelet antigens are produced by the mother. These antibodies cross the placenta and destroy fetal platelets – as a result, there may be serious bleeding *in utero*. The mechanism is similar to Rh hemolytic disease of the newborn (Section 11).

Drug-Induced Thrombocytopenia

Drug-induced autoimmune thrombocytopenia is initiated when the drug binds to platelet surface proteins (typically GPIIb/IIIa or GPIb/IX/V), inducing a conformational change. Exposure of neoepitopes in the structurally altered protein induces an immune response with formation of autoantibodies – the Fab portion of the IgG antibody binds to a complex of the drug and the platelet protein. Thrombocytopenia develops when Fc receptors on macrophages engage the Fc portion of the platelet-bound antibody. Drugs typically involved in this idiosyncratic reaction include sulfonamides, quinine/quinidine, and gold. (Heparin-induced thrombocytopenia is discussed in Section 25).

Non-Specific Immune Reactions associated with viral and bacterial infections and drug exposure may induce thrombocytopenia. Antibodies produced under these circumstances are directed against the antigenic configuration of the drug or infectious agent, not against a platelet antigen. The formation of antigen-antibody complexes induces a conformational change in the Fc portion of the antibody that then binds non-specifically to the Fc receptors expressed on platelet membranes. The platelets bound to these Ag/Ab complexes are targeted for phagocytic removal. As the antibody is not directed against the platelet, platelets are removed as "innocent bystanders". This may be a normal mechanism for clearing immune complexes from plasma, but an overload of such complexes on platelet membranes results in thrombocytopenia.

Table 30-3   Classification of Thrombocytopenia

Decreased Platelet Production
    Acquired
        Megakaryocyte hypoplasia – infections, drugs, myelodysplasia
        Ineffective thrombopoiesis – vitamin B_{12} or folate deficiency
    Hereditary
        Amegakaryocytic thrombocytopenia
        Thrombocytopenia with absent radii
        Cyclic thrombocytopenia – TPO deficiency

Increased Platelet Destruction
    Immunological
        Autoimmune
            Idiopathic – immune thrombocytopenic purpura (ITP)
            Secondary – infections, collagen-vascular disorders, drugs,
                  pregnancy, lymphoproliferative disease
        Alloimmune
            Neonatal
            Post-transfusion

        Innocent bystander: Fc receptor mediated – infections, drugs
    Non-immunological
        Thrombotic microangiopathies – disseminated intravascular
        coagulation, thrombotic thrombocytopenic purpura (TTP),
        hemolytic-uremic syndrome

Abnormal Platelet Distribution
        Hypersplenism
        Dilution of platelets by transfusion

Pseudothrombocytopenia
        In vitro platelet clumping due to EDTA/immunoglobulin

---

Pseudothrombocytopenia

This is an *in vitro* artifact that may be induced when blood is anticoagulated with EDTA. The decreased calcium concentration resulting from EDTA chelation induces a conformational alteration in platelet GPIIb/IIIa, exposing a cryptic epitope. Platelet agglutination develops when naturally occurring plasma antibodies (usually IgG) bind to this neo-antigen. Platelet clumping results in an erroneously low platelet count when determined by automated cell counting; the clumped platelets can be seen on the blood smear. This anomaly is confirmed by demonstration of a higher platelet count when blood is anticoagulated with heparin or citrate.

ESSENTIAL THROMBOCYTHEMIA

Essential thrombocythemia is a myeloproliferative disorder associated with an elevated platelet count, giant platelets, and an increased number of MKs in the bone marrow. It is a myeloproliferative clonal disorder similar to other myeloproliferative diseases. The thrombocytosis may be associated with either thrombosis or hemorrhage.

PHARMACOLOGICAL PLATELET INHIBITORS

(1) **Inhibitors of prostaglandin-mediated platelet activation.** Aspirin (ASA) acetylation of the enzyme cyclooxygenase-1 (COX-1) blocks prostanoid synthesis. The structural configuration of cyclooxygenase includes a long channel through which arachidonic acid gains access to the activation site of the enzyme; acetylation of a serine residue in this channel blocks the access of arachidonic acid to the site. As platelets are end-stage cells that do not synthesize protein, acetylation suppresses cyclooxygenase-1 activity and synthesis of aggregation-promoting TxA_2 for the life of the platelet. Inhibition of TxA_2 synthesis is the principal antithrombotic mechanism of aspirin. The antithrombotic effect of low dose aspirin depends on its irreversible inhibition of platelet cyclooxygenase while there is continuing resynthesis of this enzyme and production of PGI_2 by the endothelial cell.

Other non-steroidal anti-inflammatory drugs (NSAIDs) compete reversibly with arachidonic acid for binding to the COX-1 active site but, unlike ASA, do not induce permanent inactivation of the enzyme. As a result, inhibition of platelet function by these agents is of shorter duration than with ASA.

(2) **Inhibitors of ADP-mediated activation.** Ticlopidine and clopidogrel irreversibly inhibit the $P2Y_{12}$ receptor for ADP, thus inhibiting ADP-dependent platelet aggregation. $P2Y_{12}$ is a G protein-coupled receptor that inhibits adenylyl cyclase activity. Interference with the function of this receptor results in an increase in the level of cAMP.

(3) **Phosphodiesterase inhibitors** function by blocking the degradation of cAMP, an

inhibitor of platelet aggregation. With the increase in cAMP, there is diminished platelet activity. The phosphodiesterase inhibitor in clinical use is dipyridamole.

(4) **Antagonists of ligand binding to $\alpha_{IIb}\beta_3$ (GPIIb/IIIa).** Abciximab is the Fab fragment of a humanized murine monoclonal antibody (Section 17) that blocks the GPIIb/IIIa integrin site on the platelet membrane, interfering with fibrinogen and vWF binding and platelet aggregation.

————— ••••◉◉••• —————

SUGGESTED READING

Alberio L, Dale GL. Platelet-collagen interactions: membrane receptors and intracellular signalling pathways. Eur J Clin Invest, 29:1066-1076, 1999.

Ballmaier M, Germeshausen M, Schulze H, et al. *c-mpl* mutations are the cause of congenital amegakaryocytic thrombocytopenia. Blood 97:139-146, 2001.

Bennett JS. Novel platelet inhibitors. Annu Rev Med 52:161-184, 2001.

Bevers EM, Comfurius P, Dekkers DWC, Zwaal RFA. Lipid translocation across the plasma membrane of mammalian cells. Biochim Biophys Acta 1439:317-330, 1999.

Brass LF. More pieces of the platelet activation puzzle slide into place. J Clin Invest 104:1663-1665, 1999.

Clemetson KJ. Primary haemostasis: sticky fingers cement the relationship. Curr Biol 9:R110-R112, 1999.

Cramer EM. Megakaryocyte structure and function. Curr Opin Hematol 6:354-361, 1999.

Hollopeter G, Jantzen HM, Vincent D, et al. Identification of the platelet ADP receptor targeted by antithrombotic drugs. Nature 409:202-211, 2001.

Huizing M, Anikster Y, Fitzpatrick DL, et al. Hermansky-Pudlak syndrome type 3 in Ashkenazi Jews and other Non-Puerto Rican patients with hypopigmentation and platelet storage-pool deficiency. Am J Hum Genet 69:1022-1032, 2001.

Kahr WHA, Zheng S, Sheth PM, et al. Platelets from patients with the Quebec platelet disorder contain and secrete abnormal amounts of urokinase-type plasminogen activator. Blood 98:257-265, 2001.

Kaushansky K. The enigmatic megakaryocyte gradually reveals its secrets. BioEssays 21:353-360, 1999.

Kim AS, Kakalis LT, Abdul-Manan N, Liu GA, Rosen MK. Autoinhibition and activation mechanisms of the Wiskott-Aldrich syndrome protein. Nature 404:151-158, 2000.

Kulkarni S, Dopheide SM, Yap CL, et al. A revised model of platelet aggregation. J Clin Invest 105:783-791, 2000.

Long MW. Thrombopoietin stimulation of hematopoietic stem/progenitor cells. Curr Opin Hematol 6:159-163, 1999.

López JA, Andrews RK, Afshar-Kharghan V, Berndt MC. Bernard-Soulier syndrome. Blood 91:4397-4418, 1998.

Marnett LJ, Rowlinson SW, Goodwin DC, Kalgutkar AS, Lanzo CA. Arachidonic acid oxygenation by COX-1 and COX-2. J Biol Chem 274:22903-22906, 1999.

Mistry N, Cranmer SL, Yuan Y, Mangin P, et al. Cytoskeletal regulation of the platelet glycoprotein Ib/V/IX-von Willebrand factor interaction. Blood 96:3480-3489, 2000.

Mondoro TH, White MM, Jennings LK. Active GPIIb-IIIa conformations that link ligand interaction with cytoskeletal reorganization. Blood 96:2487-2495, 2000.

Nimer SD. Essential thrombocythemia: another "heterogeneous disease" better understood? Blood 93:415-416, 1999.

Oh J, Liu ZX, Feng GH, Raposo G, Spritz RA. The Hermansky-Pudlak syndrome (HPS) protein is part of a high molecular weight complex involved in biogenesis of early melanosomes. Hum Mol Genet 9:375-385, 2000.

Rizvi MA, Shah SR, Raskob GE, George JN. Drug-induced thrombocytopenia. Curr Opin Hematol 6:349-353, 1999.

Roth GJ. A new "kid" on the platelet thrombin receptor "block": glycoprotein Ib-IX-V. PNAS 98:1330-1331, 2001.

Ruggeri ZM. Old concepts and new developments in the study of platelet aggregation. J Clin Invest 105:699-701, 2000.

Shattil SJ, Kashiwagi H, Pampori N. Integrin signaling: the platelet paradigm. Blood 91:2645-2657, 1998.

Shotelersuk V, Dell'Angelica EC, Hartnell L, Bonifacino JS, Gahl WA. A new variant of Hermansky-Pudlak Syndrome due to mutations in a gene responsible for vesicle formation. Amer J Med 108:423-427, 2000.

Storey EF, Sanderson HM, White AE, et al. The central role of the P_{2T} receptor in amplification of human platelet activation, aggregation, secretion and procoagulant activity. Br J Haematol 110:925-934, 2000.

Vijayan KV, Goldschmidt-Clermont PJ, Roos C, Bray PF. The $P1^{A2}$ polymorphism of integrin $\beta3$ enhances outside-in signaling and adhesive functions. J Clin Invest 105:793-802, 2000.

ENDOTHELIUM

"Something there is that doesn't love a wall."
Mending Wall – Robert Frost

The cells, proteins and other constituents of the blood engage in physiological processes that cannot be divorced from the conduits through which they flow. The endothelial barrier between the circulation and the surrounding tissue is not a passive membrane – it influences vascular flow, hemostasis, and the movement and migration of the cellular elements of the bloodstream; it is responsive to stimuli originating in the circulating blood and neighbouring tissues. These are discussed in detail in the relevant Sections; in this Section, the interrelationship of these multiple roles is examined as they operate in juxtaposition to one another.

Endothelial Cell-To-Cell Junctions (Figure 31-1)

The endothelium is a confluent monolayer of cells linked to one another by a variety of molecular interactions including tight junctions and adherens junctions. These structures, located at the lateral cell-cell borders, control transendothelial permeability and the movement of leukocytes into extravascular tissues.

Tight junctions are present in the vessels of the blood-brain barrier and in the large arteries, but not in the postcapillary venules that are the primary site of leukocyte migration. The intimate contact between the endothelial cells (ECs) produced by tight junctions is most pronounced at the vascular surface of the intercellular cleft. They essentially seal the endothelial surface. Components of tight junctions include a group of surface proteins without transmembrane domains that cluster at the cytoplasmic face of the contact area, and transmembrane proteins (occludins) which associate laterally with those of the neighbouring cell and intracellularly with the actin filament system.

Adherens junctions provide the structural base for interendothelial stability. They are formed by the cadherin adhesion proteins. Cadherins preferentially adhere to neighbouring cells expressing the identical cadherin molecule (homophilic adhesion) – clusters of these molecules at sites of cell contact form the adherens junctions. Cadherins are single-pass transmembrane proteins; the cytoplasmic tail associates with cytoplasmic structural proteins, α and β catenins, which in turn mediate linkage to the actin/myosin cytoskeleton. The adherens junctions are of primary importance in regulating the permeability of the microvasculature. Permeability is increased by a variety of agonists: thrombin, histamine, vascular endothelial growth factor (VEGF), and activated neutrophils adherent to the endothelium. Induction of intracellular signaling by these agents results in phosphorylation of the catenins and myosin, followed by

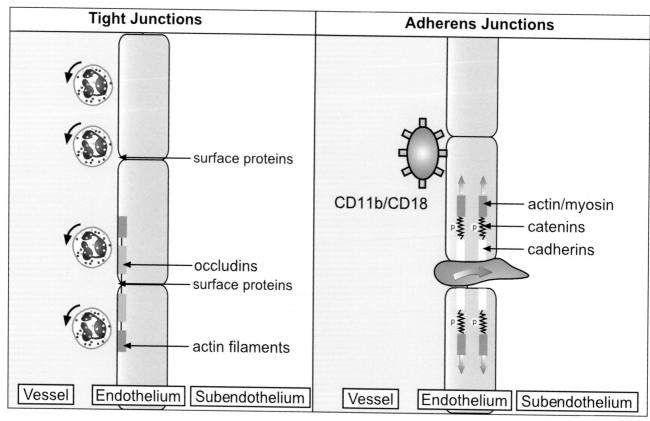

Figure 31-1 Endothelial Cell Junctions

dissociation of the cadherins and disruption of the adherens junctions. The increased permeability of the endothelium allows passage of fluid and proteins into the tissues and leukocyte migration through the vessel wall to the site of inflammation or injury.

Endothelial Cell Heterogeneity

The endothelial surface is not uniform – it varies, from organ to organ and site to site, in morphology and in response to external stimuli. Endothelial cells lining major arterial vessels and capillaries of the central nervous system are flat with tight intercellular junctions. In the spleen and bone marrow sinusoids, the endothelium is discontinuous, permitting cells to pass through the intercellular gaps. In high endothelial venules (HEV), ECs are tall and cuboidal. HEVs are present in the postcapillary circulation in lymphoid tissue that are sites for lymphocyte homing and recirculation. The ECs in arteries, veins and the microvasculature differ in their expression of both promoters and inhibitors of coagulation. (Heterogeneity also may govern the sites to which tumors metastasize). In the bone marrow, the ECs constitutively secrete cytokines that regulate hematopoiesis and control traffic in and out of the marrow. The functional properties of ECs undergo profound alterations in response to a variety of external stimuli. This change in phenotype, referred to as activation, involves complex molecular interactions that occur in response to various forms of stress and injury: inflammation, hypoxia, toxins, and mechanical stress.

Endothelial Cells as Regulators of Vascular Hemodynamics (Figure 31-2)

A number of products synthesized by ECs regulate blood flow and blood pressure. These include the vasodilators nitric oxide and prostacyclin, and the vasoconstrictor endothelin-1. Platelet activating factor (PAF) enhances vasoconstriction by inducing release of thromboxane A_2 from platelets.

Nitric Oxide (NO) is generated through the oxidation of arginine to citrulline by endothelial nitric oxide synthase (eNOS). It is produced both constitutively and in response to a variety of surface receptor stimuli (eg, thrombin and ADP) and to shear stress. In addition to its role as a vasodilator, NO serves a vasoprotective role: it inhibits platelet adhesion, activation,

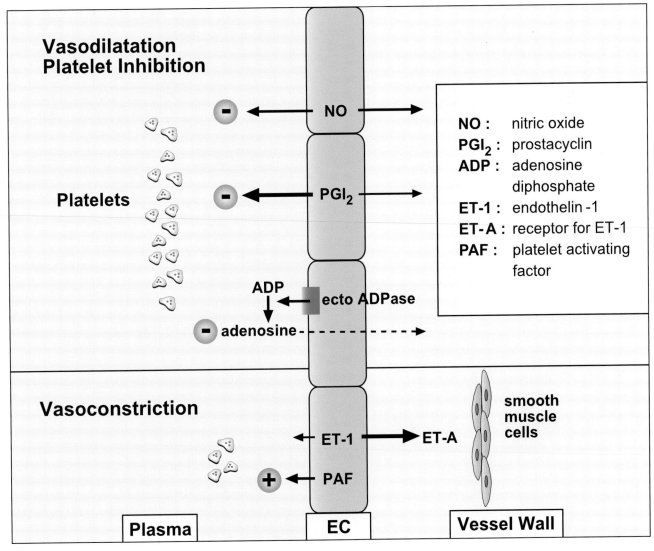

Figure 31-2 Endothelial Vasoregulation

aggregation, and the expression of platelet P-selectin; it reduces EC expression of adhesion molecules and adhesive interactions with neutrophils. These functions protect normal endothelium from platelet deposition and from injury by oxidants released from activated neutrophils. NO has an important role in maintaining cardiovascular homeostasis – regulating systemic blood pressure and vascular remodeling.

Prostacyclin (PGI$_2$) is an eicosanoid derived from arachidonic acid (Section 30). Cyclooxygenase converts arachidonic acid to prostaglandin G$_2$ (PGG$_2$) and prostaglandin H$_2$ (PGH$_2$). In platelets, PGH$_2$ is converted by **thromboxane synthase** to thromboxane A$_2$ (TxA$_2$), a potent platelet activator and vasoconstrictor. In ECs, PGH$_2$, generated by the same initial sequence, is converted by **prostacyclin synthase** to prostacyclin. PGI$_2$ functions, synergistically with NO, as an inhibitor of platelet aggregation and as a vasodilator; the PGI$_2$ receptor is present on platelets and on vascular smooth muscle cells. PGI$_2$ is not produced constitutively but is induced by a variety of agonists and by shear stress at sites of vascular perturbation. Most PGI$_2$ is secreted into the plasma where it inhibits platelet aggregation; PGI$_2$ also binds to smooth muscle cells in the vessel wall, countering the vasoconstrictive activity of TxA$_2$.

Endothelin-1 (ET-1). The endothelins are 21-amino acid peptides synthesized by a variety of cells. Three members of this family have been identified but only ET-1 is produced by endothelium. It has a role in the maintenance of basal vasomotor tone. Stimuli, such as hypoxia or shear stress, induce RNA transcription and secretion of ET-1 within minutes of exposure to the stimulus. Although some ET-1 is secreted into the plasma, the major portion moves to the abluminal side of the EC in juxtaposition to the vascular smooth muscle cells where it binds to ET-A, a G protein-linked receptor expressed on these cells (Figure 31-3). Binding of ET-1 results in increased intracellular calcium levels which, in turn, induce vasoconstriction. The ET-1 secreted into the plasma can prime neutrophils for endothelial adhesion; it may contribute to endothelial damage in pre-eclampsia and disseminated intravascular coagulation (DIC).

Endothelium and Platelets (Figure 31-2)

Platelets are discouraged from adhering to normal intact endothelium by EC production of NO, PGI$_2$ and a membrane-associated ectonucleotidase, ecto-ADPase. The membrane bound ecto-ADPase degrades extracellular ADP released from stimulated platelets, thus inhibiting ADP-induced platelet aggregation. Adenosine, the metabolic product of ADP degradation, largely remains in juxtaposition to and associated with the surface of the EC where it functions as an inhibitor of platelet aggregation and as a vasodilator.

When endothelium is denuded, there is an immediate response to the injury as platelet glycoprotein surface receptors adhere to subendothelial components: to fibronectin (via platelet GPIc/IIa), to collagen (via platelet GPIa/IIa), and to vWF (via platelet GPIbα). These interactions result in platelet activation: ADP is released and a configurational alteration of platelet GPIIb/IIIa facilitates binding of fibrinogen and vWF. The net result is platelet recruitment and aggregation with formation of a platelet thrombus (Section 30).

Endothelium and Leukocyte Trafficking

Leukocytes must leave the bloodstream to enter specific tissues. In areas of inflammation, the stimulated endothelial cells actively participate in leukocyte recruitment through a highly regulated process. As neutrophils enter the inflammatory area, the activated ECs display the glycosylated ligands that interact with the constitutively expressed L-selectin on leukocyte microvilli. An on-off adhesive contact between L-selectin and its ligand results in neutrophil tethering and rolling along the vessel wall in the direction of flow. Due to the shear forces in the circulating blood, adhesion bonds dissociate at the cell's upstream end and new bonds form downstream. This results in the rolling motion that serves as an "automatic braking system" countering the effects of shear stress. P-selectin stored in the envelope of the Weibel-Palade bodies of the EC moves to the cell surface and engages the leukocyte in tighter binding. This is augmented by E-selectin interaction with its leukocyte ligand. The vasoactive phospholipid PAF is co-expressed with P-selectin on the surface of activated ECs. (PAF was first described as an

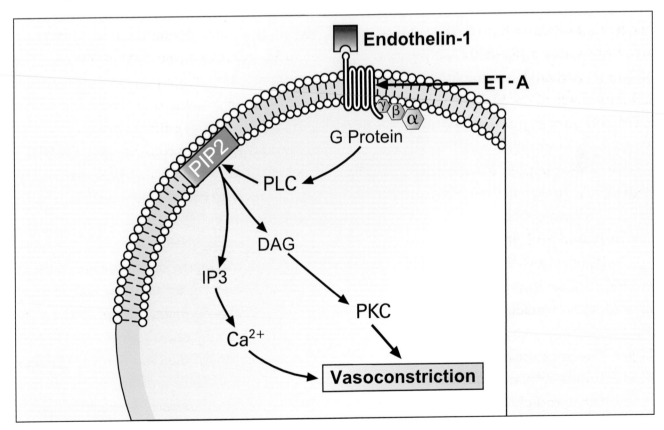

Figure 31-3 Endothelin-1 Signaling

inducer of platelet aggregation and release of granule contents, hence its name). PAF binding to the neutrophil via a G protein-coupled receptor induces inflammatory responses: adhesive activity of the surface integrins, oxygen radical generation and granule secretion. In addition, chemokine-binding to specific neutrophil receptors initiate intracellular signals that stimulate the cytoplasmic domain of the CD11b/CD18 integrin. Primed CD11b/CD18 interacts with the intercellular adhesion molecules (ICAM-1 and ICAM-2) on the EC surface to reinforce leukocyte binding. As the surface integrins adhere to the endothelial surface, the neutrophil crawls to the intercellular junction where PECAM-1 (platelet-endothelial cell adhesion molecule) initiates migration into the subendothelial tissues (Sections 3 and 7).

A similar process governs lymphocyte homing and recirculation. Lymphocyte homing to peripheral lymph nodes and Peyer's patches takes place in the specialized high endothelial venules. Memory cells move to specific inflammatory sites in response to cytokines and chemokines released by activated tissue cells (Section 18).

Endothelium and Anticoagulants (Figure 31-4)

The thromboresistant surface maintained by normal quiescent endothelium depends upon its ability to prevent platelet adherence and clot formation. Factors expressed on the surface of ECs regulate and limit coagulation (Section 25).

Thrombomodulin (TM) is a high-affinity endothelial thrombin receptor that binds locally generated thrombin. Thrombin bound to TM undergoes a change in specificity from a procoagulant to an anticoagulant protease that activates the protein C pathway. TM also is involved in clearance of thrombin: ATIII rapidly inhibits thrombin bound to TM – the inactive complex dissociates from TM and is removed from the circulation by the liver.

Endothelial protein C receptor (EPCR) is expressed at high levels in large vessels, at lower levels in capillaries. Protein C activation by the thrombin/TM complex on the endothelial surface is augmented many fold when protein C is bound to EPCR. In a complex with protein S on the endothelial surface, activated protein C degrades factors Va and VIIIa. Deficiencies of protein C, protein S, and EPCR are associated with an increased risk of thrombosis (Section 25).

Heparan sulfate and heparin-like proteoglycans, on the surface of ECs, augment antithrombin III inhibition of serine proteases, including thrombin, factors IXa and Xa. Proteoglycans also are secreted into the subendothelial matrix where the heparans bind chemokines to produce high concentrations in juxtaposition to inflammatory foci – the chemokines prime neutrophil activation at these sites.

Tissue factor pathway inhibitor (TFPI) produced by ECs inhibits the extrinsic pathway of the coagulation cascade (Section 25).

Endothelium and Procoagulants

The normally anticoagulant endothelial surface can be perturbed at sites of vascular

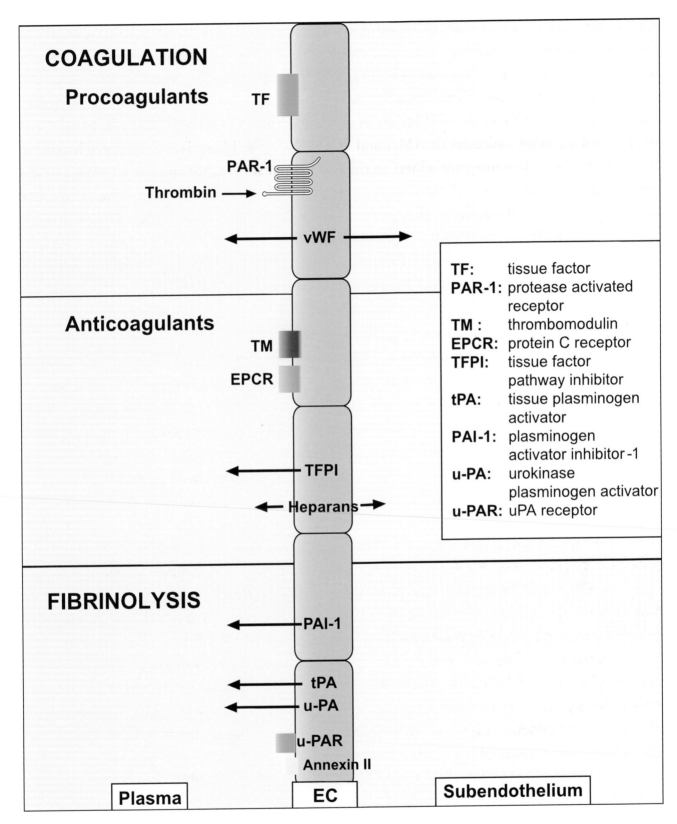

Figure 31-4 Endothelial Regulators of Coagulation and Fibrinolysis

injury. The result is exposure of potent thrombogenic agents in the subendothelium and procoagulants on the surface of ECs.

Tissue factor (TF) functions as a cofactor of VIIa to initiate the extrinsic pathway of the coagulation system (Section 24). Expression of TF on the plasma membrane of activated endothelial cells is induced in the vicinity of vascular injury by specific agonists such as thrombin and endotoxin, triggering local generation of coagulation proteases

Thrombin receptor PAR-1 (protease activated receptor-1) is displayed on the EC surface. Thrombin binding induces intracellular signaling that results in activation of the endothelial cell: upregulation and surface expression of P-selectin induces leukocyte rolling along the vessel wall; enhanced production of PAF activates platelets and leukocytes in the vicinity.

von Willebrand factor (vWF) is a glycoprotein synthesized by ECs and stored in intracellular organelles, the Weibel-Palade bodies (Section 27). vWF is synthesized as large multimers and stored in this form or released into the circulation where the multimers are degraded to smaller units by a specific plasma metalloproteinase. VWF has two roles: it stabilizes factor VIII in the circulation and it is an adhesive protein that interacts with platelet surface receptors. Stored vWF is released following endothelial injury and in response to stimuli such as thrombin, histamine and epinephrine, or by therapeutic administration of DDAVP (desmopressin).

Endothelium and Fibrinolysis

Tissue plasminogen activator (t-PA) and its inhibitor PAI-1 (plasminogen activator inhibitor-1) are synthesized in the microvasculature by endothelial cells. Secretion of t-PA is upregulated in response to thrombin, hypoxia, exercise and other forms of stress. PAI-1 expression is enhanced following exposure to inflammatory stimuli, and is secreted in juxtaposition to thrombi. Binding sites for both plasminogen and t-PA are present on the endothelial surface — t-PA cleavage of plasminogen generates the active fibrinolytic enzyme plasmin. u-PA (urokinase plasminogen activator) also is expressed by activated ECs. The u-PA receptor, u-PAR, is expressed on ECs engaged in tissue repair and angiogenesis. u-PA bound to its receptor on ECs is protected from inactivation by PAI-1 and PAI-2 (Section 29).

CLINICAL CORRELATES

Sites of Thrombotic Disease

Perturbation of the endothelium by mechanical or chemical factors converts the normally non-thrombogenic surface to a prothrombotic surface. The vulnerability to thrombotic disease and location of thrombi vary in both macrovascular and microvascular sites. Patients, with congenital deficiencies of protein C, protein S, or ATIII, or with the molecular variants factor V Leiden and prothrombin 20210A, characteristically present with deep vein thrombosis of the lower extremities. In antiphospholipid antibody-associated thrombotic disease and thrombotic thrombocytopenic purpura (TTP), small vessels in both the arterial and venous systems are vulnerable (Sections 24 and 25).

Red Blood Cell Adhesion

The normal phospholipid asymmetry of red blood cell membranes is maintained by an active process requiring ATP and a translocase enzyme. In some pathological states associated with red blood cell damage the asymmetry is lost – exposure of phosphatidylserine on the outer surface of the membrane increases adherence to the endothelium. The loss of membrane asymmetry in sickle cells with subsequent increased adherence to endothelium probably plays a role in the vaso-occlusive events in sickle cell disease.

Leukocyte Adhesion

EC injury that occurs in vasculitis of varying etiology is the result of pathological leukocyte adherence to the vascular wall. Lymphocyte adherence with cytokine release may occur in immune-mediated endothelial injury: in systemic lupus or graft-rejection following organ transplant. There is evidence that ECs can process and display antigen, becoming specific targets for cytotoxic lymphocytes. ECs may sustain damage in viral disease or from bacterial endotoxins. Overwhelming infection may result in immune injury of the endothelium and development of purpura fulminans; in the experimental counterpart, the Shwartzman reaction, endotoxin induces upregulation of ICAM-1 on the endothelial surface and subsequent neutrophil adhesion and cytokine release.

Hereditary Hemorrhagic Telangiectasia (HHT)

HHT is an autosomal dominant disease expressed as vascular dysplasia with recurrent hemorrhage from vascular lesions in skin and mucous membranes. Patients present with epistaxis, gastrointestinal bleeding, neurological and pulmonary manifestations due to arteriovenous malformations. The vascular lesions consist of direct arteriovenous connections without an intervening capillary bed. Two germline mutations with similar phenotypes have been identified. The molecular defects occur in two distinct endothelial receptors for transforming growth factor β (TGF-β). In HHT-1 the defect is a mutant gene for the TGF-β receptor **endoglin**. In HHT-2, there is a mutation in the TGF-β receptor **ALK**1. The TGF-β family comprises a large number of structurally related polypeptide growth factors that regulate an array of cell processes including development, homeostasis, and repair of almost all tissues, including endothelium. Both mutants disrupt TGF-β signaling during angiogenesis. Endoglin and Alk1 probably act in the same pathway since mutations in either result in HHT. The autosomal dominant nature of HHT suggests these two receptors are crucial for normal vessel formation.

●●●●◉●●●●

SUGGESTED READING

Abdalla SA, Pece-Barbara N, Vera S, Tapia E, Paez E, Bernabeu C, Letarte M. Analysis of ALK-1 and endoglin in newborns from families with hereditary hemorrhagic telangiectasia type 2. Hum Mol Genet 9:1227-1237, 2000.

Butcher EC, Picker LJ. Lymphocyte homing and homeostasis. Science 272:60-66, 1996.

Chen S, Springer TA. An automatic braking system that stabilizes leukocyte rolling by an increase in selectin bond number with shear. J Cell Biol 144:185-200, 1999.

Cines DB, Pollak ES, Buck CA, Loscalzo J, Zimmerman GA, McEver RP, et al. Endothelial cells in physiology and in the pathophysiology of vascular disorders. Blood 91:3527-3561, 1998.

Levin ER. Endothelins. N Engl J Med 333:356-363, 1996.

Ostrovsky L, King AJ, Bond S, Mitchell D, Lorant DE, Zimmerman GA, et al. A juxtacrine mechanism for neutrophil adhesion on platelets involves platelet-activating factor and a selectin-dependent activation process. Blood 91:3028-3036, 1998.

Preissner K, Nawroth PP, Kanse SM. Vascular protease receptors: Integrating haemostasis and endothelial cell functions. J Pathol 190:360-372, 2000.

Rosenberg R, Aird WC. Vascular-bed-specific hemostasis and hypercoagulable states. Mechanisms of disease. N Engl J Med 340:1555-1564, 1999.

Schafer AI. Vascular endothelium: In defense of blood fluidity. J Clin Invest 99:1143-1144, 1997.

Springer TA. Traffic signals on endothelium for lymphocyte recirculation and leukocyte emigration. Annu Rev Physiol 57:827-872, 1995.

Zimmerman H. Nucleotides and CD39: Principal modulatory players in hemostasis and thrombosis. Nature Medicine 9:987-988, 1999.

INDEX

836